MCAT Psychology and Sociology

Content Review

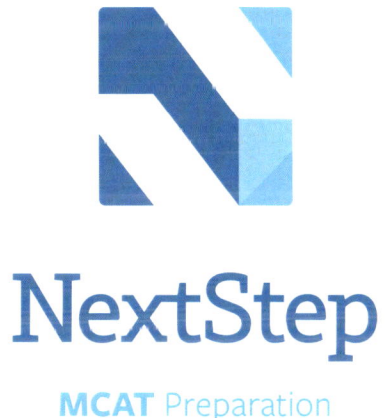

Copyright 2019 by Blueprint Education Subsidiary Holdings LLC

All rights reserved. This book or any portion thereof may not be reproduced nor used in any manner whatsoever without the express written permission of the publisher, except for the use of brief quotations in a book review.

Printed in the United States of America

Third Printing, 2019

ISBN 978-1-944935-38-2

Blueprint Education Subsidiary Holdings LLC
6080 Center Drive
Suite 520
Los Angeles, CA 90045

MCAT is a registered trademark of the American Association of Medical Colleges (AAMC). The AAMC has neither reviewed nor endorsed this work in any way.

Revision Number: 2.0 (2019-07-01)

This page left intentionally blank

This page left intentionally blank.

This page left intentionally blank.

This page left intentionally blank.

STOP! READ ME FIRST!

Welcome and congratulations on taking this important step in your MCAT prep process!

The book you're holding is one of Next Step's six MCAT review books, and contains concise content review with a specific focus on the science that you need for MCAT success. To get the most out of this book, we'd like to draw your attention to some distinctive aspects of our book set and their role in MCAT prep.

First and foremost, **books are not enough** for MCAT prep. Realistic practice is absolutely essential, and should include both MCAT-targeted practice questions and an ample number of full-length practice exams that simulate the MCAT itself.

Second, our **books reflect our experience**—as 520+ MCAT scorers, as tutors and instructors with years of experience, and as veteran writers and communicators. This makes our books unlike many other MCAT review products, which provide a dry, factual overview of scientific knowledge without MCAT-specific context. Instead, our books recognize that the **MCAT is primarily a test of thinking**—and more specifically, a test that reflects how the American Association of Medical Colleges encourages future physicians to think. The "MCAT Strategy" sidebars throughout the book call out specific points to be aware of as you study, and in general, our approach to presenting science is informed by how science is tested on the MCAT—that is, in a way that draws upon passages, builds connections across subject areas, and prioritizes an understanding of fundamental principles. In a nutshell, it's our hope that by studying with these books, you can benefit from our team's unparalleled MCAT expertise.

Third, after completing a chapter, we urge you to test your knowledge with **online practice materials,** including both the online end-of-chapter questions, and the other practice materials that Next Step offers.

We wish you the best of luck on your MCAT journey,

The Next Step MCAT Team

TABLE OF CONTENTS

1. Experimental Designs and Methods 1
2. Biological Basis of Behavior. 17
3. Sensation and Perception 43
4. Consciousness 67
5. Cognition and Language 83
6. Emotion, Stress, Memory, and Learning 101
7. Motivation, Attitude, and Personality 125
8. Psychological Disorders 145
9. Social Psychology 155
10. Social Interactions 177
11. Social Structures 193
12. Demographics and Social Inequality 213

Image Attributions and Index 235

This page left intentionally blank.

Experimental Designs and Methods

CHAPTER 1

0. Introduction

Scientific experiments will be present throughout your MCAT prep journey, as 75% percent of questions in each science section are based on passages, and many of those passages will directly present the results of experiments. Furthermore, some questions may directly ask you about aspects of experimental design (especially on the Psychological, Social, and Behavioral Foundations of Behavior section, which we'll refer to as "Psych/Soc" from now on for the sake of brevity). Therefore, it pays to become familiar with the basic conceptual and terminological toolkit that scientists use to discuss aspects of research design at the beginning of the study process.

1. Types of Variables

All research studies explore some kind of relationship between two or more phenomena that exist in nature or in society. The term **variable** is used to refer to those phenomena, because such phenomena must show some kind of variation in the real world in order for them to be interesting from a research perspective.

At the simplest level, a study investigates the relationship between an **independent variable** and a **dependent variable**. In an **experimental study**, the researcher manipulates the independent variable, and then observes how the dependent variable changes in response to those manipulations. For example, researchers might analyze a certain chemical reaction by changing the pH of the reaction environment to investigate how pH affects the rate or yield of the reaction. Keep in mind that the *dependent* variable *depends* on the independent variable. Another important consideration to understand about the relationship between independent and dependent variables is that the dependent variable cannot happen earlier in time than the independent variable.

However, it is not always possible to manipulate the independent variable in an experimental setup directly. Consider a study investigating whether type 2 diabetes increases the risk of cardiovascular disease. For practical and ethical reasons, it would be impossible to induce type 2 diabetes in some people, withhold treatment, and watch what happens. Therefore, another strategy is needed, such as observing people with type 2 diabetes and comparing their rate of cardiovascular disease development to that of people without type 2 diabetes. However, in any analysis of this relationship, type 2 diabetes would still be the independent variable and cardiovascular disease would be the dependent variable, because the goal would be to explore how cardiovascular disease risk depends on type 2 diabetes status. In graphs, the independent variable is almost always presented on the x-axis and the dependent variable is presented on the y-axis, making it easy to visualize how the dependent variable shifts as a function of the independent variable. However, it is preferable to understand how the terms independent variable and dependent variable reflect an underlying logical relationship between two parameters, rather than memorizing facts about how these variables tend to be presented visually.

Since reality is complicated, other variables may be relevant to the relationship that we set out to explore. Such complications can be described using the concepts of confounding, mediating, and moderating variables.

A **confounding variable** is a third variable that affects both the independent variable and the dependent variable. By doing so, it potentially obscures the true relationship between the independent and dependent variables. As textbook writers are almost universally coffee drinkers, one of our favorite examples here is the relationship between coffee consumption and cardiovascular disease, something that has been a topic of recurrent concern. The initial studies of this relationship were conducted several decades ago, and showed some evidence of an association between coffee drinking and heart disease. However, at that time, cigarette smoking was more common than it is now. As we know, cigarette smoking is directly and causally associated with cardiovascular disease, and at the time, it also happened to be the case that cigarette smoking was more common among coffee drinkers than among non-coffee drinkers. This overrepresentation of smoking among coffee drinkers could either exaggerate the relationship between coffee drinking and cardiovascular disease, or even generate an apparent relationship where no real cause-and-effect relationship exists at all. The latter is the consensus in modern research, so if you're a moderate coffee drinker, don't worry about it. The key point, though, is that a confounding variable is specifically defined as one that has a relationship with both the independent and the dependent variable.

> **MCAT STRATEGY > > >**
>
> When faced with a challenging experimental passage, the first step in understanding it is to identify the independent and dependent variables, followed by clarifying the role of any other variables that may be present.

Given the importance of this point, and the frequency with which it causes misunderstandings, let's consider a further example: In a genetically inherited condition known as familial hypercholesterolemia, a mutation causes extremely high cholesterol levels, often resulting in death from cardiovascular disease at very young ages in individuals homozygous for the mutation. Therefore, familial hypercholesterolemia is certainly a risk factor for cardiovascular disease. However, could we say that it is a confounder in the possible relationship between coffee drinking and cardiovascular disease? In order for that to be the case, familial hypercholesterolemia would also have to have some relationship with coffee drinking, which seems unlikely. Therefore, familial hypercholesterolemia is not a confounding variable. The risk of cardiovascular disease may be influenced by many different factors, some of which might be confounding variables with regard to the impact of coffee drinking, and others of which might not be. Again, a confounder must affect both of the variables implicated in a relationship.

A **mediating variable** provides a mechanistic link between an observed relationship between two variables. Mediating variables can be visualized as being in between the independent and dependent variables. Mediating variables are often relevant for relationships that are statistically robust, but fail to make sense in a direct cause-and-effect kind of way. A real-world example is provided by a 2018 study published in JAMA that explored the relationship between county-level median household income and the mortality rate from cancer. The researchers found a strong relationship, in which lower levels of income were associated with higher mortality rates from cancer. That finding doesn't make very literal causal sense, in that cancer cells don't check on a person's income before undergoing malignant transformation. Instead, the researchers found that the majority of this relationship could be explained by the availability of quality health care, smoking, and food insecurity. That is, poverty is associated with factors that are themselves more directly related to cancer.

A **moderating variable** modulates the intensity of a certain relationship. So, for instance, a relationship may exist between workplace stress and symptoms of anxiety or depression. Healthy coping strategies like exercise or meditation might not remove that relationship entirely, but it's possible that they could reduce the intensity of that relationship; that is, in people who engage in healthy coping behaviors, the impact of workplace stress on psychological outcomes like anxiety or depression might be less severe. Graphically, we can view a moderating variable as affecting the arrow that we might draw to connect the independent and dependent variables.

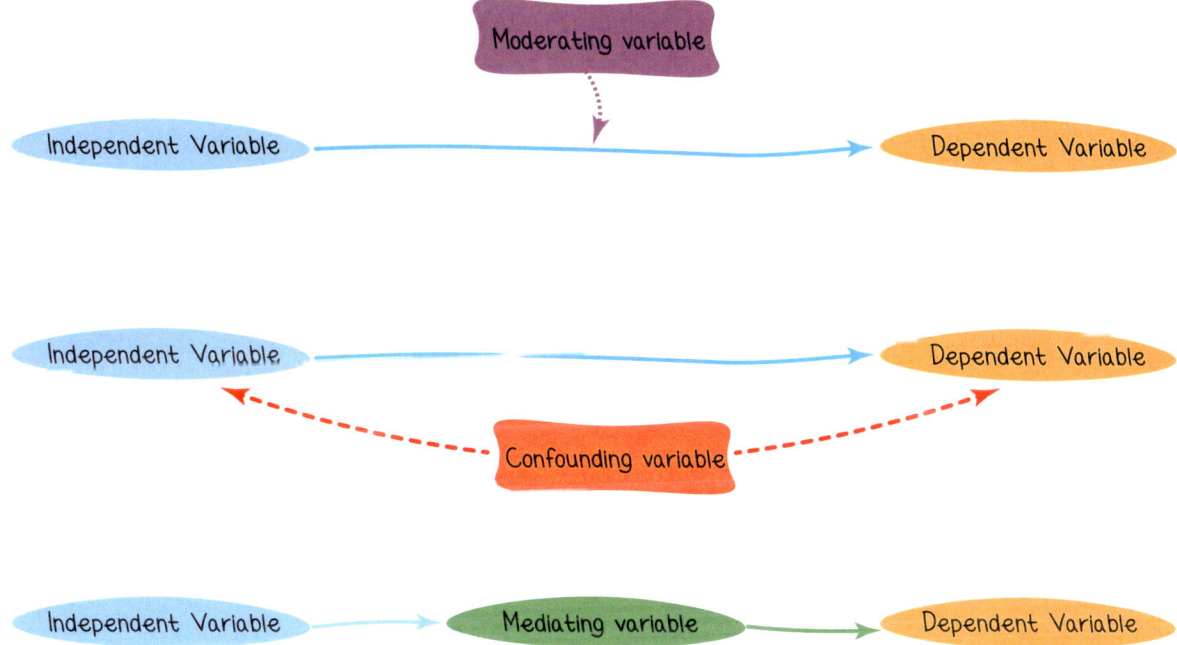

Figure 1. Types of variables

Once we decide, on a conceptual level, what it is that we want to investigate, that goal must be translated into something that we can measure in a practical way. That process is known as **operationalization**. In some cases, operationalization is fairly straightforward; for instance, regarding coffee drinking and cardiovascular disease, self-reported coffee consumption could probably be linked to medical records on cardiovascular disease. Of course, there could be some issues with the reliability of self-reported data, but the basic idea is fairly clear. Operationalization can often be more difficult, however, in psychology experiments. For example, in a study exploring how environmental cues (e.g., being in a light or dark room) affect participants' levels of energy when carrying out a task, it would be necessary to measure levels of energy. For example, researchers could measure the speed at which participants carry out some task, or their efficiency. Any variable in an experiment may need to be operationalized in a non-obvious way, and the validity of an experiment may be affected by whether that operationalization is carried out skillfully or not.

However, assessing the reasonableness of the operationalization of a variable requires understanding how that variable fits into the logic of the experiment. This point underscores the necessity of thoroughly understanding the concepts of independent and dependent variables, as well as applying them to the concrete details of any experiment under analysis.

2. Types of Studies

After identifying variables of interest, researchers must choose a study design. Many different types of study design exist, but the most basic distinction is between **experimental studies** and **observational studies**. In experimental studies, the researchers directly manipulate an independent variable, at scales that can range from cell culture in a lab to administering various drugs or treatment strategies to humans. In observational studies, researchers carefully analyze pre-existing patterns of variation to obtain information on significant relationships. Additionally, depending on how researchers measure variables of interest, studies can be classified as **quantitative**, if numerical measures are used, **qualitative**, if verbal or open-ended measures are used, or **mixed-methods**, if both of those tools are combined.

I. Experimental Studies

Experimental designs may seem simple, in that at their core, they involve doing something and observing what happens. However, conducting high-quality experimental research that yields valid scientific data requires a little bit more care in terms of the setup. First, controls are needed to assess the impact of an intervention. Controls can be negative or positive. **Negative controls** do not receive the treatment or intervention of interest, although in research on humans or animals, they might receive a placebo or sham treatment (e.g., a sugar pill instead of a pharmacologically active drug). Negative controls are crucial in order to demonstrate whether an intervention actually has an effect. For example, imagine researchers identify some interesting molecule that might cure the flu. If patients with the flu who receive the drug get better, can we conclude that we now have a cure for the flu? Not so fast, because the vast majority of patients with the flu will recover anyway. Therefore, it is necessary to compare patients with the flu who take the new, possibly-miracle drug, to patients with the flu who take nothing—or a placebo—and just suffer through it, and see whether a statistically significant difference emerges.

Positive controls, in contrast, receive a treatment that is known to induce the outcome of interest. For example, researchers interested in evaluating a new drug that induces apoptosis might construct an experiment that includes a positive control group, which receives a known apoptotic agent. Positive controls serve several purposes. One is that they confirm the adequacy and competency of the experimental procedures. For instance, if you conducted an experiment and nothing happened, is it possible that you're just unskilled at conducting experiments? As anyone who has done bench work in a lab knows, things can go wrong in many ways. Positive controls provide some insurance against that possible interpretation. Additionally, positive controls provide a way to benchmark the effectiveness of the treatment being studied.

For results obtained using controls to be valid, the control samples or participants should be equivalent to the experimental samples or participants, and they should receive identical treatment throughout the study. This is where **randomization** and **blinding** come in. In a lab-based experimental study, it's expected that samples will be randomly allocated to control or treatment groups, and to whatever extent possible, it's also considered good practice for lab technicians or other people involved in an experiment not to know which samples are which during routine maintenance. The latter consideration is known as blinding, and it also applies in human experiments. For example, if a comparison is being made between the effects of a drug and a placebo pill, a double-blinded design is commonly used, in which neither the participants nor the researchers who interact with the study participants know who is receiving a placebo and who is receiving the compound being studied. Although that information must be stored somewhere for the data to be analyzed, participants are randomly assigned to one group or another, and the actual information necessary to ensure that the right participants receive the right pills is restricted to the least amount of people necessary (and those people never interact directly with the participants).

Pulling these threads together, an experimental study in which participants are randomized to either a treatment group or a control group is, intuitively enough, known as a **randomized controlled trial (RCT)**. An RCT is non-blinded if everyone involved knows which participants are in which group, double-blinded if neither the participants nor the researchers know which participants are in which group, and single-blinded if either the participants or the researchers, but not both, know who is in which group. That last category (single-blinded) might seem like a puzzling choice at first, but the idea is that in some studies, double-blinding isn't reasonably possible. Consider, for instance, a study exploring the efficacy of group support sessions on improving quality of life in patients with a chronic illness. There's no reasonable way to blind participants to whether they're attending a group support session or not. However, it could be possible to blind their treating clinicians to that fact. This would result in a single-blinded design.

II. Observational Studies

Experimental studies are not always feasible, for practical and ethical reasons. Returning to the example of investigating the possible connection between coffee drinking and cardiovascular disease, it would not be possible to grab a bunch of people, assign them to either drink coffee or not to drink coffee, and then track them for decades to see how many develop cardiovascular disease. Alternatively, if a new disease is emerging in the population, and scientists are trying to determine its causes, it may not be feasible to conduct experiments, in the strict sense of the word.

In cases like these, **observational designs** must be used. As we've mentioned, observational designs analyze pre-existing variation in the population. A simple example is a **cross-sectional study**, in which researchers take a set of people representative of a population, measure various things about them, and look for correlations among those measurements. Ideally, this is done with a large enough group of people to ensure appropriate statistical power, and various strategies can be used to ensure that such a sample is as representative as possible. Opinion polls are a simple example of a cross-sectional study, although such designs in medical research often incorporate a broader range of physical and medical information, enabling the analysis of topics such as the relationship between cholesterol levels and blood pressure, whether any such parameter is associated with having been diagnosed with some disease, how factors like that are related to quality of life, and so on. Such analyses are often termed **correlational studies**, because they focus on how certain variables are correlated with each other; that is, whether a high level of one variable predicts a high or low level of another variable, and vice versa.

Cross-sectional studies can be powerful, but they have some inherent limitations because they provide only a snapshot of a certain population at a certain time. Of particular importance, such studies cannot provide information about causality. For instance, a cross-sectional study that finds a link between obesity and physical inactivity could not allow researchers to determine on that basis alone whether physical inactivity causes obesity or vice versa. Additionally, a single cross-sectional study provides no information about changes over time. The latter limitation can be addressed by incorporating a **longitudinal design**, in which multiple measures are made over time. For example, a longitudinal cross-sectional design might allow an assessment, of say, whether high blood pressure in the year 2005 predicts developing heart disease by the year 2015. A distinction is made between **risk factors**, which are independent variables associated with a higher risk of a negative outcome, and **protective factors**, which are those associated with a lower risk of a negative outcome. Technically speaking, observations about risk factors and protective factors identified through a longitudinal cross-sectional study cannot conclusively establish a cause-and-effect relationship, but it would move further in that direction than is possible with measurements from just a single time point. **Cohort studies** are a subset of longitudinal cross-sectional studies, in which a group of subjects is assembled according to some organizing principle, often age, and followed up over time. Such an analysis, in which data are gathered moving forward, is known as a **prospective analysis**, whereas cross-sectional studies that look back over time are known as **retrospective**.

A final point to make about longitudinal designs is that although they're commonly associated with cross-sectional studies, it is also possible for experimental studies to be longitudinal as well, depending on the length and regularity of rounds of treatment and follow-up measurements.

Case-control studies are another important subtype of observational studies. As the name implies, case-control studies involve gathering up some "cases"—or individuals with an outcome of interest—and comparing them to "controls," or people who do not have that outcome of interest, with the goal of identifying differences between the two groups that might shed light on the phenomenon in question. Case-control designs are important in epidemiology, for investigating the cause of an emerging disease.

On an even more basic level, researchers might simply report their experiences with a certain condition or treatment. If applied to a single case, this is known as a **case study**; if applied to multiple cases, this is known as a **case series**.

Case studies and series can provide useful clinical guidance on how to recognize and treat rare conditions, even if they remain fundamentally anecdotal, and they can also sometimes provide warning for newly emerging diseases.

Now, not all studies are created equal in terms of the strength of the evidence that they produce. It's generally thought that randomized controlled trials, or RCTs, provide the strongest evidence of any study design, due to their experimental and carefully structured nature, followed by cohort studies, case-control studies, and case reports or case series. But even better than an RCT is multiple RCTs, right? **Systematic reviews** are studies in which a researcher combs through the literature on a given topic and critically assesses the outcomes of various studies; this approach is often combined with meta-analyses, in which data from multiple studies are combined and re-analyzed. **Meta-analyses** are thought to yield the strongest available evidence on a given topic, but beware—since individual studies in a meta-analysis are almost guaranteed to have used different measures, drawing direct conclusions from these can be treacherous.

We've just covered a lot of terminology, but the good news is that as you move forward with your MCAT study process, you will have the opportunity to read summaries of many studies in experimental passages, which will allow you to practice using this conceptual toolkit to understand why scientists structure their research in certain ways. You may be asked directly, especially in the psych/soc section, to identify which term is best used to describe the research design of a certain study, but even if you're not directly asked about it, it's helpful to get into the habit of critically reading and thinking through the design of any study that you encounter, in order to have a more informed sense of the insights and pitfalls of a certain study. Even clinicians who don't actively conduct research themselves must be positioned to critically assess the impact and scope of newly-emerging critical research, so these skills will serve you in good stead in the future.

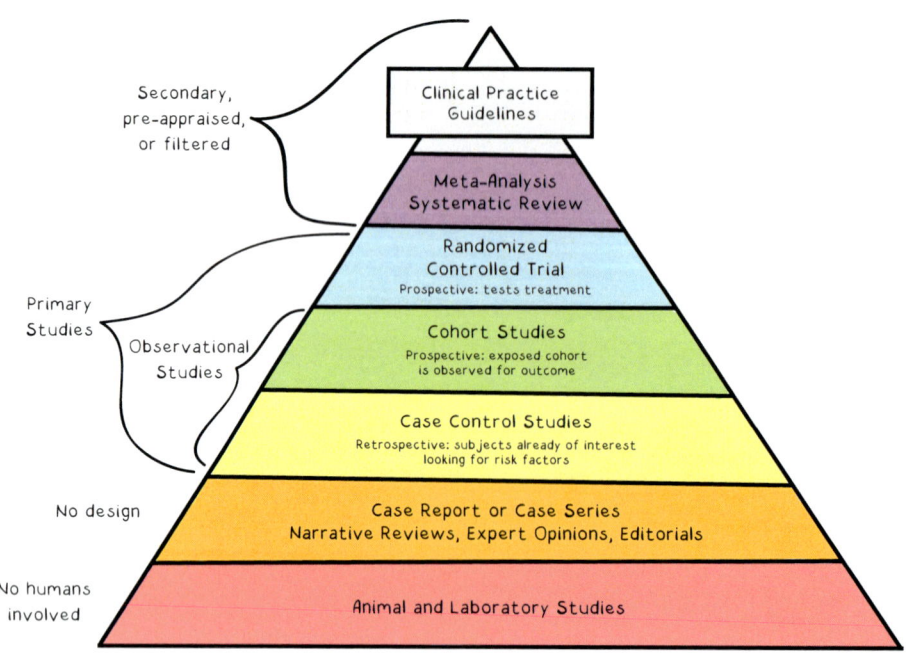

Figure 2. Hierarchy of evidence

3. Experimental Design: Pro-Tips and Pitfalls

A solid understanding of types of variables and types of study design form the basis of questions about research design on the MCAT, but there are a few additional points where more extensive expertise can pay off. In this section, we present an overview of several miscellaneous considerations helpful for honing your ability to answer questions on research design that require an analysis of subtleties beyond simply identifying the type of variable being investigated in a given study or the type of study design being used.

Institutional Review Board approval is a mainstay of modern research, and a concern for **ethical standards** lies at the core of this requirement. Recent decades have exhibited a trend towards an increased rigor in terms of research ethics, largely in response to increased awareness of the pervasiveness of research misconduct throughout the history of science.

Several codes and guidelines exist regarding **research ethics**. There's no expectation that you need to be aware of all of them, but seven principles identified by researchers at the National Institutes of Health, or NIH, provide a reasonably concise and comprehensive overview of the main factors that researchers must consider when conducting research on humans. The first principle is that research must have **social and clinical value**; that is, a study must be attempting to answer an important question. The second principle, on a related note, mandates that research have **scientific validity**. Next, the principle of **fair subject selection** indicates that participants in a study should be chosen based on the relevance for the study's scientific goals. The principle of a **favorable risk benefit ratio** mandates that the risks of study participation should be minimized, and that the benefits of the study must outweigh whatever risks are present. The principle of **independent review** states that an independent board of reviewers should assess the research proposal for any study before it starts, in order to identify any conflicts of interest and minimize any ethical concerns. The principle of **informed consent** states that participants must be informed of the purposes, methods, risks, and benefits of the study and be given the choice to participate accordingly. Finally, the very broad principle of **respect for potential and enrolled participants** includes, but is not necessarily limited to, factors such as respecting privacy, maintaining confidentiality, and monitoring participants' welfare during research.

Debate exists about whether various phenomena relating to physical and mental health are due to **"nature" or to "nurture,"** which refers to a debate regarding the extent to which genetic or environmental factors are responsible for a given outcome. Certain choices can be made in terms of research design to try to explore these issues. Perhaps most notably, studies have been conducted on twins and siblings to try to tease apart these issues, especially among twins or siblings who have been raised in different environments. Such studies, for instance, have played a major role in demonstrating the relatively high heritability of psychiatric disorders such as schizophrenia.

> **MCAT STRATEGY > > >**
>
> Of these ethical principles, the most important are the need for informed consent and the idea that research involves a trade-off between risks (or inconveniences) and benefits). However, keep in mind that experiments may still involve causing discomfort or pain to participants; doing so may be necessary to investigate the research question, and as long as participants provide informed consent, that is not necessarily an ethical problem.

A similar issue is at stake for investigating non-communicable diseases, as most saliently exemplified by cardiovascular disease, stroke, and cancer. These have become major issues in the developed world, and research increasingly indicates that both environmental factors, in the form of external factors such as pollutants or contaminants or in the form of health behaviors like smoking or physical inactivity, and genetic susceptibility play a role in the development of these diseases. In particular, genetic factors may serve to buffer, or moderate, the impact of environmental factors. For instance, if someone talks about how their grandparents lived to the age of 90-something but ate bacon every day and smoked like a chimney, that's a reference to the idea that genetic factors might protect against otherwise deleterious environmental factors. With the advent of modern genomic technologies, genetic screening has been used to try to identify genetic predictors of various health outcomes. Interestingly, though, the potential of so-called genome-wide association studies has not quite been fulfilled, for two main reasons: first, statistical power is an issue with studies exploring a tremendous amount of potential relationships; and second, the effect size of many of the relationships found through such studies is not large enough to motivate public health efforts to be taken in response. Nonetheless, this is certainly an area of ongoing research, and the goal of personalizing medicine based on genomics is still a major motivator among researchers and clinicians alike.

The ultimate goal of much biomedical research is to establish **cause-and-effect relationships.** At the end of the day, causality is a philosophical construct—in other words, it's not something we could isolate in the lab and point to—but a consensus exists about the basic factors necessary to establish a causal relationship. First, an association, or correlation, must be found between two variables. For instance, in a cross-sectional analysis, variation in one variable must predict variation in another. Then, it is necessary to establish that variation in the independent variable—as a cause—temporally precedes, or comes before, variation in the dependent variable. Finally, a plausible mechanism must be established through which the putative cause could exert the effect that we have in mind. For this final point, it may be necessary to pay careful consideration to possible mediating variables.

Mistaking a correlational relationship for a cause-and-effect relationship is a major pitfall, both in academic research, and especially in our attempts to analyze, understand, and change reality. To help understand where reasoning about correlation versus causation can go off the rails, it's helpful to think of correlation as a bidirectional, or reciprocal, relationship, where two variables tend to rise and fall in tandem, or in opposite patterns, whereas causation is a unidirectional relationship, in which changes in one variable result in changes in another. Some correlations are shown to reflect a cause-and-effect relationship; for instance, the influenza virus will cause the sickness known as influenza, adrenaline will cause sympathetic nervous stimulation, and so on. Other correlations might be pure coincidence; for instance, an enterprising researcher on the internet found a close correlation between the divorce rate in Maine over time and the rate of per capita margarine consumption. Alternatively, other correlations can reflect the same underlying cause. For instance, a strong negative correlation exists between the number of pirates in the Carribbean and the global rate of carbon dioxide emissions. That's not because pirates reduced carbon emissions, or because higher carbon emissions directly eliminated piracy, it's because the underlying phenomena of globalization and industrialization took place, resulting in both fewer pirates and higher carbon emissions.

> **MCAT STRATEGY > > >**
>
> The need to pay careful attention to when evidence supports cause-and-effect relationships is a unifying factor for all sections of the MCAT; be on the lookout to avoid causality-related errors.

4. Experimental Methods

Consider two very different experiments. The first experiment finds that children who are administered 18 milligrams of growth hormone per week grow, on average, 5.5 centimeters more than children who are not treated. The second experiment asks its participants to eat 10 chocolate-frosted jelly-filled donuts with rainbow sprinkles, and then describe what they see when looking at a Rorschach inkblot test. These descriptions are then compared to those made by a non-donut-eating control group, who enviously give the donut-eating group side-eye at the conclusion of the study. Which is the better experiment?

While the first experiment might sound more scientific than the second, neither is necessarily objectively better or worse. Instead, these experiments simply use different experimental methods. The growth hormone experiment used **quantitative methods**, which generate numerical data. In other words, quantitative methods always produce numbers as results. These results are then categorized, ranked, or used to construct fancy graphs and draw statistical conclusions.

In contrast, **qualitative methods** produce results that are not numbers. These results could be words, opinions, observations, or anything else that is not numerical. In the study of donut consumption and the Rorschach test, the results were descriptive, or qualitative, which can vary widely and cannot be easily quantified. Qualitative research is typically more open-ended and exploratory than quantitative research, and the findings obtained by qualitative research may be used later to develop a quantitative test on the same topic. If we'd asked the participants to rank on a scale from 1 to 10 how scary a particular inkblot appeared, that would be quantitative, but if we ask them what they see and write down their response, that's qualitative. We could always design a follow-up experiment in which our results are some numerical measure (such as "from 1 to 10, rate how happy this inkblot makes you feel,") rather than freeform observations.

Categorization of research methods isn't always binary. Many experiments aren't simply quantitative or simply qualitative. Instead, these studies may incorporate a mix of both methods, in what we rather uncreatively call **mixed-methods** research. For example, a study might first measure the number of chocolate-frosted jelly-filled donuts with rainbow sprinkles that each participant can eat in an hour, which is quantitative, and follow up by asking the participants to describe their feelings about eating so many donuts, which is qualitative.

Another key distinction exists between objective measures and subjective measures. Objective measures are, at least theoretically, unbiased; they are based on facts or numbers, and if performed correctly, they do not vary based on the individual measuring them. Height is a classic example; for example, a certain actor's biography lists their height as 6 feet and 1 inch and their publicist insists this is true, but a medical assistant measures them at 5 feet and 7 inches. The medical assistant's value is objectively correct, technically speaking. In contrast, subjective measures are subject to opinion, meaning that two participants could produce two different, but equally valid, sets of results. Subjective research questions could include "How comfortable do you feel right now?" or "To what extent do you think it was a bad idea to eat those donuts last week?" Since the participant's perceived level of comfort and personal definition of a bad idea are subject to that participant's internal feelings, his or her answers are subjective, not objective. Subjective questions don't really have a wrong or right answer, unless your mom asks you how her home-cooking tastes, in which case there's only one right answer.

To come full circle by returning to our initial question, we now know that our growth hormone height experiment was quantitative, since its results were numerical: height in centimeters, or inches because the US likes to do its own thing when it comes to units of measurement. Since height is not subject to bias, this measure is objective. In contrast, our experiment on the chocolate-frosted jelly-filled donut with rainbow sprinkles-eating Rorschach testers was qualitative, because its results were personal, freeform descriptions. As descriptions, these were subjective, since different participants could give very different, but equally valid, responses to the same inkblot test. Keep in mind that these don't always go together; it is possible to encounter a quantitative study design of a subjective measure, or a qualitative study design of an objective measure.

5. Validity

Imagine that you're a physician researcher designing an experiment. Assuming that you want it to be a good experiment, you'll want to ask yourself two key questions. The first question is: how do you know if your measurements are accurate? For example, if you measure a given volume as 18 mL, how can you tell that its actual volume is 18 mL, and not some completely different value?

Let's set this question aside for now, and assume that we know beyond a shadow of a doubt that our results will be accurate. This leads to a second question: how do we know that our results will apply to the "real world," rather than being entirely specific to this experiment? For example, consider a study where we observe the behavior of young children. This experiment takes place in a lab, where the children are surrounded by white walls and scary researchers. Even if our data are absolutely reflective of how the children behaved in this lab, we cannot possibly extrapolate it onto child behavior in real life, because in real life, children usually aren't in labs with intimidating scientists around them. In the case of this lab experiment, our data are not generalizable to outside situations.

We can answer both of these questions—how do we know our results are accurate and how do we ensure that they apply to non-lab, real-life situations—by assessing the study's validity. **Validity** refers to the extent to which a study's results are both genuine (which answers the first question) and generalizable (which answers the second).

Validity can be divided into three major categories: internal, external, and test validity. **Internal validity** describes the extent to which we can draw causal conclusions from the study data. In other words, did we conduct the study in such a way that we know that manipulating variable *x* caused some change in variable *y*? For example, did you know that as ice cream sales rise in US cities, so do murder rates? So, can we conclude that changes in ice cream sales caused a murder frenzy, or might those changes be due to some other factor? If we can draw causal conclusions between ice cream sales and the murder rate, our study has internal validity, but if we cannot conclusively determine that causation explains this relationship we observed, our study lacks internal validity.

In fact, it's pretty unlikely that ice cream inherently provokes people to think, "hey, wouldn't today be a great day to commit murder?" I'm pretty sure the worst thing ice cream's ever done to people is give them brain freeze. Instead, both ice cream sales and murders might increase due to a separate common factor, like the time of year. In the summer months, people tend to go outside more, leading more people to ward off the heat with a scoop of salted caramel, and also leading to more people around to murder and be murdered. Here, time of year is a confounding variable: an outside factor that we are not studying, but that impacts both variables under consideration. This confounding variable can lead to the incorrect conclusion that ice cream sales cause murders—or maybe that murders drive ice cream consumption—so this study has low internal validity. In essence, then, internal validity depends on how much we are able to minimize confounding variables. The fewer and less impactful the confounding variables, the higher the internal validity and the more likely we are to derive causal information.

External validity is more relevant to our earlier example about child behavior in a laboratory setting. It refers to the extent to which we can generalize our results onto different experimental situations or real life. Since we couldn't generalize the children's behavior in the lab to their behavior in the very different real world, that study lacked external validity.

And third and final type of validity is **test validity**, which describes how well a research design was able to test what it intended to test, rather than something else. Since test validity is so broad, it is often broken into several subtypes. The first is **construct validity**, which tells us whether our test actually assesses the "construct" we have designed it to test. For example, if we design a test to assess athletic ability, does it actually assess athletic ability, or does it assess something else? If this test only involves chess players, we'd say this study lacks construct validity, since chess performance is not an accurate assessment of athletic skill, or at least until chess is adopted by the Olympics.

Content validity is how well the test covers the full scope of content the researchers intend to measure. If our test of athletic ability only asks its participants to lift a heavy object, it has low content validity, because there are many other aspects of athletic ability, like aerobic endurance, flexibility, and hand-eye coordination.

Criterion validity describes how well our test correlates with some other well-respected criterion, like an established alternate test of the same measure. This gives us a good way to determine whether our new test can be trusted. For example, the Olympic decathlon has long been accepted as a fairly accurate assessment of overall athletic ability. That's because the decathlon has 10 events: hundred-meter dash, long jump, shot put, high jump, four hundred-meter dash, 110-meter hurdles, discus, pole vault, javelin, and the 1500-meter run. Therefore, if the results of our new test don't correlate at all with decathlon performance, our test has low criterion validity.

A final type of test validity, **predictive validity**, is slightly different from the previous three, which largely focus on current aspects of the test or study. In contrast, predictive validity measures how well our test predicts later scores on some chosen measure. Take the NFL Combine, a weeklong scouting event for college football players that's intended to predict the success of NFL players on the football field. If athletes often perform terribly in the Combine but go on to become fantastic NFL players, the initial test of the Combine has low predictive validity.

6. Reliability, Precision, and Accuracy

Reliability, precision, and accuracy: these terms are used interchangeably in casual conversation, but in science, they mean very specific things that uniquely help us describe an experiment and its results.

Reliability is the extent to which study results are consistent. It answers the question, "If we do the study again, will we see similar results?" Another way to put this is: if we do the same thing over and over again across multiple trials, do we see a strong positive correlation between the data sets?

Reliability is remarkably similar to another term that you might remember from college lab classes: **precision**, which describes how close together experimental measurements are. If the same object is measured three times, with values of 3.31, 3.33, and 3.29 millimeters, the measurements are very precise. While precision is used to refer to data points, such as these measurements, reliability refers to the study or experiment as a whole. A reliable study, then, is one that we'd expect to produce precise results. If we were to use a dartboard analogy, and our darts hit approximately the same place on the target with each throw, then we could say that the dartboard is a reliable measurement tool, and that our thrower has precise aim.

Accuracy, in contrast, refers to the closeness of a measurement to the actual, real value that we are measuring. The closer our result is to the correct value, the more accurate that result is. If the object in the previous example actually has a length of 10 feet, then our measurements of 3.3-something millimeters were precise, but astonishingly inaccurate. While it differs in meaning, accuracy is similar to precision in that it describes data points, not the overall study that obtains this data. If a measurement tool used in an experiment produces accurate data, we use the term validity. Just like a reliable experiment must produce precise results, a valid experiment is expected to produce accurate results.

Knowing this information, we can imagine four scenarios that are possible for any experiment or study. The ideal scenario is that the study is both reliable and valid. We can illustrate this by imagining a group of skydivers, all of whom want to land as close as possible to the center of a field below. A reliable study is analogous to the skydivers all landing very close to each other, while a valid study is exemplified by the skydivers landing on or very near the center - exactly where they wanted to!

However, there are a few ways this study can go wrong. The results might be unreliable, meaning that repeating the experiment yields values that are not at all consistent, or invalid, meaning that the results are also not close to the true real-life values. This would be a nightmare for our skydivers, who land scattered far away from each other (unreliable) and far from the target (invalid). A second error involves data points that are closely clustered around an inaccurate value, meaning that they are reliable but not valid. Here, our skydivers land very close together, but in the wrong location. The final possibility is perhaps the trickiest to understand. In this scenario, our results are unreliable - they're all over the place - but they are valid, because the average of our wildly inconsistent results is close to the real value. Here, our skydivers are nowhere near each other, but the average of their locations is very close to the center of the field. To sum things up, reliability and validity are distinct characteristics of a study or a process, just like precision and accuracy are distinct qualities of a data set. But a well-executed experiment and its data should have all four of these qualities.

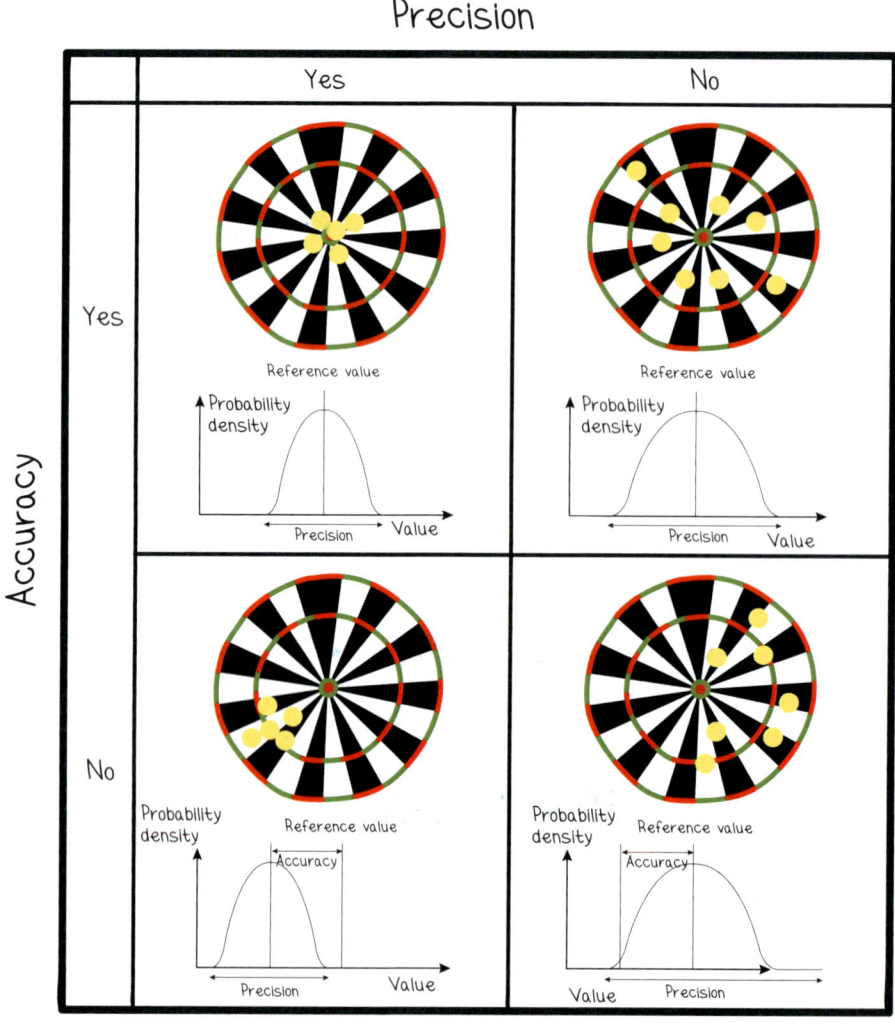

Figure 3. Accuracy versus precision

7. Survey Methods and Related Biases

While measures like validity and reliability can apply to any experiment or study, other concepts are specific to certain study methods. In particular, exam questions often focus on **survey methods**, which typically aim to collect large amounts of data from participants. Survey methods often take the form of a **questionnaire**, which is a list of questions that the researchers choose and then send to a group of participants to answer. This can't just be any random group of participants - it needs to be a representative sample, meaning that its demographics are reflective of the population the researchers intend to study.

For example, if a survey that aims to understand American exercise habits is only sent to Americans who own large dogs, the unrepresentativeness of this sample could skew the results. Maybe people with large dogs exercise more often than average because they need to walk their dogs, or maybe the kind of person who is willing to own a large dog happens to exercise more or less frequently than the kind of person who isn't. To avoid these issues, researchers should carefully choose a sample that does not deviate from the overall population on any characteristic that might affect responses. In this example, the exercise survey should be sent to participants in proportions that approximately resemble the American population as a whole. If 56% of Americans are dog owners, then, somewhere around 56% of the surveyed individuals should be dog owners as well. This concept is called representativeness.

Questionnaires are a form of self-report, meaning that the participants can choose how to answer each question without the researcher interfering or verifying the accuracy of the response. The items in a questionnaire will often take the form of a **Likert scale**. This scale consists of a statement followed by a continuum of possible responses, from 1 to 5 or 1 to 10, usually ranging from strong agreement with the statement to strong disagreement. The participant can then choose which response best matches his or her feelings.

Survey research methods are inexpensive and relatively easy to implement, and they can reach a far larger sample than a more hands-on experiment feasibly could. However, as you might expect, problems can arise when the data obtained by survey methods are biased or incorrect. Biases inherent to survey methods are termed **self-reporting bias**, also known as **response bias**. These biases occur as a natural side effect of allowing respondents to choose their own answers. Two key examples of self-reporting bias may appear on the MCAT, the first being **social desirability bias**. This is the tendency of respondents to answer in a way that they think makes them look more socially successful. For example, when survey participants are asked to self-report their salary, they might round up a little bit or add a few zeros to feel wealthier or impress the researcher. Since they'd virtually never round down, the overall data set is skewed.

The second important example of self-reporting bias is **acquiescence bias**, or the tendency to answer "yes" when asked a question, especially when you aren't sure of the answer. Have you ever been in a social situation where someone asked you if you'd seen or liked a particular movie, and you said yes without thinking? Researchers can counter this by including survey items with opposite meanings. If the participant answers similarly to both items that contradict each other, it provides clear evidence of acquiescence bias, and those items can be thrown out or otherwise accounted for. For example, if one item is "I love the Avengers movies" and a later item is "I hate the Avengers movies," and a respondent answers "strongly agree" to both, the researchers can't determine the participant's true feelings and should not draw conclusions from those responses.

Despite these challenges, survey methods have several advantages, including low cost, the ability to reach huge numbers of participants, and ease of implementation. But it's important to recognize that they can fall victim to specific biases, and great care should be taken to ensure that the surveyed sample is representative. On the MCAT, you will almost certainly be asked if you trust the results of a study, and understanding experimental flaws and biases will help lead you to judge for yourself whether a study is trustworthy.

7. Must-Knows

- Experimental studies manipulate an independent variable to observe how a dependent variable changes.
- Independent variables are manipulated (usually on the x-axis of an accompanying graph).
- Dependent variables change in response to the independent variable (usually on the y-axis).
- Confounding variables affect both the independent and dependent variable.
- Mediating variables provide a mechanistic link between two variables.
- Moderating variables change the intensity of a relationship between two variables
- Operationalization is the process of making a variable measurable.
- In experimental studies, negative controls receive effectively no treatment, and positive controls receive a treatment that is known to induce the outcome of interest.
    - Randomization and blinding help improve the validity of any study design.
    - Randomized control trials (RCTs): participants randomly assigned to either a treatment or control group.
- Observational studies analyze pre-existing variation in a population.
    - Cross-sectional studies: sample a population and measure various things about this group.
    - Case-control studies compare individuals with the outcome of interest (cases) and unaffected individuals (controls).
    - Case studies and case series: deal in depth with one or a few individuals in particular.
    - Longitudinal design: multiple measures are made over time.
        - Cohort studies: people are grouped by some organizing principle and followed through time, often age.
        - Retrospective studies analyze participants' history (backwards in time).
        - Prospective studies analyze participants moving forward in time.
- Systematic reviews and meta-analyses: combine data from many studies + critical or quantitative assessment.
- Ethical standards include: informed consent, favorable risk-benefit ratio, scientific validity, independent review, clinical value, fair subject selection, and the principle of respect.
- Experimental methods can be quantitative, qualitative, or mixed; measures can be objective or subjective.
- Validity: relates to meaningfulness of a study's results.
    - Internal validity: how well we can draw causal conclusions from the data.
    - External validity: how well experiment predicts real-world outcomes.
    - Test validity: how well design tests what it intends to (construct, content, criterion, and predictive validity).
- Accuracy: whether measure produces values close to the objectively true value; precision: whether the results are close to each other; reliability: whether the measurement can reproduce similar results
- Survey methods: often use questionnaires; this method is inexpensive but vulnerable to self-reporting bias
    - Social desirability bias: tendency to reply in a way that seems more socially successful/applicable
    - Acquiescence bias: tendency to answer "yes" to a question by default.
- Representativeness: idea that a sample should accurately reflect the population it's taken from.

End of Chapter Practice

The best MCAT practice is **realistic**, with a focus on identifying steps for further improvement. For those reasons, we recommend completing practice questions in an online setting that simulates the real MCAT interface, and taking advantage of advanced analytic features to help you determine how best to move forward in your MCAT study journey.

With that in mind, **online end-of-chapter questions** are accessible through your Next Step account.

As a further supplement, given the importance of active learning for effective studying, we also suggest that you consult the Must-Knows as a basis for creating a study sheet, in which you list out key terms and test your ability to briefly summarize them.

This page left intentionally blank.

Biological Basis of Behavior

CHAPTER 2

0. Introduction

Why do people act the way they do? This is one of the big questions we're faced with in our lives. For better or for worse, studying for the MCAT is probably not going to lead you to enlightenment in this regard, but the full name of the MCAT section that we commonly abbreviate as "psych/soc" is "Psychological, Social, and Biological Foundations of Behavior"—therefore, the MCAT does push you to think about this, at least a little bit. In this chapter, we'll focus on the biological basis of behavior, with due consideration of how this approach is distinct from psychological and sociological approaches.

1. Conceptual Approaches to Behavior

I. Biological Approaches

A biological approach to behavior refers to how genes, hormones, and neurotransmitters shape an organism's response to environmental stimuli or its own internal needs. The trope of brain surgery as a prototypical example of an intellectually challenging field underscores the complexity of biological systems. However, their complexity is what we call emergent complexity, which results from very many relatively simple processes all interacting at once. After all, a hormone or a neurotransmitter is what it is and does what it does, acting in an almost mechanical way. We don't have to worry about the self identity of melatonin, or its developmental stages, or how conflict theorists versus social interactionists might explain its effects on alertness. When studying how the nervous system and the endocrine system regulate behavior, as we'll explore in greater depth later in this chapter, it's remarkable how the individual processes don't *directly* relate to the overall output. However, every individual step is highly predictable, so our approach to studying how the endocrine and nervous systems affect behavior is essentially to account for a series of inputs and outputs, to determine how they work together, and to make a prognosis from there.

II. Psychological Approaches

Psychological approaches to behavior involve thinking about the human mind as a whole. The average adult human brain has about 100 million neurons and 100 trillion connections between those neurons. Highly complex systems tend to have a logic of their own, so in a psychological approach, we use higher-level abstractions, and talk about things like emotions, attitudes, memories, cognition, personality, and so forth. Through careful scientific work, researchers have identified associations between certain brain areas and specific psychological phenomena, but the level of precision does not permit the specific targeting of fine-tuned processes such as anger.

Therefore, in comparison to the biological approach to behavior, there's a little more wiggle room in the psychological approach. For instance, you might study Ekman's list of universal emotions (happiness, sadness, contempt, surprise, fear, disgust, and anger) and wonder about how we actually define happiness and sadness. Furthermore, an excellent question would be: what evidence supports the idea that certain emotions are universal? These are great questions, and other psychologists have indeed brought up concerns like this. However, the urge to ask questions like this must also be balanced with the fact that the MCAT is a standardized test that focuses on testing knowledge.

The question of how to engage with psychology material isn't quite as simple as memorization, though. For example, psychological development is an important sub-field within psychology, and as we'll see, psychologists love to propose various stages of development. There's Freud's stages, and Piaget's stages, and Kohlberg's stages, and Erikson's stages, and so on. On one hand, the advice to learn them, not argue with them, still applies to some extent. But on the other hand, thinking about why different psychologists chose to highlight different aspects of human development—that is, where these theories are coming from and what they're trying to explain—can help solidify your knowledge. Thus, to some extent, you can make the extra "wiggle room" of psychological approaches to behavior work for you.

That said, researchers can still carry out scientific experiments to shed light on questions about psychology and behavior. Because of the complexity of human psychology, it's especially important for researchers to design their experiments very precisely, paying careful attention to possible confounding variables, how to measure outcomes of interest, and how their findings can be interpreted. This is why the psych/soc section of the MCAT places such an emphasis on experimental design, as we'll discuss elsewhere.

> **MCAT STRATEGY > > >**
>
> Although it is necessary to memorize a lot of information for the MCAT, simply wading through a list of terms to recognize can both be exhausting and can lead to a superficial level of knowledge that is highly vulnerable to being forgotten. The best way to approach MCAT studying is to seek a balance; engage critically with the material to boost your interest and retention, but don't get too far sidetracked from the main task at hand.

III. Sociological Approaches

Sociological approaches have even more wiggle room, so to speak, than psychological approaches, because sociology deals with extraordinarily complicated systems. As we discussed, a single person is extraordinary complex, so it's mind-blowing to consider all the ways that millions, or even billions, of people interact. What's more, the approximately 7.5 billion people on Earth don't just interact with each other in a vacuum; instead, our interactions occur within the context of all of human history, within the framework of institutions shaped by our ancestors. In this light, it's amazing that we can make sense of society at all. More concretely, though, the high level of complexity associated with sociology means that many different perspectives on sociology-related issues tend to exist.

Mental flexibility is therefore critical for studying sociological approaches to behavior. For example, to answer a single question, it might be necessary to consider the perspectives of social constructionism, symbolic interactionism, functionalism, and conflict theory. However, the goal is to do so in a way that favors correctly answering that question, not seeking to reach a conclusion about which framework is objectively "correct." Instead, the goal is to cultivate the ability to think about how adherents of a given theory would try to explain a phenomenon presented in a passage or question. Doing so requires getting to the essence of each theoretical approach in a very concise way, focusing on how a given approach fits into the larger picture of all the different ways in which researchers have tried to explain society.

Another important consequence of the sheer complexity involved in sociological approaches to behavior is that it is bound to be harder to use experimental study design to explore sociological questions. We can't just build our own society from scratch to test a hypothesis, or make random changes in society just to see what happens—after all, these are people's lives we're dealing with here! For this reason, sociology tends to place a greater emphasis on retrospective study designs, where we look back and analyze things that have already happened, or cross-sectional study designs, where we try to take a snapshot of things as they exist at the present moment in time and look for relationships, or qualitative research designs, where we seek to explore people's experiences through words, not numbers. Chapter 1 contains much more detail on experimental design, but for the purposes of this chapter, it's useful to have a general sense of the different approaches that researchers can take to understand behavior.

As we launch our study of psychology and sociology, we'll be focusing on some high-level biological approaches to behavior, but having a sense of where this discussion is going in terms of building contrasts between psychological and sociological approaches will help you put all this information in context!

2. Genetics and Development

At a very nitty-gritty level, who and what we are is just a sum and product of our genes and our experiences. In this section we will first discuss the genetic aspect of behavior, then look at how we are affected by our experiences, and finally review how both genetic and environmental factors work together to create variation in behavior.

I. Genetic and Environmental Factors

The tremendous advances made in molecular genetics in the twentieth century both revolutionized our understanding of the mechanics of reproduction and development and opened up some very intriguing possibilities for psychology. This seems particularly compelling if we zoom out from just thinking about humans to examine broader classifications of life. Different types of animals—let alone plants and microbes—show very different types of behavior. For the most part, animals don't go to school, have symbolic culture, or use language, so many of these hard-coded, or **instinctual**, behaviors are shaped by genetics.

A slightly graphic example can clarify this point. Have you ever observed a cat with diarrhea? When a cat has an overwhelming need to defecate and can't make it to a litter box or soil in time, it will make ineffectual digging motions with its paws, as if it were burying its feces in sand. This behavior occurs because cats have an instinctual, or hard-wired, need to bury their waste. Even if circumstances don't allow them to actually do so, their bodies will make the attempt anyway. Instinctual behaviors are hard-wired, but behaviors can also be learned. For example, some owners have trained their cats to use toilets made for humans, which is definitely not an example of instinctive cat behavior. However, complications like this aside, it is important to have a solid understanding of the basic distinction between instinctive and learned behaviors.

However, it can be challenging to find purely instinctual behaviors in humans, because we have an astonishing capacity for **cultural learning**. For instance, think about how humans have taken hunger, which is an extremely basic physiological need, and have found ways to satisfy that need that range from healthy home-cooked food to fast food to fancy gourmet masterpieces, all of which show extensive cross-cultural variation.

The contrast that we established between cats, birds, and humans suggests that genetically coded behaviors are shaped by evolution, since the genetic code itself is subject to evolutionary pressures. That means that behaviors that promote reproductive success may be selected for. We refer to such behaviors as adaptive traits. Imagine that you're a hungry rattlesnake living in a very hot desert. Hunting at night might be the only way to reliably survive. Doing so will avoid overheating, and will enable to you to consume prey animals that are also nocturnal, like mice. Therefore, being nocturnal will ultimately help you survive and reproduce more than your fellow snakes. Therefore, this is an adaptive trait, or one that increases fitness. In contrast, because hunting in the heat of the day would pose a danger of overheating and make it difficult to find prey animals because they're all hiding from the heat too, diurnal hunting behavior would pose an elevated risk of death, and we would expect any gene that promotes diurnal hunting to be selected against. However, we must be very careful to link adaptive traits specifically to reproductive success, rather than moral or aesthetic bias about what makes a trait good or bad. Furthermore, this is a simplified view of evolution; in real populations, many harmful alleles are not lost and many adaptive ones do not significantly propagate. We therefore cannot say that any existing traits in modern animals are present only because they are adaptive.

> **MCAT STRATEGY > > >**
>
> The Psychology/Sociology section of the MCAT may expect you to apply a simplified version of evolution, in which existing, widespread behaviors are considered to be adaptive, but even in this context, "adaptive" always refers to promoting reproductive success in an evolutionary context.

The idea that behavior might be shaped by genetics is also intuitively appealing based on what we can observe in everyday life. For instance, even within a single family, different children may take after different parents seemingly at random, or parents might share stories about children having different temperaments as babies, before non-genetic factors could have had much influence. In fact, scientists believe temperament—which refers to how individuals respond behaviorally and emotionally to stimuli from the world that surrounds them—is biologically shaped. Furthermore, because temperament forms the foundations of personality, genetic factors play an important role in making us who we are.

But just as intuitively, **environmental factors** also shape people's development. At a high level, a child born to an affluent family who grows up in an excellent school district, with access to nourishing food, extracurricular opportunities, and a network of well-placed acquaintances and family friends, is likely to have a very different life trajectory from a child born in poverty who receives a substandard education, doesn't receive enough food at home, and must work from a young age. But other environmental factors can also affect development, such as stress and exposure to compounds that affect hormonal development in the body. Examples include endocrine-disrupting compounds, such as BPA from certain types of plastic and PAH from the combustion of hydrocarbons. Development is also impacted by observational learning from those around us. Therefore, it is possible both that children's attitudes and perceptions, of themselves and others, are influenced by those of their parents, and that psychologically complex family relationships affect a child's development. However, some of these possibilities are easier to measure and study than others, which is part of the excitement of studying psychology and sociology.

II. Gene–Environment Interactions and Heritability

Genetics and the environment both matter, but it's not always clear how to distinguish their effect. This issue, known as the **nature versus nurture debate**, is a thorny conundrum in several fields of science. In psychology, this mainfests in the form of research aimed at characterizing the heritability of a trait, which is defined as the proportion of how much variation in a trait (phenotype) is due to variation in the genotype. Or, in plain(er) English, how much is a trait determined by genes alone? A **heritability** of 1 would mean that all variation in a trait is explained through pure genetics, and a heritability of 0 would mean that all variation in a trait can be explained through environmental factors or chance.

Determining how heritable a trait is turns out to be surprisingly difficult, because in most cases, families share both genetic similarities and environmental similarities. Therefore, studying whether traits tend to cluster in families has some limitations. Advanced statistical techniques can help to some extent, but some special circumstances can shed light on this issue. Twin studies are extremely useful for these purposes, because identical twins, or monozygotic twins, share 100% of their genome, and non-identical twins—also known as fraternal, or dizygotic, twins—share about half of their genomes, just like any other pair of biological siblings. Another angle on this problem is to study adopted children, who have genetic similarities with their biological parents and environmental similarities with their adoptive family.

Most psychological traits have been estimated to have a heritability in the range of 0.3 to 0.6 (30 to 60%), which is to say that both genetic and environmental factors play a role in their development. Interestingly, schizophrenia has a much higher heritability, which has been estimated to be as high as 0.8. Now, this does not mean that, for instance, if your identical twin has schizophrenia, your odds of developing schizophrenia are 80%. The concordance rate for schizophrenia between identical twins is indeed quite high—somewhere in the range of 40% to 50%—but it's better to think of heritability as a number that quantifies the relative impact of genetic versus environmental variation on a trait, not as a probability estimate, and certainly not as a number that can be directly applied to an individual's situation.

Clinicians have the goal of making real, practical improvements in people's lives. So is all lost when it comes to treating highly heritable conditions? Not at all! In addition to medications and intriguing new possibilities like gene therapy, environmental interventions can sometimes be used to treat even purely genetic conditions. An example is the disorder phenylketonuria (PKU). People with PKU have a mutation that makes them unable to properly metabolize the amino acid phenylalanine. If left untreated, the phenylalanine build-up caused by PKU can result in severe cognitive impairment and death. Thus, a simple, cheap, and effective treatment is not to consume phenylalanine. Despite the numerous innovations of modern medicine, implementing a low-phenylalanine diet early in childhood remains the best way of treating this condition.

III. Mechanisms of Environmental Effects on Behavior

Experience is a mechanism through which environment influences behavior. After all, human beings are learning machines. We learn information, we learn how to behave in various situations, we learn to speak various languages depending on our culture and environment, and we even learn many preferences—for example, what you consider to be comfort food depends on where and how you grew up. Depending on which behavior we're focusing on, we might be more or less consciously aware of how experiences have shaped our behavior, but overall, virtually all human behaviors are shaped by experience.

One way that the environment influences behavior is through **gene expression**. Genes can be expressed, or transcribed, at a greater or lesser rate depending on the needs of the organism, in response to environmental or internal stimuli. It's been fairly well established that gene expression differs between people affected by different conditions, including some that might not seem very precisely defined biologically. For example, an interesting study from the late 2000s found different patterns of gene expression in older adults who reported feeling lonely and isolated versus those who felt more socially connected. However, we have not yet answered the question of how these changes in gene expression happen.

One mechanism stems from the fact that DNA sequences known as promoters initiate the expression of certain genes. There are also some genes, termed regulatory genes, that code for proteins that in turn affect gene expression through promoters or similar sites and interactions with other proteins. Researchers have proposed that variations in promoters and regulatory genes might shape behavior. Another study from the early 2000s suggested that a specific allele in the promoter for the serotonin transporter gene, *5-HTT*, makes people more susceptible to depression. A fair amount of scientific controversy ensued, and this issue can't be considered completely settled, but the mechanism itself is plausible, and is definitely worth being aware of for the MCAT.

The other possible mechanism to be aware of is **epigenetics**, or changes to the genome that do not involve changing the actual nucleotide content. The most important epigenetic change is **methylation**. As the name suggests, this involves adding a methyl group to nucleotides, generally to cytosine. This has the effect of silencing DNA, or shutting down the expression of specific genes. Methylation is a normal part of development and helps explain why different cells in our body do different things, despite having the same DNA sequence, but it also occurs in response to environmental stimuli, like stress, or even in response to exercise. Some studies have even suggested that methylation patterns can be inherited! In any case, this is a lively area of ongoing research in psychology, especially in terms of explaining the effects of chronic stress on an individual's mental health.

So, to summarize, even by just casually observing our surroundings, we can encounter huge variations in behavior. Some of that variation is clearly genetic, most clearly in the case of animal behavior. Some of that variation is learned and cultural, like differences in terms of what people consider to be comfort food, or how they dress. Much variation, though, especially in parameters that are interesting for psychology, involves a combination of genetic and environmental influences, and environmental influences frequently exert their effects by shaping patterns of gene expression.

3. Human Physiological Development

One of the most important ways in which biology shapes behavior is through the trajectory of human development. The basic pathway through which humans develop through pregnancy, infancy, childhood, adolescence, and even into old age is hard-wired, although considerable variation can occur across individuals with regard to the timing of various stages, and there is room for environmental factors to affect this process.

I. Pregnancy and Childhood

We cover the first major steps of embryogenesis and early pregnancy elsewhere, so we can jump in at around 12 weeks of **pregnancy**, at which point the fetus is still very small, but the basic architecture of the organ systems has been formed. During this period, the fetus is growing in its mother's uterus, and its umbilical cord connects it to the placenta, which is basically the fetus's point of contact with the mother. The placenta is a highly vascular bed of tissue that brings the fetal and maternal circulation in close proximity to exchange nutrients, gases, and waste products. Pregnancy usually lasts for about 37 to 41 weeks, and is divided into three trimesters. The **first trimester** is basically when the major structures of the fetus are formed, the **second trimester** is when the details get filled in and the fetus grows, and the **third trimester** involves growing and finalizing preparations for the outside world.

The specific steps of prenatal development are all pretty hard-wired, but the fact that the placenta enables two-way communication between the fetus and the mother means that there's also some room for environmental influences. Maternal malnutrition and cigarette smoking have been linked to negative effects on fetal development, and the possible impacts of psychological factors such as stress, anxiety, and depression have also been investigated.

Once babies are born, they have a set of **reflexes** that are completely hard-wired. Of course, reflexes aren't limited to babies. For example, the stereotypical part of a physical exam in which a doctor taps a patient's knee and sees if the patient's leg will jerk in response tests what's technically known as the **patellar reflex**. This is ample confirmation that reflexes are present in adult humans, too. But there's a set of important reflexes that are unique to babies, and disappear during further development.

Perhaps the most adorable of these reflexes is the **palmar grasp reflex**, which you can observe if you gently stroke your finger along an infant's palm—the baby will grab onto your finger as if it's trying to hold your hand. Two other important reflexes, the **rooting** and **sucking reflexes**, assist babies in feeding. The rooting reflex describes how a baby will search for an object that brushes against its mouth or cheek, and the sucking reflex describes how a baby will automatically start making sucking motions when something grazes the top of its mouth. Some other reflexes are named after researchers. The **Moro reflex** is a kind of startle reflex that occurs in response to sudden movement or loud sounds, in which a baby extends its arms and legs, pulls them back in, throws back its head, and cries. In the **Babinski reflex**, when the bottom of a baby's foot is stroked, the big toe bends up and the other toes fan out, whereas in healthy adults the toes curl downward. There are a few other newborn reflexes, but these are the big five.

In the first few years of life, children go through an almost unbelievable sequence of developmental steps. Of course, the timing of various milestones can vary tremendously, even within the range of normal development.

From a motor point of view, in the first year of life, a baby takes steps towards being able to navigate the world, including standing with assistance, crawling, and learning how to hold toys. From a social point of view, most interactions in the first year are focused on the primary caregiver and tend to be somewhat solitary. One notable milestone, though, is when infants start to show anxiety when interacting with strangers at around 7 or 8 months. Late in the first year of life, babies start enjoying the peek-a-boo game, which may be an indicator of important cognitive developments related to object permanence. More about that later, though. Linguistic behavior in the first year of life includes laughing, babbling, and maybe some simple words like "mama."

Between 12 and 24 months, or 1 and 2 years, children become more physically independent as behaviors like walking and climbing emerge. Other motor behaviors become more and more complex and coordinated, and this trend continues over the next few years. Two-year-olds can typically do things like basic drawing with a marker or crayon, deliberately kicking or throwing balls with an aim in mind, and stacking multiple cubes. You may have heard of the phrase "terrible twos", and indeed, two-year-olds tend to be pretty self-centered. This can be challenging for caregivers, but is also important for identity formation. Along similar lines, children at this age often like to explore boundaries involving the word "no." The age of two is also when language development blossoms, with a dramatic increase in the number of words a child uses, including pronouns like "me" and "you." By three years old, more mature behaviors emerge, like toilet training (although this also varies across cultures), the ability to carry out more complicated fine motor tasks like drawing recognizable objects, and manipulating behaviors, as well as social behaviors like taking turns and awareness of gender. Language development progresses rapidly, with more complex sentence structures emerging, as well as a dramatic increase in both active vocabulary—that is, the words that a child uses—and passive vocabulary, or the words that a child understands.

The key themes to extract from this discussion of early childhood development are that considerable variation exists in the specific timing of milestones across children, and that overall, more and more complex behaviors are developed. A final important concept here is that of the **critical period**. Experiences, either positive or negative, in early childhood can imprint themselves on a person, with implications that extend throughout the lifetime. One common area where this concept shows up is language: Humans have a hard-wired ability to learn language, but the actual language we learn—English, Chinese, Hindi, or any other of the thousands of languages spoken on earth—depends on our environment. And in fact, we have to get environmental input in order to learn to speak. There have been some really sad cases of extreme child neglect, or children who grew up in the wild, where children didn't get the early childhood language input they needed, and then had considerable difficulty learning language later in life. This suggests that the period of early childhood is critical for language development—hence the term critical period. However, this concept has been extended to include sensory perception and the formation of key psychological relationships, and even to the possibility that traumatic or stressful events early in life might have long-lasting consequences.

II. Adolescence and Adulthood

The next major developmental period is **adolescence**, which is the transition from childhood to adulthood. It is usually associated with the teenage years, although some important aspects of adolescence can start a bit earlier. There's a key point of terminology to be aware of here, though: Adolescence is a very broad term, which includes all of the cognitive, social, and behavioral changes that take place in this period, and as such, cultural understandings and conceptions of adolescence vary.

Puberty refers more specifically to the biological changes that happen during adolescence. Puberty itself is a long, drawn-out process, with landmarks including the onset of menstruation, or menarche, in females and the first ejaculation in males. Of course, some physical changes precede those events. A common timeline might be for puberty to start in females at around 10 or 11 years of age, for menarche to happen at around age 12, and for puberty to end around 15 to 17 years of age. For males, the corresponding timeline is generally pushed back by a year or so. Some research has suggested that puberty has been starting earlier in many children due to environmental influences, like hormone exposure or obesity, and variation has also been found across racial and ethnic groups. So it really depends, and these age ranges are truly just estimates.

Throughout puberty, a very wide range of changes happen to the body, in addition to the development of fertility. **Secondary sex characteristics** develop during this time, most notably including the growth of pubic hair and body hair in both sexes, the growth of breasts and wider hips in females, and facial hair and the Adam's apple in males. Sex-specific differences in fat and muscle distribution also take place as the body changes and grows These changes are orchestrated by sex hormones, most importantly testosterone and estradiol.

After adolescence we enter **adulthood**. There are no specific milestones to worry about here, although it's worth noting in passing that the part of the brain responsible for rational decision-making, the prefrontal cortex, keeps developing until age 25 or so. More specifically, the neuronal axons in the prefrontal cortex become covered with myelin sheaths, or myelinated, during this time and thus transmit signals more rapidly. This may help explain why teenagers and younger twenty-somethings are more likely to engage in what's considered reckless behavior than are older adults.

However, as adulthood continues, we age, and eventually die. **Aging** is an extremely complex process, and an entire field of anti-aging medicine exists to try to find ways to delay aging and to extend the human lifespan. One possible physiological contributor to aging is the eventual degradation of **telomeres**, which are nucleotide sequences at the end of chromosomes that protect them from losing nucleotides during DNA replication. The loss of telomeres places a hard limit on how often a cell can divide, with clear implications for aging and death. Aging involves a gradual physical decline, as people become more frail and more prone to a wide range of diseases. Some aspects of cognitive function also decline, including fluid intelligence and mental processing speed. Others though, such as crystallized intelligence, which refers to accumulated knowledge, remain stable. This is why the elderly are considered wise in many cultures!

The oldest age reliably recorded is 122 years, and life expectancy in the most highly-developed countries is creeping up above 80 years, although it tends to be higher in women than in men. Science fiction and hype in popular culture aside, most researchers don't think that dramatically extending the human lifespan is on the table, but exciting findings are emerging in terms of how to extend the healthy lifespan and improve quality of life during aging.

4. The Endocrine System and Behavior

Your first association with the endocrine system might be how glucose is regulated by the antagonistic pair of insulin and glucagon, perhaps followed by calcium and fluid regulation, which is carried out by processes with fun names like the renin-angiotensin-aldosterone system. However, in addition to its effects on glucose and fluid homeostasis, the endocrine system is one of the two physiological systems that closely regulate behavior on a biological level.

I. Principles and Anatomy

The **endocrine system** is covered in much more detail in the Biology textbook, but a quick crash course in how it works and its major components will help you understand how hormones help regulate behavior. The endocrine system is a network of organs distributed throughout the body that secrete signaling molecules, called hormones, into the bloodstream. The term endocrine refers to signaling that happens when molecules are secreted into the circulatory system, which carries them throughout the body to exert their effects. Some hormones, known as **direct hormones**, cause their target cells to make direct changes in some physiological function, while others cause other hormones to be released. The latter type are referred to as **tropic hormones**, and their existence makes it possible for, say, hormone A to cause hormone B to be released, which causes hormone C to be released, which only then causes the final physiological effect. This mechanism means that the body can exert exquisitely fine control over hormonal levels and processes, which is necessary since the endocrine system controls many vital functions.

A useful way of creating an overview of the endocrine system is to start from the top (in the brain), and move down through the body. There are two reasons for this. For one it's fairly intuitive, using our knowledge of anatomy to understand the endocrine system. More interestingly though, hormones secreted at the top of our body tend to be regulatory—that is, more likely to orchestrate the release of other hormones—while hormones secreted further down in the body tend to do the nitty-gritty work of actually affecting other cells in the body.

> **MCAT STRATEGY > > >**
>
> Although direct hormones are generally more immediately relevant for behavior than tropic hormones, understanding the signaling networks that contain tropic hormones helps provide valuable background information.

Starting from the top, the **hypothalamus** has the job of converting input from the nervous system into endocrine signals, so it's sometimes known as the bridge between the nervous and endocrine systems. As the name suggests—remember that "hypo" means "low"—the hypothalamus is located below the thalamus in the forebrain, directly above the pituitary gland. The hypothalamus releases various high-level tropic hormones, which travel down to the anterior pituitary to promote the release of other tropic hormones. For example, gonadotropin-releasing hormone (GnRH) acts on the anterior pituitary to trigger the release of luteinizing hormone (LH) and follicle-stimulating hormone (FSH), which ultimately regulate reproduction. Likewise, corticotropin-releasing factor (CRF) promotes the release of adrenocorticotropic hormone (ACTH) from the anterior pituitary, which eventually stimulates the adrenal glands to release cortisol, which is involved in stress. In yet another example of this pattern, the hypothalamus also releases thyrotropin-releasing hormone (TRH), which then causes thyroid-stimulating hormone (TSH), to be released from the anterior pituitary, which in turn promotes thyroid hormone production in the thyroid gland.

The **anterior pituitary** gland (adenohypophysis) is the next organ of note. It's located directly below the hypothalamus and, as we've mentioned, receives hypothalamic input. This input comes via hormones released into what's known as the hypophyseal portal system, which is basically a system of blood vessels connecting the hypothalamus to the anterior pituitary. It secretes some tropic hormones of its own, like LH and FSH, which exert sex specific effects on reproductive organs, ACTH, which promotes cortisol release, and TSH, which promotes the release of thyroid hormones. It also secretes prolactin, which stimulates milk production, endorphins, which reduce the perception of pain, and growth hormone.

The **posterior pituitary** gland (neurohypophysis) also receives input from the hypothalamus, but it receives this input in the form of neuronal rather than hormonal signals because it is actually composed of neurons itself. The posterior pituitary has two important outputs, antidiuretic hormone (ADH), which regulates fluid balance, and **oxytocin**, which has various effects on behavior that we'll be discussing in more detail shortly. Moving down the body, the **thyroid gland** and **parathyroid glands** are small organs located in the throat. The thyroid releases the aptly-named **thyroid hormone**, which is mostly known for its effects on metabolism, but can also influence behavior.

Moving down into the abdominal cavity, we encounter the pancreas, which is a very important endocrine organ for the body as a whole, but not a high priority for the Psych/Soc section. In contrast, the **adrenal glands** are worth dwelling on. These are two small glands located on top of the kidneys, and they're divided into distinct portions: The adrenal cortex and the adrenal medulla. The **adrenal cortex** secretes **cortisol**, which mediates the chronic stress response, while the **adrenal medulla** secretes **epinephrine and norepinephrine**, which are involved in the acute stress response. Finally, the **ovaries** in females and the **testes** in males release **estrogen** and **testosterone**, respectively. These two sex hormones are of great importance to the study of behavior.

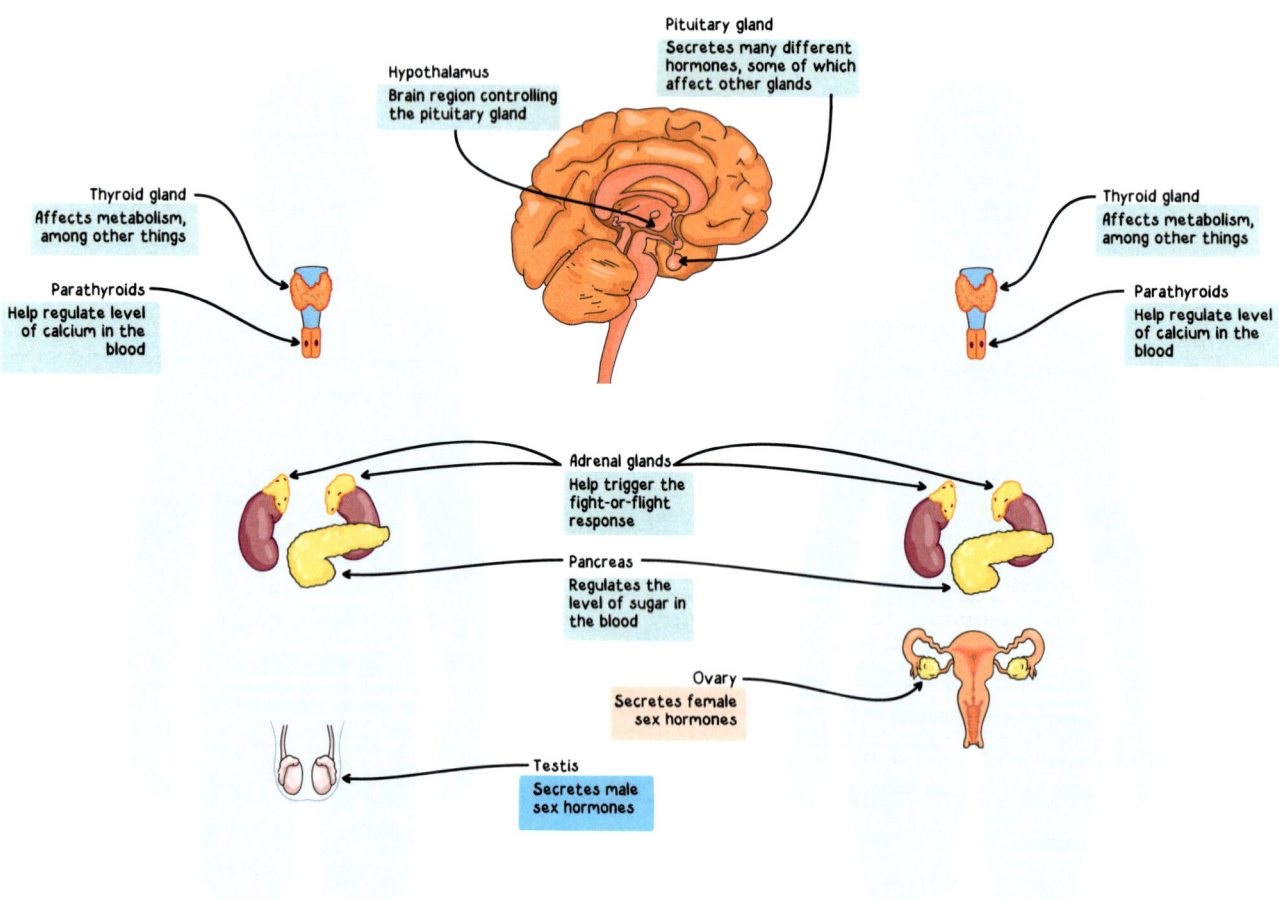

Figure 1. Endocrine organs

II. Behavioral Effects of Hormones

Now let's get to the pertinent question: How does the endocrine system affect behavior? This is a huge question—you can find entire textbooks with titles like *Behavioral Endocrinology* and journals with names like *Hormones and Behavior*—but some highlights are relevant for the MCAT.

We just mentioned the sex hormones, **estrogen** and **testosterone**. These hormones help coordinate reproductive processes and orchestrate the myriad changes that happen during puberty, as well as the maintenance of secondary sex characteristics. From a behavioral point of view, they also help promote libido—or interest in sexual behavior—and testosterone is also associated with complex changes in social behavior. A number of interesting studies have investigated how short-term stimuli can affect levels of these hormones. For example, winning a competition, or even just seeing one's favorite team win, can increase testosterone levels, whereas losing can decrease those levels. While we often associate estrogen with females and testosterone with males, that's an oversimplification: Both sexes secrete some of each hormone, but estrogen tends to predominate in women and testosterone in men.

Oxytocin is another hormone that does a frankly amazing number of things. If only we could be as productive as our hormones! Physiologically, oxytocin is best known for promoting uterine contractions during labor, which is a famous (and testable) example of positive feedback—basically, more oxytocin causes more contractions, which cause more oxytocin to be released, and so on, until childbirth. However, this hormone also has a surprisingly wide range of behavioral effects, most of which seem to be clustered around bonding, affection, and mood. In reference to these effects, oxytocin has been called the "cuddle hormone" or "love hormone." The effects of oxytocin promote bonding, empathy, and trust. It has also been reported to have antidepressant properties, and oxytocin levels have been found to spike after orgasm. **Prolactin** is kind of like oxytocin's cousin hormone, in that it also has a well-known physiological effect related to reproduction, along with a wide range of other behavioral effects. Physiologically, prolactin helps induce lactation for breastfeeding. Behaviorally, prolactin modulates the stress response, anxiety, and depression, and dysregulation of the prolactin system has been suggested as a possible contributor to postpartum depression. These effects are very complicated, though, and can be influenced by many factors. So the science here is far from settled, but the possibilities are very intriguing.

Next, **melatonin** is a hormone produced by the pineal gland in the brain that regulates wakefulness. More specifically, melatonin is thought to induce sleep as part of human's circadian body clock, so it has been studied as an insomnia treatment and as a potential way to help night-shift workers and travellers cope with out-of-sync sleep cycles. The science is still out on this issue, though. Interestingly, blue light—like from phones and computer screens—suppresses melatonin production, so there's some reason to think that our nocturnal electronics habits might be hurting our sleep by impairing our body's ability to produce melatonin at the right time. For this reason, special apps have been developed that block the waves of blue light coming from our devices at night.

Hunger is another important behavioral cue, and it turns out that hunger is also mediated by hormones, in particular a dynamic trio called **leptin**, **ghrelin**, and the enigmatically named **neuropeptide Y**. Leptin and ghrelin basically form a tag team of hormones with antagonistic effects. This antagonism is a theme we will revisit in more depth in our review of the endocrine system. Leptin reduces hunger—that is, it tells the body it's okay to stop eating, and even better, it can go ahead and expend energy. Interestingly, it's primarily released by adipose, or fat, cells. Ghrelin is the opposite; it promotes hunger. It's released by cells in the gastrointestinal tract when your stomach is empty, which you can remember by thinking of how when your stomach *g-g-growls*, you're producing *g-g-ghrelin*. Both leptin and ghrelin act on the hypothalamus. Interestingly, emerging research is suggesting that leptin and ghrelin have a whole range of additional roles on top of regulating hunger, ranging from reproduction, the immune system, and obesity in the case of leptin, and including learning, mood, sleep, and reproduction for ghrelin. In the same spirit, neuropeptide Y is best known for stimulating appetite to increase food intake, but research into other possible effects is ongoing.

Hormones also mediate the stress response. **Epinephrine** and **norepinephrine**, which are secreted by the adrenal medulla, are responsible for the acute stress response—also known as the **fight-or-flight response**. Interestingly, these compounds, and especially norepinephrine, can also be secreted from some neurons, making it both a hormone and a neurotransmitter. In contrast, the long-term stress response or **chronic stress response** is mediated by **cortisol**, a hormone released from the adrenal cortex. It causes some physiological effects, most notably an increase in blood sugar levels, but it's also a prime candidate as a biological basis for the various psychological effects of chronic stress.

The final hormone we'll mention here is **thyroid hormone**. Thyroid hormone is best known for promoting metabolism. However, it is also needed for proper neurological development, and interestingly, both abnormally low levels of thyroid hormone, known as hypothyroidism, and abnormally high levels, known as hyperthyroidism, have some psychological symptoms along with physical symptoms. Patients with hypothyroidism can present with fatigue and depression, while symptoms of hyperthyroidism include irritability.

Now, we've covered a lot of ground in just a few pages, so let's step back and re-orient ourselves: The takeaway is that hormones shape behavior in many ways, some of which are relatively well understood and some of which are still being figured out. Some of the most important behavioral domains regulated by hormones include reproductive behavior, bonding, alertness, hunger, stress, and mood— pretty big stuff! This is not to say that hormones are the only factors that shape these behaviors, but the scientific consensus is that they do play an important role, so it's worth having a high-level sense of which hormones are associated with each of those domains.

5. Mechanisms of the Nervous System

This is a long chapter. Take a breather. You've probably been studying for a while. Close your eyes and relax for a minute.

If you did any of that, you just observed how the nervous system can affect behavior: Actions that we take consciously are mediated by the nervous system. Let's break that idea down a little more by figuring out how. The light waves entering your eye as you read this are converted into electrical signals by photoreceptors, and those signals are passed along several cells until they travel to your visual cortex in the occipital lobe. At this point, your prefrontal cortex jumps in to make a decision, then signals are sent from your brain down the tracts of your spinal cord to your motor neurons, which eventually release neurotransmitters into neuromuscular junctions to move the muscles that help you stretch (or roll your eyes at the author). We're only scratching the surface here, but the basic rhythm of a stimulus leading to a perception leading to a response will occur again and again as we study psychology. In this section, we'll cover the essential features of the nervous system that explain how we respond to stimuli.

I. Principles and Anatomy

Neurons are the key functional cells of the nervous system. The anatomy of a neuron is covered in greater depth in our Biology textbook, but the basic idea is that the main body of the cell, the soma, has projections known as dendrites that receive input from other nerves or other specialized sense organs. At rest, an **electric potential difference** of about -70 mV exists across the membrane of a neuron. That electric potential difference can get smaller in response to various stimuli, and if it reaches about -55 mV, that **depolarization** causes a signal and a cascade, known as an **action potential**, to start. The action potential then travels down the long, thin axon. At the end of the axon, the axon terminal, the action potential causes neurotransmitters to be released into the **synapse**, which is the space between one neuron and another neuron or its target cell.

CHAPTER 2: BIOLOGICAL BASIS OF BEHAVIOR

As a first step when tackling something complicated, it's often a good idea to try to distill the problem to its simplest form and then layer on complications. The simplest examples of how neurons affect behavior are reflexes, which are completely automatic behaviors that occur in response to certain stimuli. A particularly good example, because it's both simple and familiar, is the **patellar reflex**, which occurs when the patellar tendon—just below the kneecap—is struck by a hammer. This causes the quadriceps muscle to flex, jerking the leg up. The way this works is that the reflex hammer stretches a sensory neuron that is specialized at sensing mechanical input. This neuron extends all the way back to the spinal cord—parenthetically, neurons can be well over a meter long—where it releases a neurotransmitter into its synapse with a motor neuron. That causes the motor neuron to send a signal back down to where it connects to the quadriceps muscle. This synapse between motor neuron and muscle is called the neuromuscular junction, and this is where the neuron releases a different neurotransmitter—this time, acetylcholine— to cause the muscle to contract. The patellar reflex is one of the simplest and clearest examples of structures known as **reflex arcs**, which are simple neural pathways that control reflexes.

As a point of terminological hygiene, **sensory neurons**, which carry information about stimuli to the central nervous system for processing, are known as **afferent neurons**, while **motor neurons**, which carry signals to react from the central nervous system to the target cell, are known as **efferent**, as they elicit the effect. These two words, afferent and efferent, are a source of confusion for many students because they sound the same, and we can actually use that word, same, as a mnemonic where "sensory" is equivalent to "afferent" and "motor" is equivalent to "efferent."

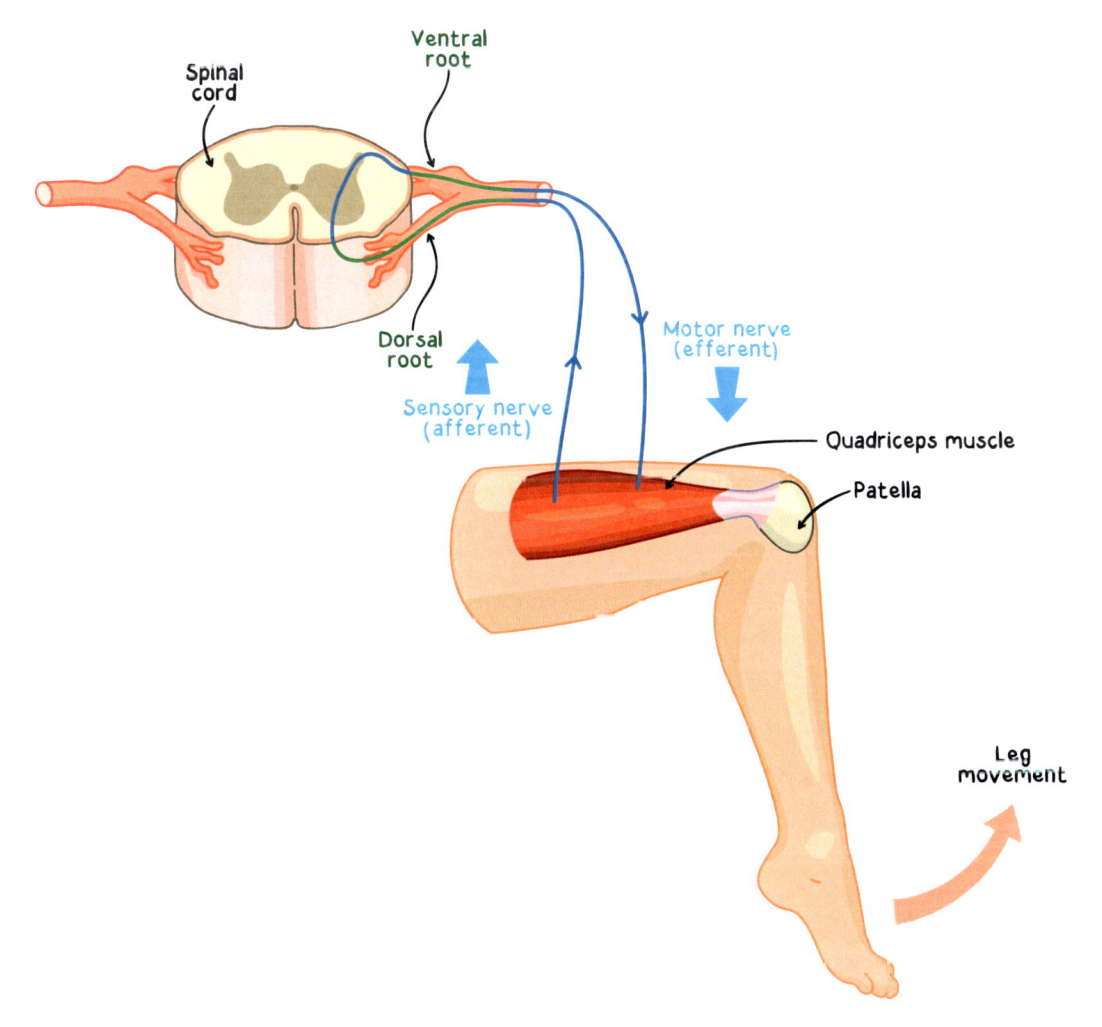

Figure 2. Patellar reflex

Now let's dig a little bit deeper into the concept of neurotransmitters. We mentioned that an action potential is triggered when a neuron is depolarized from its resting membrane potential difference of -70 mV to a potential of about -55 mV. Neurotransmitters have the ability to push this balance in one direction or another. If a neurotransmitter binds receptors on a neuron and has the effect of depolarizing that neural membrane by making the membrane potential difference less negative—say, pushing it to -65 mV—then it's making it easier for another signal to come in and push the neuron over its depolarization threshold (-55 mV). Such a neurotransmitter is called **excitatory** because it depolarizes the target neuron, making it more likely to send a signal. The converse can also occur. If a neurotransmitter instead makes the membrane potential difference even larger—say, pushing it down to -75 mV—this hyperpolarization makes it harder for other excitatory stimuli to depolarize the neuron enough to elicit an action potential. Not surprisingly, since such a neurotransmitter would inhibit the generation of an action potential, we would call it **inhibitory**. Keep in mind here, by the way, that neurons generally receive input from multiple sources—even though it can be convenient to use a simple model of one neuron affecting the next in isolation, reality is typically more complex. In these cases, it is the sum of the depolarizing and hyperpolarizing input on a neuron that determines whether it will fire an action potential.

On a mechanistic level, neurons bind to specific receptors that cause ion channels to open up, which in turn allow certain ions to flow in ways that either reduce or increase the potential difference.

MCAT STRATEGY > > >

Although you won't be tested on rote knowledge of receptor subtypes, it's important to be aware of the concept of receptor specificity in case it comes up in a passage. Plus, this topic may help give you an appreciation for why neuroscience is not traditionally considered an easy topic!

The specificity of some cell types to some neurotransmitters is part of what allows different neurons to do different things: A neuron that expresses a receptor for serotonin will respond to serotonin signaling, and one that doesn't, won't. To make things even more interesting, a given neurotransmitter can have different receptor subtypes, which can be expressed in different areas and do different things. For example, some serotonin receptors trigger an excitatory effect, and others trigger an inhibitory effect, meaning that it wouldn't exactly be accurate to call serotonin either excitatory or inhibitory.

II. Key Neurotransmitters

For the MCAT, there's about a half dozen key neurotransmitters that you should be aware of, some of which we've already mentioned in passing while sketching out the patellar reflex arc. Let's quickly review their main functions.

Let's start with **acetylcholine**. As we mentioned, this neurotransmitter is responsible for activating muscle contraction at the neuromuscular junction—that is, wherever motor neurons synapse on target muscle cells. So whenever you move a muscle, acetylcholine is at work. Acetylcholine also is the neurotransmitter used to communicate signals between the central nervous system and the autonomic nervous system, which controls involuntary, unconscious behaviors. Within the autonomic nervous system, acetylcholine is also used to send signals from neurons of the parasympathetic nervous system—responsible for the "rest and digest" response—to their target tissues. So, in a nutshell, acetylcholine's job is communication, both between the nervous system and other body tissues, and between different divisions of the nervous system.

Next, we'll cover a pair of neurotransmitters that you can think of as having opposite effects: glutamate and GABA. **Glutamate** is an excitatory neurotransmitter. That is, it depolarizes postsynaptic neurons, pushing them closer to the action potential threshold. Interestingly, glutamate is the most common neurotransmitter, and about 90% of neuronal connections in the brain involve glutamate. In contrast, **GABA**, or gamma-aminobutyric acid, is an inhibitory neurotransmitter. Therefore, it hyperpolarizes postsynaptic neurons, pushing them further away from the action potential threshold.

Dopamine is another heavy-hitting neurotransmitter with several important effects. Most notably, it's involved in reward pathways, with implications for addiction, in part because many psychoactive drugs increase dopamine levels, resulting in euphoria. It's also involved in mediating certain motor functions, and as a result, the loss of dopamine-secreting neurons in a part of the brain called the substantia nigra leads to Parkinson's disease, a neurodegenerative condition that typically starts with tremors and leads to further impairments in motor function.

Serotonin is another important multifunctional neurotransmitter. It functions in the brain to regulate mood, appetite, and sleep, and it also regulates intestinal movement in the gastrointestinal tract. Serotonin is notable for its potential role in the biological underpinnings of depression, with a current hypothesis being that depression reflects low serotonin levels. An important class of antidepressants known as selective serotonin reuptake inhibitors, or SSRIs, boosts the functionally available levels of serotonin in synapses by preventing serotonin from being taken back up by neurons. Instead of generating more serotonin, these drugs keep serotonin in the synapse longer, allowing the brain to get more bang for its buck from each serotonin molecule.

Now, have you ever heard of the runner's high? The feeling of bliss after working out is thought to be mediated by **endorphins**, a category of neurotransmitters that suppress pain and can produce a euphoric response. Interestingly, they function similarly to opioids, and the name endorphin itself is designed to reflect this by being a combination of *endo*, meaning internal, and *orphin*, as in morphine, like the opioid painkiller. On a somewhat related note, **norepinephrine** is the main neurotransmitter involved in the acute stress response, also known as the fight-or-flight response, which enables us to run by elevating our heart rate and blood pressure. This is mediated by the sympathetic division of the autonomic nervous system. The neurotransmitter **epinephrine**, or **adrenaline**, is closely related to norepinephrine and has similar physiological effects.

Two key concepts—**agonists** and **antagonists**—are key to understanding the logic of attempts that researchers have made to modify or target neurotransmitter signaling.

An agonist is a compound that activates a certain receptor, causing some kind of response. Therefore, we can say that serotonin is an agonist of the various subtypes of serotonin receptors. But where it gets interesting is that other compounds can also activate those receptors, through a process that you can crudely think of as mimicking serotonin. For example, several psychedelic and hallucinogenic drugs stimulate a certain serotonin receptor subtype, making them serotonin receptor agonists. Certain agonists do not evoke as strong of an effect as the original substance, and these are called partial agonists. In contrast, antagonists have the opposite effect. They bind a receptor, but do not activate it or cause a response. By doing so, they prevent the receptor from being bound by an agonist; in other words, the antagonist stops a neurotransmitter or drug from being able to exert its effects on that receptor. For example, we mentioned that serotonin regulates intestinal movement, and it turns out that some serotonin receptor antagonists help treat chemotherapy-induced nausea by preventing serotonin from acting on its receptors there.

6. The Peripheral Nervous System

The nervous system is intricately organized, with different structures corresponding to different functions. Practically speaking, we often focus on these structures because they contain the key to understanding and possibly even manipulating how the nervous system modulates behavior. For the MCAT in particular, it's essential to know what a given structure does, so that you can predict what might happen if it's activated or deactivated.

The highest-level division of the nervous system is between the **peripheral nervous system** and the **central nervous system**. The central nervous system is the **brain** and the **spinal cord**, and the peripheral nervous system is everything else. That is, the peripheral nervous system includes nerves that shuttle sensory information from body tissues to the central nervous system for processing, as well as the nerves that extend out from the central nervous system and send motor impulses.

In this section, we'll discuss the peripheral nervous system, which, at least from the point of view of the MCAT, is far simpler. The peripheral nervous system is divided into the **somatic nervous system** and the **autonomic nervous system**. The somatic nervous system is responsible for carrying out voluntary activities, so it contains the efferent—or motor—neurons that innervate our skeletal muscles and allow us to move our bodies consciously, as well as the afferent—or sensory—neurons that take in information from our environment that helps us make decisions about what to do. Parenthetically, some sources only include motor neurons in the somatic nervous system, and instead view sensory neurons as an independent component of the peripheral nervous system. For our purposes and the MCAT, understanding their respective functions is much more important than the decision of how exactly to classify sensory nerves.

In contrast to the somatic nervous system, the autonomic nervous system is responsible for unconscious activities. You can remember this because *autonomic* sounds like *automatic*. More specifically, the autonomic nervous system handles stuff like digestion, heart rate, breathing rate, whether our pupils dilate or constrict, and urination. The autonomic nervous system itself is also divided into two main components: the **sympathetic nervous system** and the **parasympathetic nervous system**. Broadly speaking, these push the activity of the autonomic nervous system in opposite directions (act antagonistically) depending on what's most appropriate.

Let's start with the sympathetic nervous system, which is responsible for the **fight-or-flight response** to acute stress. This response occurs when a person is faced with an immediate threat, and it involves multiple organs. Its effects all contribute to the goal of mobilizing the body's resources to deal with an emergency now, while putting off anything that can wait. The heart rate increases, and the blood vessels in the skeletal muscles dilate, or widen. Epinephrine is also released, increasing blood glucose levels. The bronchioles in the lungs dilate, allowing more air to be processed. These effects all combine to give more resources to the skeletal muscles, allowing quick and forceful movements to resolve the threat. Simultaneously, the pupils in the eyes dilate, making vision more sensitive. Sweating helps dissipate any extra heat you generate while dealing with the crisis at hand—that is, while either fighting or fleeing. An interesting consequence of sweating is that it increases skin conductance, which can be used in psychological experiments—and lie detectors—as a measure of stress. The responses we've listed so far largely involve stimulation—faster heart rate, more air inhaled, higher blood glucose—but the sympathetic nervous system response also involves deprioritizing things that aren't essential, like digestion: If you're in a life-or-death emergency, you can probably wait to extract all the nutrients from that burrito you had for lunch. So the blood vessels supplying the gastrointestinal tract constrict, meaning that less blood gets to those tissues. The rate of peristalsis, the contractions that push material through the digestive tract, also decreases. The fight-or-flight response has some behavioral effects too. For instance, you might experience tunnel vision, in which your vision might focus just on objects within your central visual field; you might also experience some shaking, and sexual arousal becomes less likely. The common theme here is that the fight-or-flight response is the time to focus on essential responses to an emergency and to deprioritize everything else!

CHAPTER 2: BIOLOGICAL BASIS OF BEHAVIOR

The parasympathetic nervous system, in turn, is responsible for the **rest-and-digest response**, which is basically the opposite of the fight-or-flight response. Most notably, the blood vessels supplying your muscles constrict, while the vessels supplying the digestive tract dilate, and this combination results in more blood supply for digestive activities. Parasympathetic activation also causes your pupils to constrict. More generally, parasympathetic nervous activity promotes digestion, the related activities of salivation, urination, and defecation, and also lacrimation (or tear production) and sexual arousal. If you step back and think about it, you might notice that these parasympathetic activities, especially digestion and its related processes, are pretty essential to life. So in that context, perhaps it's not surprising to learn that in reality, both the sympathetic and parasympathetic nervous systems tend to be active at any one time. In most circumstances, it's more about the balance between the two than it is about one or the other.

Interestingly, the autonomic nervous system also has a third branch, called the enteric nervous system. This is basically a separate system of nerves that regulates the activity of the gut. It does get some input from the sympathetic and parasympathetic nervous systems, but it can act independently of them.

> **MCAT STRATEGY > > >**
>
> For the MCAT, there are two essential skills related to the peripheral nervous system: knowing the terminology inside and out, and being able to predict the causes and effects of sympathetic versus parasympathetic nervous system activation.

So, to summarize, the peripheral nervous system has two basic jobs: (1) getting stuff done in the body, whether consciously, as in the somatic nervous system, or unconsciously, as in the autonomic nervous system, and (2) letting the brain know what's happening, most notably through sensory nerves.

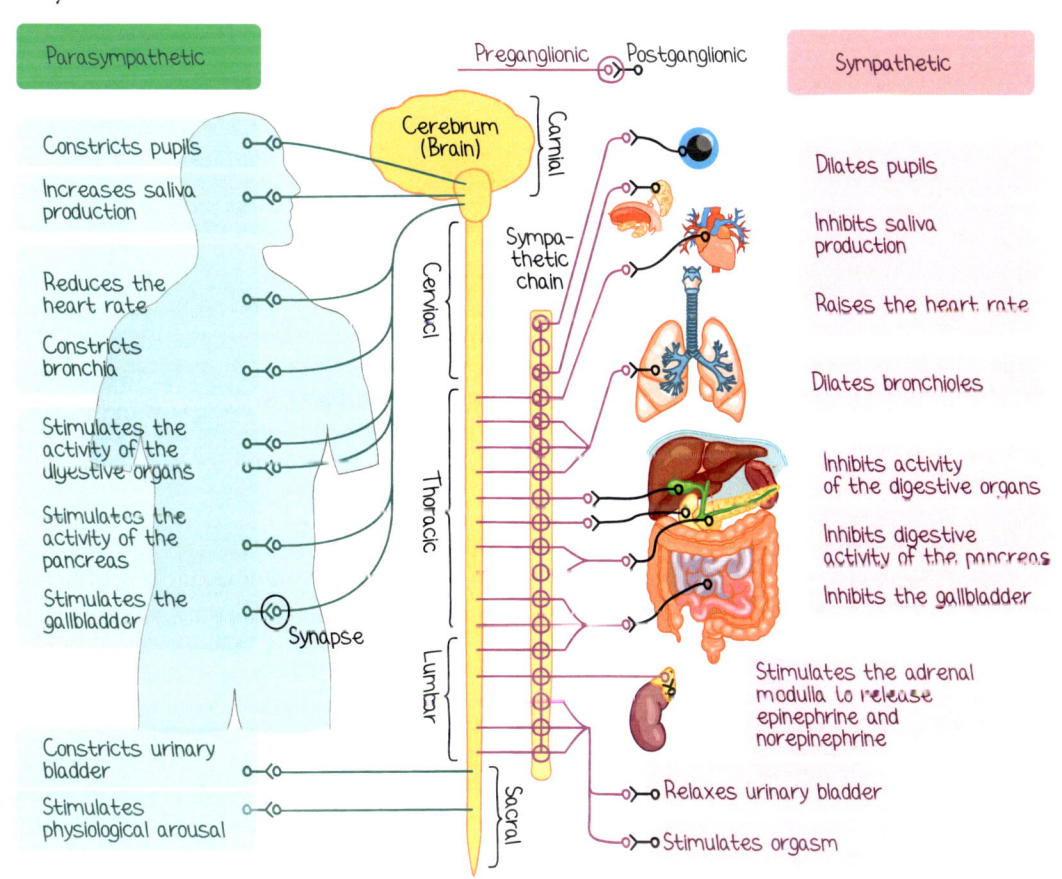

Figure 3. Parasympathetic vs. sympathetic activation

7. The Central Nervous System

If the major jobs of the peripheral nervous system are to get things done and to let the brain know about what's happening, then the major job of the central nervous system is to decide what to do. The central nervous system includes both the brain and the spinal cord.

Based on findings from developmental biology, the brain can be divided into the **hindbrain**, **midbrain**, and **forebrain**. As the name suggests, the hindbrain is located at the lower back of the brain. The forebrain actually corresponds to most of the brain by volume, and the relatively small midbrain is located in between the two. From a functional point of view, broadly speaking, the hindbrain corresponds to more basic, evolutionarily conserved functions, the forebrain handles more advanced functions, and the midbrain is somewhere in between.

To break these regions down further, let's start with the hindbrain. The **cerebellum** is the most visually remarkable component of the hindbrain, because it forms a distinct structure at the base of the brain. Its basic job is to make coordinated movement happen. That is, it integrates signals that come from elsewhere in the nervous system and makes sure that the resulting output is smooth, finely-tuned, and coordinated. Therefore, people who experience damage to the cerebellum will often show difficulties with balance, gait, and coordinated tasks.

The other two structures of the hindbrain, the **medulla oblongata** and the **pons**, extend continuously up from the spinal cord. The medulla oblongata controls autonomic functions, such as breathing, heart rate, and blood pressure, and the pons is basically a relay station through which signals are transmitted between the cerebellum, medulla, and the rest of the brain. The pons also contains clusters of neurons that deal with functions such as sleep, respiration, swallowing, taste, bladder control, and balance.

The **midbrain** is located above and in front of the hindbrain, and contains various structures that are involved in functions like motor control, sleeping and waking, and temperature regulation. The **inferior and superior colliculi** help process auditory and visual input, respectively, even though the midbrain is not the primary location of audiovisual cognition in the brain. Additionally, the **substantia nigra** in the midbrain contains neurons that communicate using dopamine to help coordinate voluntary movements. In Parkinson's disease, dopaminergic neurons in this region degenerate.

The midbrain is lumped together with the medulla oblongata and pons of the hindbrain to form a structure known as the **brainstem**, which looks like what it's named for; that is, it's a continuous extension of the spinal cord that forms the physical support for the brain. The brainstem also contains a complex set of structures known as the **reticular activating system**, or RAS, which modulates alertness and arousal.

Next, the **forebrain** contains many other structures that are important for understanding behavior. The forebrain is divided into the diencephalon, which developmentally gives rise to the thalamus, hypothalamus, pineal gland and posterior pituitary gland, and the telencephalon, which gives rise to the cerebrum. The thalamus relays sensory and motor signals and regulates sleep and alertness, while the hypothalamus is the bridge between the nervous and endocrine systems. As we've discussed, the pituitary gland releases several important hormones.

The **cerebrum** is the largest structure of the brain. In turn, the cerebrum is divided into the **cerebral cortex** and **subcortical structures**. The cortex is the thin, outer layer of the brain that is divided into right and left hemispheres. The subcortical structures include areas such as the olfactory bulb, which is involved in detecting odors, the hippocampus, which consolidates short-term memory into long-term memory, and the basal ganglia. The basal ganglia participate in a broad range of miscellaneous functions, including eye and other voluntary movements and procedural and habitual learning.

These subcortical structures that we just mentioned—the olfactory bulb and basal ganglia, as well as the hypothalamus and hippocampus—are part of the **limbic system**, which is actually not a single structure, but rather a grouping of various structures involved in emotion, memory, and motivation. The **amygdala**, which is involved in episodic memory, attention, and emotion, is another important structure of the limbic system. Finally, the **nucleus accumbens** is involved in reward, motivation, and learning, making it a neurological structure implicated in addiction.

Moving on from the limbic system, the cerebral cortex is divided into four lobes. The **frontal lobe** is involved in voluntary movement, memory processing, planning, motivation, and attention. In other words, it's the part of your brain that's responsible for adulting. The **parietal lobe**, which is located just behind the frontal lobe, is involved in sensory processing, with the exception of vision, which is processed in the **occipital lobe**, located at the very back of the brain. Finally, the **temporal lobe** is where meaning happens. More specifically, it's involved in making visual memories, in attaching meaning to information, and in language.

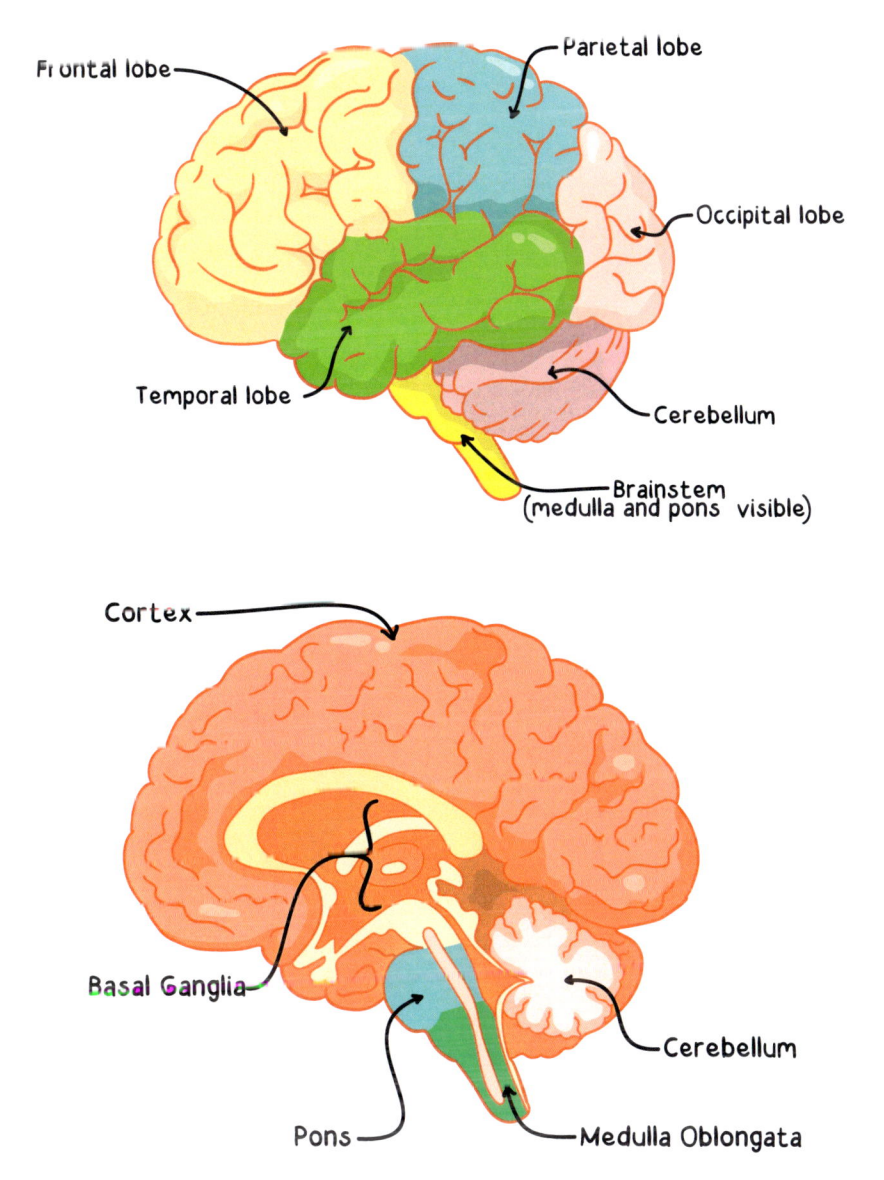

Figure 4. The brain

This four-lobe division of the cerebral cortex is just a high-level classification, kind of like how a country could be divided up into regions. But just as within each region of a country, there are notable cities, attractions, and so on, the cerebral cortex contains a myriad of various structures. You're not expected to know most of them for the MCAT, except for a few very important ones. Most crucially, **Wernicke's area** is a part of the temporal lobe that is involved in language comprehension, while **Broca's area** is a part of the frontal lobe that is involved in language production—that is, in actually speaking.

Interestingly, Broca's area and Wernicke's area tend specifically to be in the left cerebral hemisphere. This is the case for the overwhelming majority of right-handed people, and even for most left-handed people. This reflects the broader phenomenon of **lateralization**, or the tendency for the left and right hemispheres of the brain to specialize in different functions. One hemisphere is generally dominant, and the dominant hemisphere is inversely linked to handedness. The majority of people are right-handed, and that correlates to dominance of the left hemisphere. As we'll see in more detail when we cover vision, the hemispheres also specialize in terms of which eye they process visual input from. Some researchers have looked into how lateralization affects higher-level cognitive processes too. But it's important to note here that many ideas about the left brain and the right brain in popular culture are extremely exaggerated, like the proposal that the left brain is associated with analytical, logical, rational thought, while the right brain is associated with intuition, imagination, and creativity. It's really just not that simple.

Having completed this review of brain areas, an interesting question to think about is how exactly it works that different brain areas have different functional specializations. To some extent, for our purposes, the answer to this can be just because. But you should be aware that one contributing factor to differences in functionality between different brain areas or groups of neurons is the fact that different neurons can express different neurotransmitter receptors. So one neuron might respond more to serotonin and less to dopamine compared to another, for example. Or it might have a different subtype of receptor, and scaling up these differences from the level of individual neurons to larger brain areas can help explain why different parts of the brain do different things.

The **spinal cord** is considered part of the central nervous system, but essentially functions as the link between the central and peripheral nervous systems. The spinal canal contains bundles of sensory, or afferent, neurons that relay sensory information from the periphery to the central nervous system for processing. It also contains motor, or efferent, neurons that trigger muscle contraction elsewhere in the body so we can take action based on what we observe in the environment. Both the brain and the spinal cord are protected by **cerebrospinal fluid,** or CSF. The brain and spinal cord are also protected by tough membranes, known as meninges, and bones - the skull for the brain, and vertebrae for the spinal cord.

You'll have the opportunity to study **vertebrae** in much greater depth in medical school, so for now you should focus on a few takeaway points about them. Possibly the most important aspect of the structure of a vertebra is that it has a hole in the middle for the spinal cord to run through, although it is also notable that vertebrae have a clearly distinguishable anterior, or front-facing side, as compared to the posterior, or back-facing side. The anterior side is also called ventral, because it faces your stomach (as "venter" means "abdomen" in Latin), and the posterior side is also called dorsal (because "dorsum" means "back" in Latin). A very important takeaway from all this is that motor nerves are located ventrally and sensory nerves are located dorsally. A helpful mnemonic for keeping track of what's going on with nerves is *SAME DAVE*, which stands for: *sensory* neurons are *afferent* neurons, *motor* neurons are *efferent* neurons, *dorsal* location for *afferent* neurons, and *ventral* location for *efferent* neurons. This mnemonic links two often-confusing pieces of terminology with an important anatomical fact.

The spine is subdivided into regions that contain anatomically slightly different vertebrae. Starting from the top, the **cervical spine** corresponds more or less with your neck, and it contains 7 cervical vertebrae, numbered C1 through C7. The **thoracic spine** corresponds roughly with your back, and it contains 12 thoracic vertebrae, labeled T1 through T12. The **lumbar spine** is located in the lower back, and its 5 lumbar vertebrae are numbered L1 through L5. Then, the **sacrum** is at the base of the spinal cord, and the 5 sacral vertebrae, S1 through S5, actually fuse in early adulthood. Finally, the spinal cord ends with the **coccyx,** or tailbone.

CHAPTER 2: BIOLOGICAL BASIS OF BEHAVIOR

An interesting fact about the vertebrae is that the nerves leaving them at any particular level, say C7, are very specific in terms of which parts of the body they control and process sensory input from. For instance, different parts of the hand are innervated by three distinct nerves, with different origins and courses. What's more, the entire exterior of the human body is divided into dermatomes, which are areas of skin that are innervated by the branches of specific nerves, corresponding to entrance into the spinal column at the height of specific vertebrae. This connection allows doctors to predict the effects of injury to specific vertebrae, or conversely, to use a patient's symptoms to assess where the spinal cord may have been damaged.

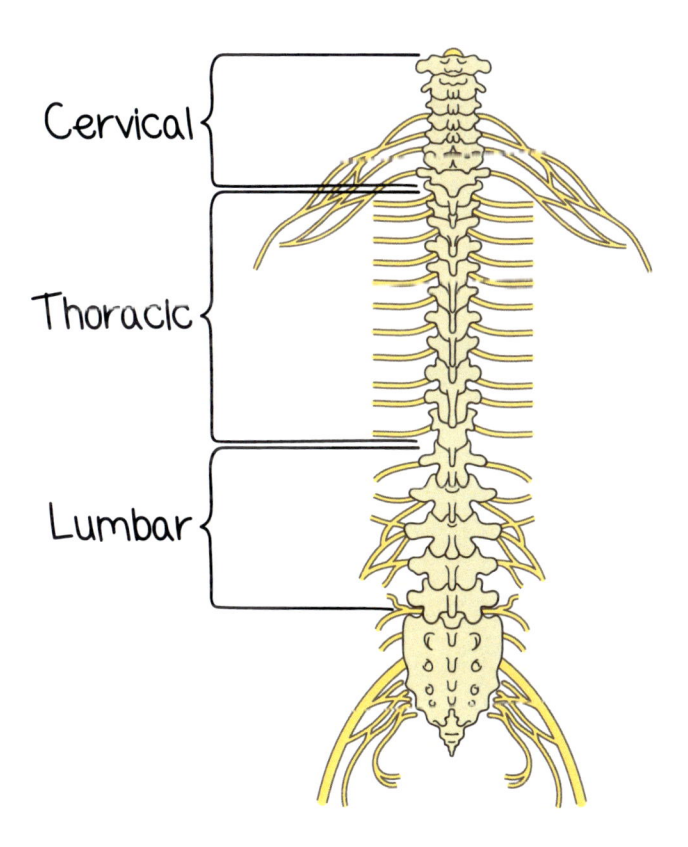

Figure 5. Divisions of the spinal cord

8. Methods of Studying the Brain

We've now discussed a dizzying range of functions of the nervous system—but how do we know so much about the central nervous system anyway? We've just presented a long list of brain structures, telling you that that one structure does one thing, another structure does something else, and a third structure is implicated in various other phenomena. But how did scientists actually figure this out?

> **MCAT STRATEGY > > >**
>
> Methods of studying the brain are important for the MCAT for two reasons: first, because the Psych/Soc section can directly ask you which technique is most appropriate for which purposes; and second, because understanding the methods used in experimental passages saves time.

We mentioned the idea that injuries to certain vertebrae in the spinal cord cause predictable defects. The idea that we can learn about the function of structures from localized injuries has been immensely influential in neuroscience: A famous historical case occurred in 1848, when a man named Phineas Gage was working on a railroad, and then in an accidental explosion, an iron rod was driven through his brain, passing through his frontal lobe. Physically, Gage made a mostly complete recovery, but his personality was radically altered, causing him to become impatient, erratic, and profane. This case became famous and launched research into the functional responsibilities of various brain areas.

Over time, the careful analysis of many patients with many different brain injuries has shed considerable light on the workings of the brain. However, this approach can only take us so far. For ethical reasons, having to damage a brain area to find out what it does is severely limiting. A broader methodological toolkit is therefore necessary. The next best thing, experimentally speaking, is to directly stimulate specific parts of the brain, either using electrodes or chemical agents, and then measure the effects either behaviorally or through some kind of imaging technique. If ethically appropriate, some of these techniques can be used in humans, although animal experiments are another option.

Since neurons communicate with each other through electrical signaling, one way to figure out what's going on in the brain at a specific time is to measure its electrical activity. This technique has been honed over several decades. **EEGs**, or **electroencephalograms**, measure brain activity through electrodes placed on the scalp. Different patterns of activity, for instance, correspond to different stages of sleep. Furthermore, while EEG is often used as a very crude tool, poor at localizing the source of signals, in the right experimental settings, electrical activity can be measured even down to the level of individual neurons.

In more recent decades, several non-invasive methods of imaging brain structures have been developed, with specific strengths and weaknesses. **Computed tomography (CT)** involves taking X-ray photographs in 360 degrees and assembling the resulting images with the help of computer programs to view structures three-dimensionally as a series of two-dimensional slices. In contrast, **magnetic resonance imaging (MRI)** uses strong magnetic fields to image structures within the body. The choice between CT and MRI depends on several factors - for instance, MRI is better at imaging soft structures and does not involve a dose of ionizing radiation, which is a downside of CT imaging, but it is also more expensive, time-consuming, and involved for the patient. However, what CT and MRI have in common is that both techniques are good for imaging static structures.

Going a step forward, some imaging techniques can be used to visualize brain activity. **Positron emission tomography (PET)** works by radiolabeling glucose, usually as fludeoxyglucose (FDG), which emits positrons as it decays. The detector is then used to determine where these decay events occur. The areas where more decay occurs are those where more glucose is being metabolized, which corresponds to more intense neural activity, since glucose is what neurons use for fuel. Some common uses of PET neuroimaging include diagnosing diseases such as tumors, strokes, and some kinds of dementia, as well as in analyzing functional changes associated with various psychological conditions. However, in many contexts, **functional MRI (fMRI)** is now preferred. The fMRI method relies on differences in magnetic properties between oxygenated hemoglobin, which is predominant in arterial blood, and deoxygenated hemoglobin, which is predominant in venous blood, to allow the visualization of blood flow. This, in turn, enables us to zoom in even closer and measure brain activity, either to get a snapshot of the brain or to observe changes as subjects perform various tasks. Brain imaging is very much an area of ongoing research, and in medical school, you'll have the opportunity to learn a lot more about the relevant mechanisms, the pluses and minuses of various imaging techniques, and cutting-edge developments in this field. Nonetheless, the basic facts that we've presented about the major techniques scientists use to learn about the brain will provide a foundation for understanding a broad range of research into brain function - and, of course, for succeeding on the MCAT.

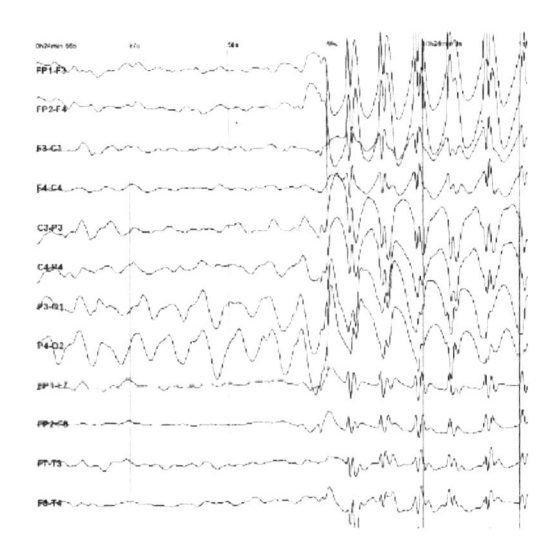

Figure 6. EEG

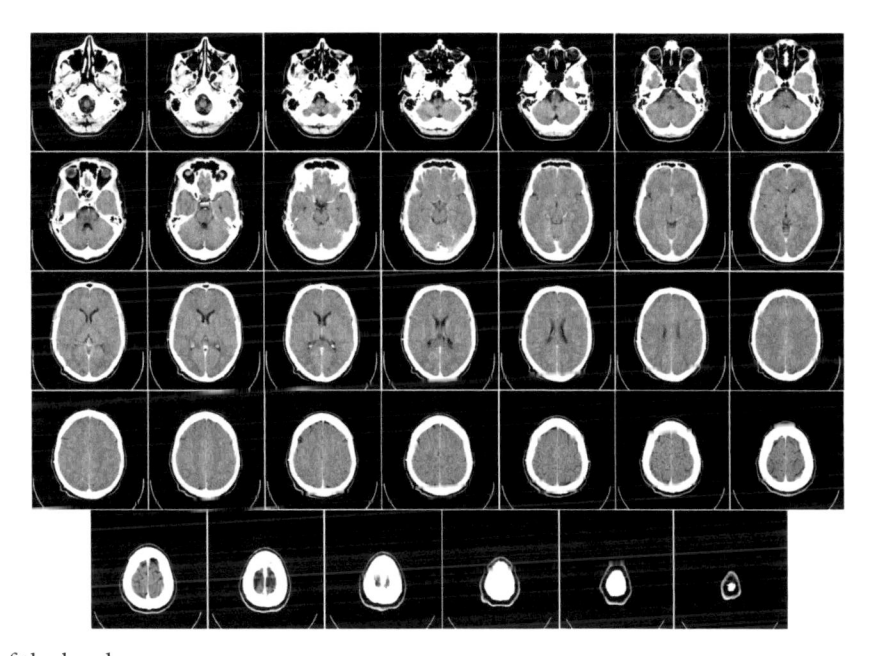

Figure 7. CT scan of the head

9. Must-Knows

- Behavioral science on the MCAT is broad, but not deep: It won't be worth taking apart the smallest details of every theory or model!
- Biological approaches: mechanistic processes that lead to behaviors.
- Psychological approaches: more interested in kinds of behavior that an individual may exhibit (normative/ abnormal, positive/ negative). Studied through observations of behavior and controlled experiments.
- Sociological approaches focus on the behavior, organization, and feelings of groups.
- Genetics influence behavior, most notably in the form of instinctual (hard-wired) behaviors.
  - Adaptive traits contribute to the fitness (mean lifetime reproduction) of an organism.
- Newborns have rooting, sucking, palmar grasp, Moro, and Babinski reflexes; first year of life = caregiver focus, stranger anxiety at 7-8 months; 1-2 years: complex motor behavior, identity formation, egocentrism.
- Critical periods: experiences can imprint on children for life.
- Other life stages: puberty/adolescence (=biological/cultural), adulthood, aging (w/ telomere degradation)
- Endocrine system regulates both behavior and physiology by secreting hormones into the bloodstream.
  - Hypothalamus: major regulatory center, releases tropic hormones CRF, TRH, GnRH > anterior pituitary
  - Anterior pituitary: releases ACTH, TSH, FSH, LH, prolactin, GH; posterior pituitary: contains neurons that release ADH and oxytocin
  - Other endocrine glands: thyroid, parathyroid, pancreas, adrenal cortex/medulla, gonads (ovaries/testes)
  - Important hormones:
    - Oxytocin: bonding, empathy, and trust
    - Prolactin: lactation; implicated in postpartum depression
    - Leptin (satiety), ghrelin (hunger), neuropeptide Y (appetite): regulate hunger
    - Epinephrine/norepinephrine: acute stress response
    - Cortisol: chronic stress response
    - Thyroid hormone: metabolic rate, neural development
- Nervous system: faster response to environmental stimuli; reflexes = completely automatic responses
- Afferent (sensory) neurons send signals to the CNS, efferent (motor) neurons synapse at neuromuscular junctions and cause muscle contraction by the release of acetylcholine.
- Receptors on the dendrites of neurons respond to neurotransmitters. One receptor type is usually responsive to only one neurotransmitter.
  - Resting membrane potential of a neuron is -70 mV (= charge difference across the membrane).
  - Excitatory neurotransmitters INCREASE this potential, making it less negative (=depolarization).
  - Inhibitory neurotransmitters DECREASE this potential, making it more negative (=hyperpolarization).
  - Chemicals interacting with receptors are agonists (stimulate response) or antagonists (block receptor).
- Peripheral nervous system = all nerves except brain and spinal cord > somatic and autonomic NS
  - Autonomic nervous system (ANS) > sympathetic nervous system and parasympathetic nervous system
  - Enteric nervous system = branch of the nervous system modulated by, but not part of, the ANS
- Central nervous system (CNS): brain and spinal cord
  - Hindbrain: cerebellum, pons, medulla oblongata
  - Midbrain: substantia nigra, superior and inferior colliculi
  - Brainstem: midbrain, medulla oblongata, and pons
  - Forebrain: largest region, divided into diencephalon (thalamus, hypothalamus, posterior pituitary, and pineal gland) and telencephalon
  - Spine: cervical (7 vertebrae), thoracic (12 vertebrae), lumbar (5 vertebrae), sacral (5 vertebrae; fused in adults) regions, and coccyx; nerves innervating specific body areas originate at distinct levels.
- Brain imaging techniques: electroencephalograms (EEG) measure activity through electrodes as waveforms, computed tomography (CT) = X-rays taken in 360° and assembled; magnetic resonance imaging (MRI) uses magnetic fields and is especially useful for soft tissues; functional MRI (fMRI) measures perfusion of brain regions; positron emission tomography (PET) uses radiolabeled glucose to measure metabolic activity.

End of Chapter Practice

The best MCAT practice is **realistic**, with a focus on identifying steps for further improvement. For those reasons, we recommend completing practice questions in an online setting that simulates the real MCAT interface, and taking advantage of advanced analytic features to help you determine how best to move forward in your MCAT study journey.

With that in mind, **online end-of-chapter questions** are accessible through your Next Step account.

As a further supplement, given the importance of active learning for effective studying, we also suggest that you consult the Must-Knows as a basis for creating a study sheet, in which you list out key terms and test your ability to briefly summarize them.

This page left intentionally blank.

Sensation and Perception

CHAPTER 3

0. Introduction

Sensation and perception ultimately form the basis for our behavior; therefore, it is necessary to clearly distinguish between these concepts. Sensation refers to the physical reality of the signals that our sensory organs pick up and send to be processed in the nervous system. Perception, as the name itself suggests, has to do with how we interpret those signals - that is, what we actually experience subjectively. For example: imagine you look out a window and see a tree in front of another building across the street. On a strictly sensory level, light waves of various wavelengths are striking your retina in various patterns, causing signals to be transduced to your brain. On a perceptual level, you can organize those patterns of color into shapes that you recognize as a tree and a building. Or imagine you're listening to a new hit song: On a purely sensory level, sound waves are colliding into your ear with various pitches, amplitudes, and rhythms, and some of those impacts are transformed into signals that are then sent to your brain. On a perceptual level, you recognize that mismash of sound waves as music, and either enjoy it or not, depending on your taste in music.

1. Sensory Receptors

In both of those examples—looking at a tree and listening to a new hit song—the first step in sensation involved a kind of interface between our body and the world surrounding us. This is where **sensory receptors** come in. This term refers to specialized dendrites of sensory neurons that respond to various kinds of physical stimuli by generating action potentials that are sent upstream towards the central nervous system for further processing. Within the peripheral nervous system, such neurons are bundled together into **nerves** (collections of axons) and **ganglia** (collections of cell bodies).

Sensory receptors communicate four properties to the central nervous system. Two are pretty obvious: **location**, or where a stimulus is coming from, and what type of stimulus it is, also known as **modality**. Somewhat less obviously, sensory receptors also communicate information on **intensity**, through the frequency of action potentials produced by a stimulus, and **duration**, or how long a stimulus lasts.

A broad distinction is also made between **exteroceptors**, which respond to stimuli from the outside world, and **interoceptors**, which respond to stimuli from inside the body. This might not seem obvious at first, since when we think of sensation, things like vision, smell, taste, and hearing immediately come to mind - all of which involve contact with the outside world, but it's also possible to sense painful stimuli from within the body. Furthermore, the body has to have some way of sensing less obvious things, like dehydration or overhydration, so that it can respond accordingly.

With that in mind, let's review the various types of sensory receptors in our bodies. These map fairly directly onto our senses, so this will also function as a quick review of the physical basis for each sense.

I. Chemoreceptors

Olfactory receptors, which are involved in the sense of smell, and taste receptors, also known as **gustatory receptors**, are similar in that they respond to chemical stimuli (making them **chemoreceptors**). However, an important difference is that olfactory receptors respond to volatile chemicals, or those in the air, while taste receptors respond to chemicals in food, which are technically dissolved - either in the food itself or in your saliva. Another interesting difference is that olfactory receptors are sensitive to a dizzying range of different compounds, to the point that trying to count the number of different smells that exist in the world would be a virtually impossible task, whereas taste receptors are much more limited. Usually, we classify tastes as savory, sweet, bitter, salty, and sour, and these perceptions correspond to distinct receptors. It's also been proposed that specialized taste receptors can transmit information about carbonation and fat content, although those have yet to enter the list of generally-recognized categories of taste.

> **MCAT STRATEGY > > >**
>
> The names of each category of sensory receptors gives you a clue about what they do (e.g. chemoreceptors sense chemicals). Use this to your advantage while studying!

II. Photoreceptors and Hair Cells

Turning to our other senses, **photoreceptors** are responsible for vision, and as the name implies, they respond to specific wavelengths of electromagnetic radiation, or light. For hearing, **hair cells** in the inner ear convert pressure signals from sound waves into action potentials. Interestingly, hair cells also use their ability to respond to pressure to sense rotational acceleration. The basic idea here is that structures in the inner ear known as semicircular canals contain a fluid called endolymph, which moves in response to rotational acceleration, and the resulting movement of endolymph places pressure on hair cells located on a structure referred to as the crista ampullaris. These hair cells then respond, sending information about rotational acceleration to the nervous system.

III. Mechanoreceptors

The last of our major senses is touch, and the receptors responsible for touch are known as **mechanoreceptors**. As the name suggests, these receptors respond to mechanical stimuli. Interestingly, distinct types of mechanoreceptors in the skin specialize in detecting specific types of touch stimuli. For instance, structures known as tactile corpuscles detect light touch, while Merkel nerve endings specialize in responding to sustained pressure. Deeper pressure beneath the surface of the skin is detected by Ruffini endings, and there are even specialized structures known as Pacinian corpuscles that respond to high-frequency vibrations. For our purposes, the point is NOT to memorize all these types, but just to understand that underlyingly, the body specializes in detecting touch stimuli to a remarkable extent.

IV. Other Receptors

Although we often lump our perceptions of temperature and pain under the general rubric of touch, there are actually separate receptors that are responsible for those sensations. Receptors that detect variation in temperature are, intuitively enough, known as **thermoreceptors**, and these receptors can specialize in detecting either warm or cold temperatures. Receptors that detect pain are known as **nociceptors** (think "noxious"). Some nociceptors respond to mechanical input, like if the skin is hit or cut. Others respond to thermal stimuli (after all, burns and extreme cold can *hurt*). Still others respond to chemical stimuli. The most famous example of this is capsaicin, which is responsible for spiciness.

As we mentioned earlier, interoceptors are sensory receptors that provide information about what's going on within the body. Those that detect pressure, like on the walls of blood vessels, are known as **baroreceptors**. Technically, these are a subset of mechanoreceptors, but they're worth making a special note of since sensing blood pressure is such an essential physiological function. A separate class of receptors, known as **osmoreceptors**, detect the concentration of solutes in blood and trigger responses when the blood either becomes too dilute or too concentrated.

Finally, receptors called **proprioceptors** are present in and around muscles, tendons, and joints, and are responsible for giving us a sense of the relative position of the parts of our body in space. This is known as **kinesthetic sense**.

V. Stimuli

An important distinction is made between proximal and distal stimuli. Since "proximal" and "distal" are just technical terms for "near" and "far away," respectively, a **proximal stimulus** is what a sensory receptor detects, while a **distal stimulus** is the object in the environment that causes those signals. Consider what happens when you look at a tree: the proximal stimulus is a bunch of light waves hitting your eyes, and the distal stimulus is the physical object with bark, leaves, and so on, that absorbs certain wavelengths of light and reflects others.

2. Sensory Thresholds and Weber's Law

Can you imagine paying attention to *everything, at all times*? Taken to an extreme, that would be absolutely debilitating for our ability to function in the world. In fact, the inability to tune out certain kinds of input is a characteristic of various psychological conditions, and it can be a tremendous problem for people affected by those disorders. This consideration underscores the fact that sensory processing involves much more than just memorizing a list of the various neurons that detect different types of sensory stimuli. Our bodies are constantly bombarded with stimuli from the outside world, so what do we actually notice?

A helpful way of approaching this question is to analye all the various points in the path between our sensory receptors and our conscious experience where we discard or filter out information. Therefore, as a first step towards answering the question "what do we notice?", which is a very big question, let's start by answering the somewhat simpler question of "what don't we notice?"

The very first step in the sensory pathways—that is, when sensory neurons respond to input—is also our very first opportunity *not* to notice something. For example, the mechanoreceptors in our skin that respond to touch are actually quite sensitive, but there are limits. Imagine wearing a lab coat over a long-sleeved shirt when a fruit fly lands on your arm in a genetics experiment gone wrong. Do you actually feel the fruit fly? Probably not. Technically, yes, the addition of the mass of the fruit fly on top of your lab coat on top of your long-sleeved shirt does create a slight change in the pressure on your skin, but that change is extremely tiny: too small for the mechanoreceptors on your skin to respond to. This idea is called the **absolute threshold**: The level of intensity that a stimulus must have in order to be picked up by sensory neurons. Practically speaking, experimenters often investigate this by looking for the lowest level of a stimulus that research participants can pick up at least 50% of the time. The crucial point is that the absolute threshold is a yes-or-no phenomenon; if a stimulus doesn't hit that threshold, then as far as our bodies are concerned, it may as well not even exist. However, what happens if it does exceed that threshold is a little bit more complicated.

Have you ever heard of subliminal messages, such as if a brand of a product, like a certain kind of carbonated beverage, is included in a video, movie, or TV show, with the goal of priming you to want that product, even if you never consciously notice it? Alternatively, the creators of a TV show or movie might sneak in a frame or two containing a certain message, with the idea that your unconscious mind might pick up on it even if it goes by too fast for you to consciously notice. There is actually some scientific backing to this idea, although not as much as advertisers might hope. Brain imaging studies have shown that the central nervous system can respond, on some level, to stimuli that we don't perceive consciously. The real-world significance of this remains a topic for further research, but it's certainly an intriguing possibility, and more to the point, it means that we need to add a new concept to our toolkit: the **threshold of conscious perception**. As the name suggests, this is the threshold that a stimulus must cross in order for us to be able to consciously perceive it at all.

The difference between the absolute threshold and the threshold of conscious perception can be confusing at times. One reason for this is that the experimental design used to investigate the absolute threshold often tries to minimize any other influences. For example, in the first major set of experiments designed to investigate the absolute threshold for vision, participants were kept in absolute darkness for over half an hour to make sure they were at maximum sensitivity to light stimuli, and then the scientists very carefully determined exactly how many photons to shine in participants' eyes, at which angles, for certain durations, and so on. As a point of contrast, to better understand the threshold of conscious perception, consider the example of embedding a frame of video with a scary image on it in an unrelated video. It's common for video to be shown at 30 frames per second, so a viewer would be exposed to that image for one-thirtieth of a second, or about 33 milliseconds. On one hand, this is more than enough time to perceive a visual stimulus in isolation; that is, if you were made to sit in a completely dark room for half an hour like those poor participants in the studies conducted on the absolute threshold of vision, and then shown a frame of video for 33 milliseconds, you'd definitely notice that you saw something. However, on the other hand, in the context of the other 29 frames per second that you're seeing, your brain will create a coherent visual narrative that wouldn't even include that weird extra subliminal frame. Hopefully, this example helps illustrate how a stimulus can be above the threshold of absolute perception while still remaining below the threshold of conscious perception.

In addition to detecting whether a stimulus is present or not, it's also important to detect changes in the intensity of a stimulus. Have you ever heard of the story of the boiling frog? The idea is that if a frog is placed directly into boiling water, it will immediately jump out to escape, but if it's placed in cool water that is then warmed very gradually, the frog will never notice the increasing temperature of the water, and will be boiled to death without ever trying to escape. This story is both grim and false, at least as applied to literal frogs in literal pots of water, but it's commonly used as a metaphor about the dangers of gradual change, and does point to the very important, and true, fact that some changes in stimuli can be too small to notice.

The **just-noticeable difference**, or **JND** for short, is one of the most intuitively named concepts you'll ever encounter in psychology. It's the smallest change in the magnitude of a stimulus that we can perceive as being different - which is why it's also sometimes called the difference threshold. So for example, let's consider weights. It might be easy to tell the difference between a 5-pound dumbbell and a 50-pound one, but distinguishing between a bag that weighs 10.0 pounds and one that weighs 10.1 pounds, would be very difficult to do with more accuracy than random guessing. The technical term for this kind of

> **MCAT STRATEGY > > >**
>
> If the JND proves difficult to master, try to make up examples of your own!

testing, by the way, is **psychophysical discrimination testing**. In such experiments, researchers test whether research subjects can tell the difference between two stimuli and then link those findings to the actual physical properties of the stimuli being studied.

Anyway, imagine someone who can reliably, but barely, tell the difference between 10 pounds and 11 pounds. Is that person's difference threshold for weight 1 pound? That might seem tempting at first, but it's worth pausing to try to extrapolate that reasoning to other cases. What about very tiny weights? Telling the difference between one-eighth of a pound and half a pound should be pretty easy. And for much larger weights, it would be very hard to reliably distinguish 100 pounds from 101 pounds. Therefore, it is necessary to think about difference thresholds in terms of proportions, rather than absolute values.

This is where **Weber's law** comes in. Weber's law states that for any given sensory input, the just-noticeable difference will be a constant proportion of the original input. For example, being able to detect 10% differences in weight would mean being able to detect the difference between 10 and 11 pounds, as in the example above, because 11 pounds is a 10% increase from 10 pounds. For smaller masses, we'd expect to be able to distinguish between 1 pound and 1.1 pounds, because going from 1 pound to 1.1 pound is a 10% increase, and for larger masses, between 100 pounds and 110 pounds, because going from 100 to 110 pounds is a 10% increase. However, we would *not* be predicted to be able to distinguish between, say, 100 pounds and 105 pounds, because that would only be a 5% difference.

However, Weber's law does break down at the extremes. It works fairly well for stimuli that are clearly within the range of what we might encounter on a day-to-day basis, but not ones that are either so faint as to be nearly undetectable or so large as to overwhelm our ability to process them. To return to our example of weight, and a 10% just-noticeable difference, the reasoning that we provided above would not apply for tiny weights on the level of milligrams. For instance, only a lab wizard could tell the difference between a 1 mg sample of sodium bicarbonate and a 1.1 mg sample. At the other end of the spectrum, it would be very difficult to tell the difference between a 10,000 pound weight and an 11,000 pound weight. Both would seem immovable, large and not very different from each other. So even though the MCAT may most commonly ask you about viable applications of Weber's law, keep in mind that it stops working well at the extremes of sensory input.

In our experience, Weber's law seems to immediately click for about half of the students that encounter it, but winds up being tricky for the other half -- and sometimes remarkably tricky. There are a couple of reasons why Weber's law can be challenging. First, and most importantly, we most often reason quantitatively in terms of absolute units, not percentages, so it can take a little bit of mental effort to switch over to percentage mode. Second, solving problems with Weber's law does definitely require good mental math skills. But it's a key testable concept within this topic area, so it's worth making it a priority to master, even if that means making some extra time to practice it.

MCAT STRATEGY > > >

What's the point of considering these extreme edge cases of Weber's law? It's good practice because the MCAT emphasizes your understanding of models, their predictions, their applications, and their limitations. With every new model you learn, or old model you review, consider what it was made for, what it's good at, and what its limitations are.

3. Signal Detection Theory and Adaptation

Finely-honed experiments are all well and good, and have yielded important insights into how our senses work, but our real-world experiences of senses and perceptions are very different from being in a laboratory where everything is closely controlled and distractors are minimized. Imagine being in a setting with a lot of background noise and visual stimuli, but with the potential need to react quickly to certain stimuli. Some real-world contexts might include being on a busy city street, where it would be necessary to respond quickly if a car accident or emergency takes place, or on a more positive note, you might need to recognize and say hello to a friend you run into. Or imagine that you're in the wilderness, and specific noises, or even the sudden lack of noise, or tiny little visual signals might indicate the presence of a dangerous predator.

As is often the case in life, we need to find a middle ground. For instance, a hiker whose reaction to every little rustle of the leaves is "OMG A BEAR IS ATTACKING" is unlikely to succeed as a hiker. On the other hand, reacting to actual bear-like growling by thinking "huh, my stomach's rumbling really loudly today, guess it's time to break out the energy bars" might not be very favorable for one's life expectancy. Therefore, on a subconscious level, as part of daily life, or even consciously, if we're given the task to look for something, our brain is constantly filtering through noise, or random background input, to try to accurately identify any signals that we need to respond to. **Signal detection theory** deals with this balance.

Some specific terminology is associated with signal detection theory. Let's return to the example of trying to figure out whether there's a bear in our immediate surroundings, and examine the various possibilities. We can even set up a table to do so. Logically speaking, there either is or isn't a bear present. We can create rows in the table for these possibilities, which we label as "Bear Actually Present" and "Bear Actually Absent". And in either case, we can either perceive the bear as present or not, and we can therefore label the columns as "Bear Perceived" and "Bear Not Perceived". Let's run through the various possibilities. If a bear actually is present, and we perceive it as present, then we're in luck - we can start taking precautionary measures to avoid ending up as bear lunch. In signal detection theory, correctly detecting something that is actually present is referred to as a **hit**. But if a bear is present, and we don't perceive it, then we're in trouble. Intuitively enough, missing something that's actually there is known as a **miss** in signal detection theory. Now what if there isn't a bear present? If we perceive a bear as present because of noise when it's not actually there, we're going to pointlessly freak out. This is known as a **false alarm** or **false positive**. Finally, if no bear is present, and we don't perceive a bear as present, then life is good, we can continue our hike in peace. This is known as a **correct rejection**. All things being equal, we want to maximize hits and correct rejections, and to minimize misses and false alarms.

	BEAR ACTUALLY PRESENT	**BEAR ACTUALLY ABSENT**
BEAR PERCEIVED	Hit	False Alarm / False Positive
BEAR NOT PERCEIVED	Miss	Correct Rejection

Table 1. Signal detection theory

Of course, life is not all bears and bushes: Dangers come in varying degrees, as do rewards or other outcomes. Sometimes success or failure is literally a matter of life and death (as with the bear) and sometimes it may not matter much, like when a friend gets a new haircut and you don't notice: They'll probably live and your friendship won't be irreparably damaged. This is why we need signal detection strategies: A schema where we decide on the ideal sensitivity of our signal detection based on the costs and rewards for hits, misses, false alarms, and correct rejections.

The question of how we make that decision is very deep, and is also relevant for researchers in artificial intelligence. However, for our purposes, in addition to focusing on the classification of possible outcomes, we should just be aware that the specific outcomes of signal detection can vary across people and even within an individual depending on his or her psychological state and the general context. Think about it this way: some people are obviously more vigilant and perceptive than others, and if you think about your own experiences, you're probably going to be more likely to interpret a creak on the stairwell as something ominous if you're alone at home, late at night, then you are in the middle of the day if friends are over.

CHAPTER 3: SENSATION AND PERCEPTION

Here's a final thing to think about regarding signal detection theory. We worked through an example of recognizing a bear in the woods. What if we replaced "bear" with "cancer" and "forest" with "medical imaging"? All of a sudden, things have taken a much more serious turn, and signal detection theory sounds a lot like the process that physicians use to diagnose disease. That similarity is not accidental, and it's one of the reasons why the MCAT expects you to be aware of the concepts of signal detection theory: As a way of laying the groundwork for the much more detailed study of diagnostic procedures that you'll do in med school.

> **MCAT STRATEGY > > >**
>
> Hopefully the examples of bears and cancer are memorable, but if you have trouble remembering the basic concepts of signal detection theory, we suggest that you develop further examples of your own. Doing so can also help check your work!

One of the most amazing things about perception is how many things we manage to ignore. When you get caught up in an engaging story or TV show, you might tune out almost all other sensory input, and even in the course of daily life, we don't usually notice the temperature of the room, the sensation of clothes on our skin, familiar background scenery, background noise, and so on, unless we specifically choose to pay attention to them. Of course, individuals show variation when it comes to this, but we really do have a remarkable ability to get used to stimuli. The technical term for this is **sensory adaptation**.

To some extent, structural diversity in sensory receptors contributes to adaptation. Some receptors adapt slowly to stimuli and continue to send action potentials as long as a stimulus is present. Receptors like this are known as tonic receptors, and some examples include sensors for stretching and pain. In contrast, phasic receptors send a quick burst of action potentials in response to a stimulus, and then stop. Some examples include receptors linked to hair follicles, which respond rapidly to being brushed or moved, but then adapt quickly.

Now that we've covered signal detection theory and adaptation, in addition to other major topics relating to sensation and perception, we should have a pretty good sense of the mechanics of how our body translates physical input from the world around us into perceptions, some of which we are consciously aware of, and some of which we ignore. These general principles lay the groundwork for exploring how our brain organizes perceptions more specifically.

> **MCAT STRATEGY > > >**
>
> Isolated terms can be hard to remember confidently. Try this: As captain of a starship, you've got to quickly fire your PHASIC receptors to fight off dangerous attackers, but you can take your time and slowly sip a gin and TONIC receptor.

4. Perceptual Organization

So far, we've mostly been talking about perception in yes and no terms, but our day-to-day experiences involve much more interesting things like shapes, colors, textures, voices, and music. Therefore, how we assemble and organize individual perceptions into meaningful units is a major question.

I. Bottom-Up and Top-Down Organization

There are two basic ways of building meaningful units of perception: **bottom-up processing** and **top-down processing.** Bottom-up processing is a natural extension of how we've been talking about sensation and perception so far; it refers to a pattern in which our brain starts with individual pieces of sensory information coming in and assembles them into a coherent whole. Top-down processing, on the other hand, refers to a scenario where the brain decides ahead of time what it's looking for, and then assembles the individual pieces of sensory information together in a way that supports that picture.

Technically speaking, bottom-up and top-down processing coexist for all of our senses, so it's helpful to use a variety of examples. A somewhat common experience is hearing a familiar song not at its beginning, but a few seconds in—basically, just enough for the beat to be slightly off—and then waiting for a moment or two while processing this raw sound, but then once you recognize the song, it all clicks into place? In that situation, your brain starts off in bottom-up processing mode, and then switches into top-down mode once you recognize the song.

Reality TV provides a good example of something similar with smell and taste. Some reality TV shows have a challenge where aspiring chefs are blindfolded, taste various ingredients, and have to identify what they're tasting. The results are surprisingly unreliable, with carrots being mistaken for cloves of garlic and the like, embarrassing nearly every participant regularly. This taste test is an example of bottom-up processing. As the identity of the real food item is revealed, top-down processing kicks in, and the contestant realizes what the food actually was, and says to themselves "oh, of course that was a carroty taste, not garlic…". Oh well!

To flip these examples and focus on top-down processing going wrong, consider the experience of looking for an object you misplaced in a familiar room, but missing it right even though it's right in front of you, because your eyes probably skimmed over the object several times without actually perceiving it, because you could not conceive of it being there. This basic phenomenon, that our expectations can literally prevent us from seeing things that are in front of our face, plays a role in topics as diverse as optical illusions and the potential unreliability of eyewitness testimony in some circumstances. That said, for the purposes of the MCAT, the main goal of these examples is to help you cement the difference between top-down and bottom-up processing.

II. Gestalt Processing

Another fact about human perception that is easy to overlook, but fascinating when you think about it, is that we are usually only partially exposed to the objects that we sense, but we automatically infer information about the whole object. For this discussion, we'll focus on how this concept applies to vision, because that's by far the most common set of examples used to illustrate these points, but in principle, everything we're saying could be extended to other senses.

There are certain properties that we're more or less hard-wired to use in terms of perceptual organization. Take depth perception, or the ability to perceive a third spatial dimension, or near versus far, in addition to up versus down and left versus right. A classic experiment is to close one eye and try to do basic everyday things like pick up an object on the desk next to you. It gets pretty tricky, right? This points to the degree to which **binocular cues**, or the existence of two eyes that pick up on light from slightly different angles, help us perceive depth. That said, it's not

CHAPTER 3: SENSATION AND PERCEPTION

impossible, just harder, to do things with one eye closed, which in turn underscores the importance of **monocular cues**, like relative size, perspective, which objects are in front of or behind each other, and brightness to infer depth. Other features we're primed to look for in our input include motion, shape, and constancy.

A school of psychologists in the late 19th and early 20th centuries tried to explain how we can build a perceptual whole that is distinct from the sum of its parts. This field of study was most prominent in Germany, so it's known by the word "Gestalt," which means "form in German. The key aspects of Gestalt theory for the MCAT have to do with the Gestalt principles of grouping.

Image A: A square made out of several small circles

Image B: Three horizontal lines (principle of proximity)

Image C: Three vertical lines (principle of similarity)

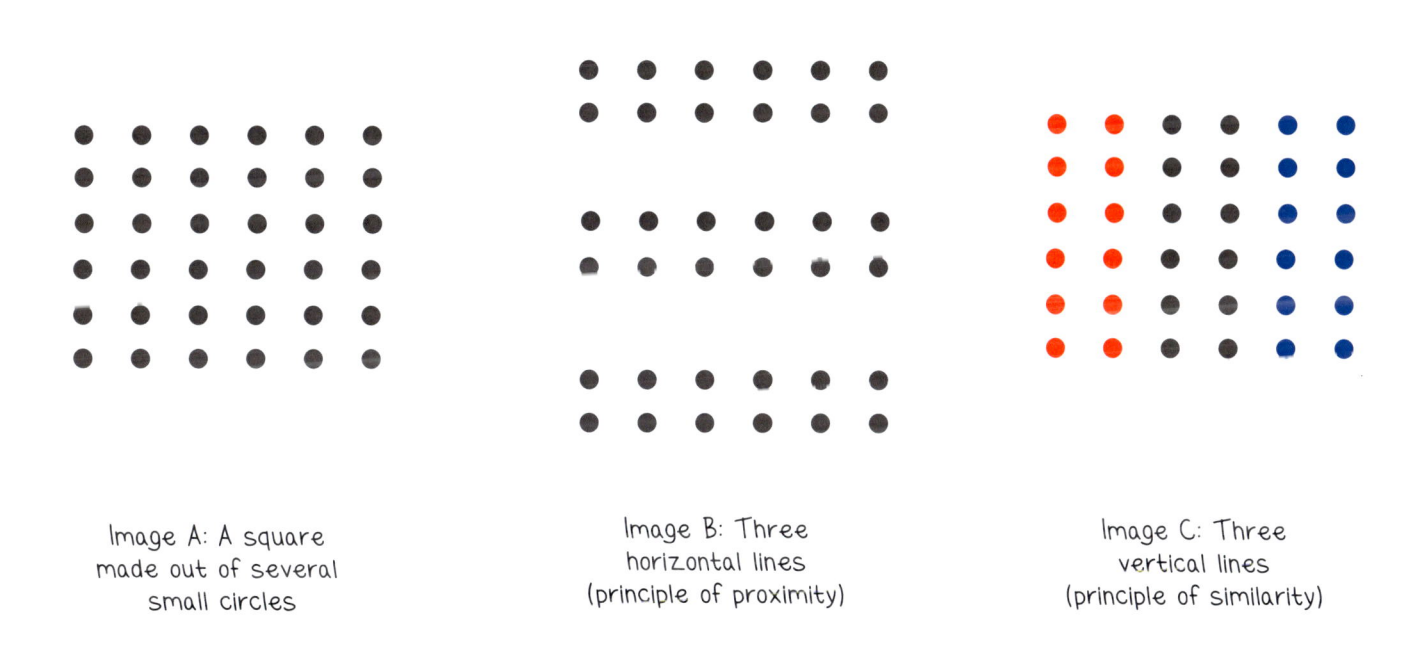

Figure 1. Gestalt principles of proximity and similarity

Let's start with a simple example. Look at the left-most shape (image A) in the above image: what is it? Our most immediate perception is that it's a square, although if we take a closer look at it, we'll notice that it's actually made up of several smaller circles. Now, look at the center image (image B), which we obtained by taking image A and splitting up the circles into three groups that form three horizontal lines, which is what we primarily perceive. This example illustrates the **principle of proximity**, which states that we perceive objects or shapes that are close to each other as forming groups. Next, let's return to image A, but make the columns on the left side of the square blue, and the columns on the right side red. Now what we see, in image C on the right, is a set of three vertical rows - like the French flag, as it happens. What this illustrates is the **principle of similarity**, which states that objects that are similar in some way will be perceived as belonging to a group.

51

Let's switch gears from our lovely square and look at these two intersecting lines. All things being equal, we're more likely to perceive these as two lines running from left to right. This is due to the **principle of good continuation**, which states that if multiple objects intersect or overlap, we tend to perceive them as relatively few uninterrupted objects, and that we tend to perceive lines or curves as extending without sharp changes. We can see this more clearly by using color to indicate the two lines, with a roughly horizontal red line on top of a roughly horizontal black line.

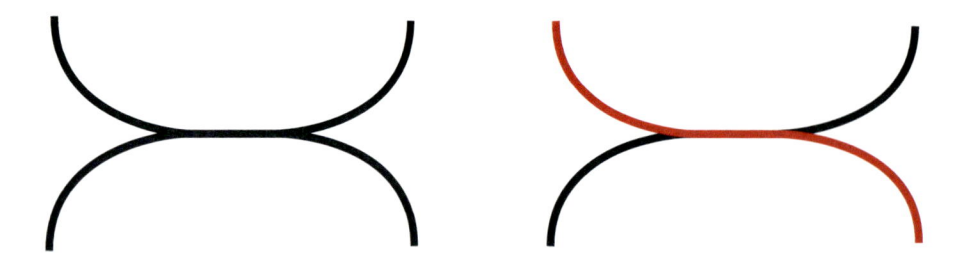

Figure 2. Gestalt principle of good continuation

However, at least in theory, we could also view this drawing as containing one line that starts in the upper left and then bends to the lower left, and one that starts in the upper right and bends to the lower right, as is shown in the left-hand side of Figure 3, which is reminiscent of chromosomes. Theoretically, we could also see this drawing as being composed of four shorter lines that converge at a center point, as in the right-hand side of Figure 3 below.

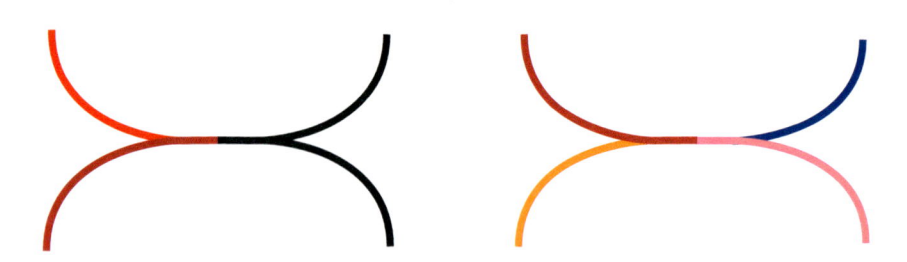

Figure 3. Interpretations violating the Gestalt principle of good continuation

This example illustrates a few important points about Gestalt principles. One is that they don't apply in isolation. So by switching the colors to make these lines look like chromosomes, we can use the principle of similarity to overrule the principle of good continuation. The role of context is crucial here. If you see the original image, just in black and white, right after being immersed in studying genetics, you might be more likely to perceive them as lining up like chromosomes. It's not really possible to catalog all the different ways that context can shape your perceptions, but we definitely bring our own expectations to the table when we perceive things, and sometimes it makes a real difference.

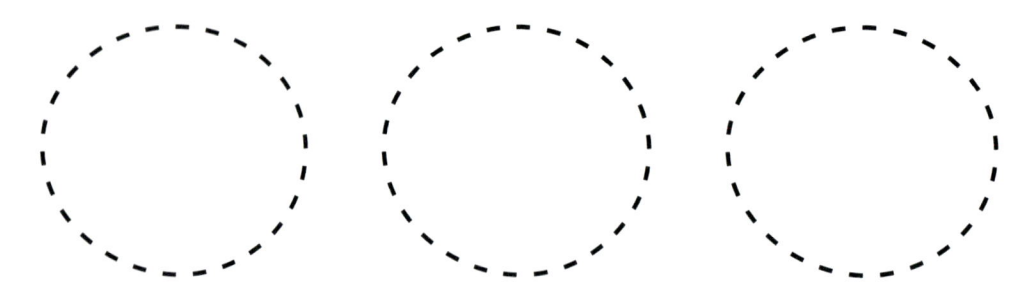

Figure 4. Gestalt principle of closure (showing three shapes we interpret as circles)

Another important Gestalt principle is the **principle of closure**, which states that we infer the presence of complete shapes even when they're incomplete. A classic example is a circle with a broken outline; we have no problem whatsoever interpreting this as a circle, and it would be hard to look at such a shape and say, "why, of course that's just a collection of random slightly curved line segments."

Finally, the **principle of symmetry** states that symmetrical objects are more likely to be perceived as part of a whole than asymmetrical objects. So, consider the two pairs of objects in Figure 5, where the left one contains a pair of shapes with symmetry about the vertical axis, while the right one contains two non-symmetrical shapes. We're more likely to use the principle of symmetry to interpret the left pair of shapes as a single unit than we are to do so with the right pair. As it happens, this principle is applied fairly often in user interface design for websites and software.

Option A: Vertical line of symmetry makes us perceive this pair as a single unit.

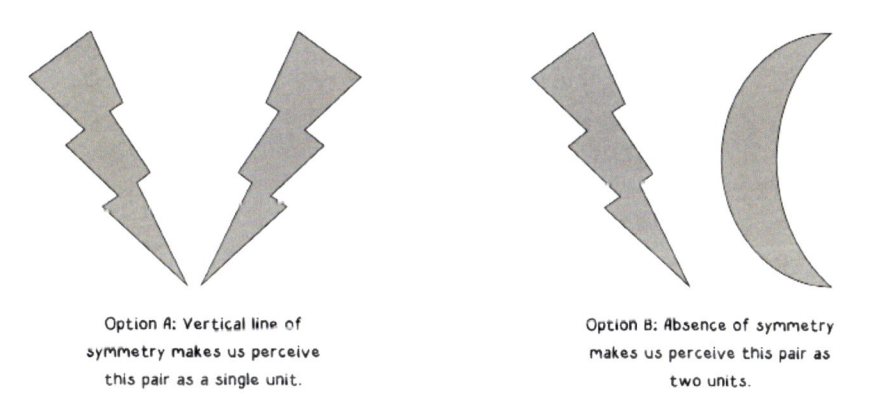

Option B: Absence of symmetry makes us perceive this pair as two units.

Figure 5. Gestalt principle of symmetry

Sometimes the Gestalt principles are referred to as "laws," so don't be surprised if you see them referred to that way, although "principle" may be preferable because context can make a difference, and there's room for multiple principles to interact. The common thread of the Gestalt principles is the **law of Prägnanz**, which is another German term. Prägnanz translates as "pithiness," meaning concise and meaningful. The logical link between all of the Gestalt principles is that we try to find simple and meaningful ways to represent objects that we perceive as wholes, not just as random parts. And that's really what perception is about. Of course, we have some more work to do in terms of tracing the specific ways that we process different types of sensory input, but the broad principles of how we perceive and filter sensory input apply across the board.

5. Structure and Function of the Eye

The anatomy of vision starts with the eye, which contains an intricately organized set of structures that detect visual stimuli, convert them to action potentials, and send them to the brain via visual pathways. It's easy to drown in detail when it comes to the eye; instead, though, we want to prioritize: We'll start with the simplest model of the eye necessary to understand why it works the way it does, and then we'll fill in anatomical details as we go.

At its most basic, the eye is a system for turning certain wavelengths of light into action potentials. The **retina**, which is located at the back of the eye, carries out this function. It contains millions of photoreceptors, which are classified as **cones** or **rods**. Cones are responsible for perceiving color and fine detail. Interestingly, there are three different types of cones that specialize in perceiving different wavelengths, which in turn correspond to different hues of color. The short-wavelength type specializes in sensing blue, with a wavelength of about 420 nm, while the medium-wavelength type specializes in sensing green at at about 530 nm, and the long-wavelength type is most sensitive to red, at about 570 nm. There are about 6 million cones in the retina, and they tend to be concentrated in its central area - most specifically, the fovea, which is a small central pit in the retina that only contains cones, but also the macula, which is the central region around the fovea.

Rods do not sense color; instead, they specialize in sensing visual input in low-light conditions. As such, they're responsible for night vision. They're highly sensitive to small changes in visual input, but do not really pick up on detail well. They contain a compound called **rhodopsin**, which is a pigment and a photoreceptor protein that is extremely sensitive to light. There are many more rods than cones - around 120 million rods, versus 6 million cones - and they tend to be distributed more densely *away* from the center of the retina, so that peripheral vision is best for seeing dimly-lit objects at night.

> **MCAT STRATEGY > > >**
>
> A useful mnemonic for distinguishing cones and rods is that cones, which start with a C, sense color, which also starts with a C. The overlap in the first letter also helps us remember that rods contain rhodopsin.

The other key aspect of how the eye works is that it focuses incoming light rays to converge on the retina, so that the retina can form an accurate, crisp, and clear image. The main structures responsible for this are the **lens** and the **cornea**. Both structures are located at the front of the eye. The cornea is the very first thing that light passes through to enter the eye. It's a clear and remarkably tough structure that's best known for protecting the eye from external injuries, but it also helps focus incoming light. The lens then finishes the job of focusing light. It's an ingenious little structure that can change shape with the help of tiny ligaments attached to its rim to help the eye focus on objects at various distances, a process called **accommodation**.

This is the bare minimum. If you know nothing else about the eye, be able to trace the path through which light is focused by the cornea and lens, and then hits the retina. In the retina, cones are predominantly located in the central areas of the **fovea** and **macula**, and they have the job of sensing color and fine detail, while the more numerous rods, which are distributed towards the periphery of the retina, pick up on low-light stimuli. Rods also take a while to become active and useful after you've been in bright places for a while - this process is called **dark adaptation** and is the reason you see better in the dark after a few minutes. This is also why night guards who smoke cigarettes, a source of light, always get knocked out in movies: They can't see anyone. Most MCAT questions on vision are answerable based on just the above. But other anatomical structures of the eye do come up as well in the context of various physiological phenomena, so it will be worth expanding our knowledge beyond the very basics.

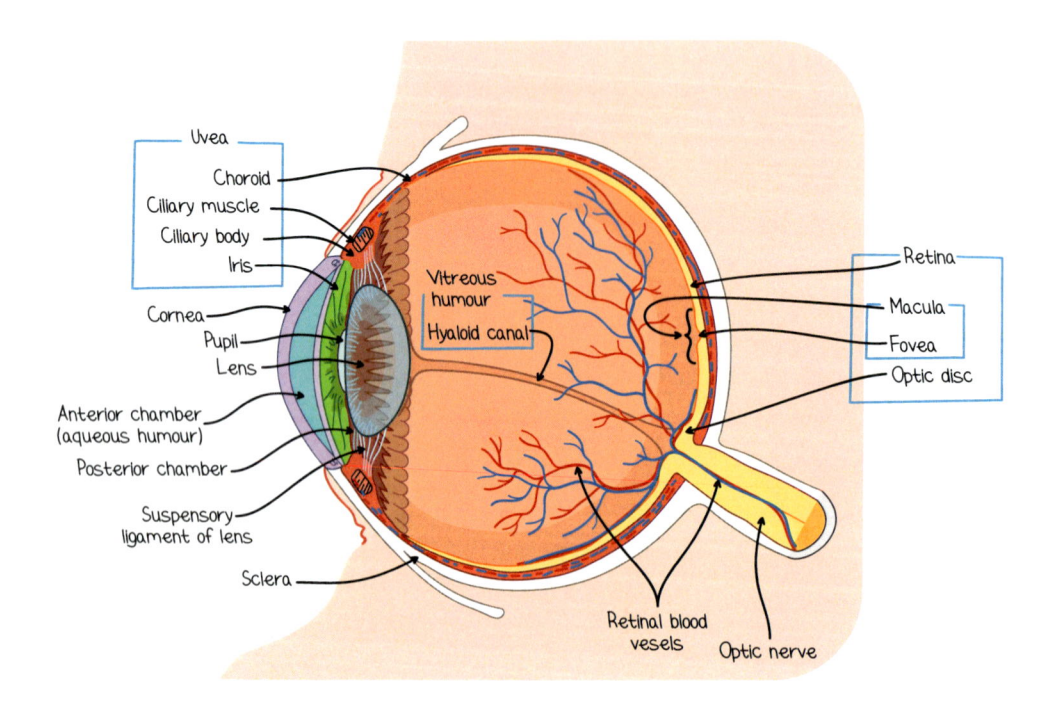

Figure 6. Structure of the eye

As you can see from our sketch of the eye, the cornea is contiguous with the external surface of the eye, and the lens bisects the interior of the eye into two unequally-sized components. In front of the lens is a structure called the **iris**, which is the part of the eye that we refer to when we say that someone has blue eyes or brown eyes. The iris has a hole in its center known as the **pupil**, which is what actually lets light into the eye; meanwhile, we can think of the iris as a sun umbrella that blocks the light that's not supposed to get into the eye. The iris is connected to two muscles, called the **dilator pupillae** and the **constrictor pupillae**. As the name suggests, one of these muscles has the job of dilating the pupil, which means pulling the iris back to make the pupil bigger and let more light in, and the other is responsible for constricting the pupil, which means extending the iris to make the pupil smaller and let less light in.

The most obvious function of dilation and constriction of the pupil is as an adaptation to help the eye deal with varying levels of light. And indeed, our pupils constrict in bright daylight and dilate in the dark. However, this response is also regulated by the sympathetic and parasympathetic nervous systems. When the sympathetic nervous system kicks in, as part of our fight-or-flight response, we dilate our pupils, making us hypersensitive to visual input that might help us handle whatever crisis caused the fight-or-flight response. Correspondingly, our pupils constrict during the parasympathetic, "rest-and-digest" response.

We also mentioned that the lens can change its shape to optimize its focus. The **ciliary muscle**, which is part of a larger structure known as the ciliary body, which adjusts the lens via the suspensory ligaments.

So now we can see that the lens, iris, pupil, and various accessory muscles and ligaments divide the eye into two high-level parts. The **anterior chamber** is the smaller, front-facing area, and the larger space towards the back of the eye is known as the **posterior chamber**. The anterior chamber contains a fluid called the **aqueous humor**, and the posterior chamber contains a gel-like, viscous fluid known as the **vitreous humor.**

Finally, let's return to the outer edge of the eye. We haven't said a lot about it besides just noting that the cornea is contiguous with it. As is often the case in anatomy, it's a little more complicated. Remember how we said that the retina is located at the back of the eye? Well, it's centered at the back of the eye, but actually extends along the inner surface of the posterior chamber. Beneath the retina lies a layer of dark, vascular tissue full of melanin called the **choroid**, which supplies the retina with blood and absorbs excess light. The choroid forms a continuous layer with the iris, which makes sense given its location as the middle layer. Then, the outermost layer of the eye is known as the **sclera**, which is contiguous with the cornea and is best known for being the structure that accounts for the white color of the eye. In addition, the eye itself is protected from the elements by a thin layer of epithelium called the **conjunctiva** - a very small, translucent film that lies in front of the cornea and sclera and is in charge of keeping your eyes lubricated.

To summarize: The eye is a fairly complicated structure, but the key is to understand how it does its job of focusing light, and then to learn the high-level structural divisions of the eye from a functional perspective, and only then to worry about the details of lower-priority structures.

6. Visual Processing

There's more to know about the retina than the fact that cones and rods are responsible for sensing light. The retina is a surprisingly complex structure: There are a few steps that happen between when a light ray hits the retina and when an action potential is sent off through the optic nerve to be processed in the brain. Cones and rods don't connect directly to the optic nerve; instead, they synapse onto neurons known as **bipolar cells**, which are called "bipolar" because they have a distinctive shape with a single dendrite and axon emanating to each side from a central body. Each bipolar cell accepts input from several cones or rods, and this is the first of many steps in the visual pathway where information is integrated. Then, in turn, bipolar cells synapse with **ganglion cells**, which are the neurons of the optic nerve. Bipolar cells serve as an in-between step in the retina.

Making matters more complicated still, sets of cells exist that mediate this process at each stage, functioning in a sort of horizontal way to further integrate input. And intuitively enough, the cells that step in at the transition between photoreceptors and bipolar cells are actually called **horizontal cells**. They inhibit photoreceptors, helping the eye to adjust to high- versus low-light conditions, and also synapse onto bipolar cells too. Similarly, the second stage of this process, where bipolar cells synapse on ganglion cells, is mediated by yet another set of cells, known as **amacrine cells**. Okay, so now we've packaged and processed visual input, which runs through the optic nerve. The next step is a little convoluted. It involves thinking a lot about left and right, so if this is a challenge for you, it's time to review whatever mnemonic you learned in elementary school to tell left from right. Take a second to orient yourself. Now imagine a thin barrier extending from your nose, dividing everything in front of you into left and right. These are known as visual fields. Next, let's divide each retina into left and right halves. Now, how does this left/right division in your eyes relate to the left/right division in your visual field? We start with light rays that bounce off of objects and from there trace a straight path, only getting refracted slightly on entering our eye. Knowing that, a light ray that bounces off of something in your left visual field will hit the right side of the retina in each eye, and vice versa.

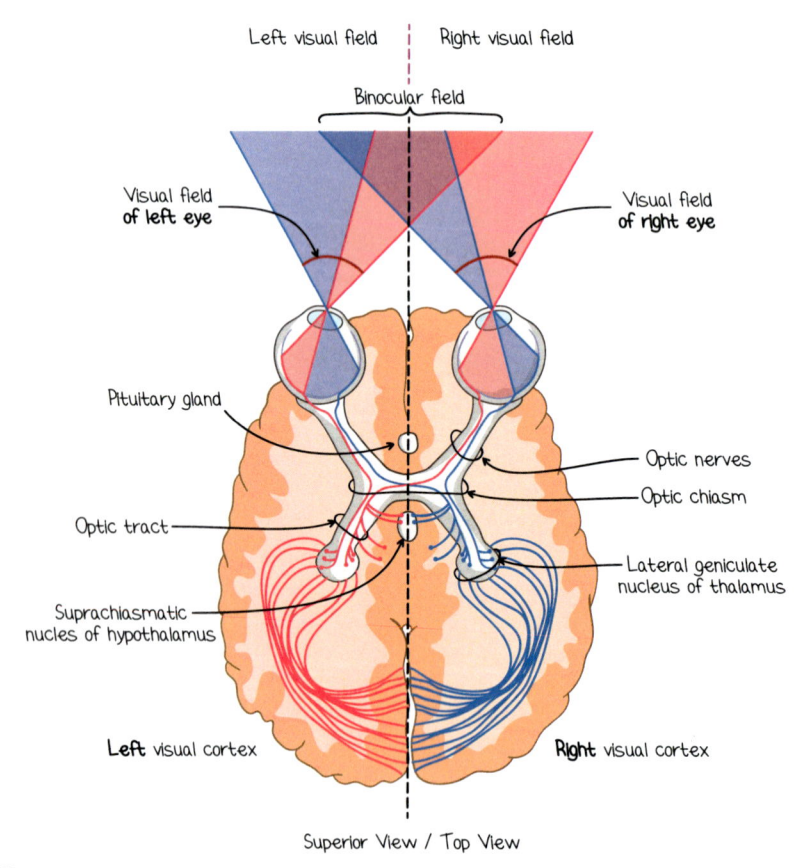

Figure 7. Visual pathways

Next, we can visualize the optic nerves as having a total of four components: one for each half of each eye. As we move towards the brain, the optic nerves cross at a location called the **optic chiasm**. Here, the segments of the optic nerve coming from the innermost halves of both eyes—sometimes called the **nasal sides**, because they're closest to your nose—cross over and get shunted to the opposite side of the brain. So, in other words, the input that hits the right side of your left eye gets processed in the right hemisphere, and conversely, the input that hits the left side of your right eye gets processed in the left hemisphere. Meanwhile, input coming from the outer halves of each retina— the halves that don't face your nose and are called **temporal sides**—stays on the same side of your brain. The input that hits the left side of your left eye stays on the left and is processed in the left hemisphere, and the input that hits the right side of your right eye stays on the right and is processed in the right hemisphere. Another way of looking at this is that the left-facing halves of both eyes get processed on the left, and the right-facing halves of both eyes get processed on the right, and some crossover is needed to make this happen. Take a moment to recreate our drawing of the visual fields above, and the two portions of each optic nerve. Then place an imaginary object in one visual field and trace the fate of light bouncing off it, hitting your retina and where that information goes. Convince yourself that what we've shown you is true before moving on!

Now that the optic nerve has reached the optic chiasm, we refer to these bundles of axons carrying visual information as the **optic tract**. The optic tract runs through the **lateral geniculate nucleus**, sometimes abbreviated as the **LGN**, which is a structure contained in the thalamus that acts as the main relay station for input from the retinas and is responsible for sending signals to the **superior colliculus**, which controls the visual startle response and the appropriately named visual cortex of the occipital lobe, which is where conscious visual perception is formed.

The LGN is an interesting structure because it contains some specialized types of neurons that sense very specific types of input. In particular, there are **magnocellular neurons** present, which got their name because they're big, and **parvocellular neurons**, which are small. These two types of neurons have roughly opposite functionalities, because there's an inherent tradeoff between what's called **temporal resolution**, the ability to pick up changes, and **spatial resolution**, or the ability to see things in detail. Magnocellular neurons specialize in detecting motion, which you can remember by the overlap in the first letter in magnocellular and motion, but aren't good at picking up details. The opposite holds for parvocellular neurons, which are great for picking up details.

> **MCAT STRATEGY > > >**
>
> Pay close attention to the logic of terms when studying! The existence of a lateral geniculate nucleus suggests that there may be a medial geniculate nucleus. It's also part of the thalamus, but it routes auditory information to the auditory cortex, while also sending signals to the inferior colliculus, which is responsible for the auditory startle response. Building connections like these will help you solidify the material.

While we're on the topic of motion, it's worth noting that our perceptions of motion and depth are deeply linked through a phenomenon known as **motion parallax**. This term describes the fact that objects that are close to us move further across our visual field than objects that are far from us, and this fact is one of the cues that we use to perceive depth. For example, imagine that you're driving in a mountainous region. Buildings by the side of the road rush by very quickly, whereas the far-off mountains seem to move very slowly as you drive by.

These observations underscore the fact that we're constantly picking up on many categories at the same time as we perceive things. For instance, upon seeing an ambulance roaring down the road with sirens blazing, we automatically monitor parameters like color, shape, timing and motion. Our ability to do this is known as **feature detection**, and the process by which we integrate all that simultaneous input is known as **parallel processing**. However, more specific tasks (e.g., looking for a lost set of keys in a room, or an animal that we're hunting in the woods) require a more systematic, deliberate search. Such a perceptual strategy, where we consciously look in one place after another and analyze stimuli in order, is called the **serial processing model**.

7. Hearing and Vestibular Sense

Hearing is similar to vision in that it involves a complicated anatomical system for translating stimuli into vivid subjective experiences. Hearing and vision also tend to be the two senses that the MCAT most frequently tests in detail. So, given these similarities, we'll take a similar approach to studying these two senses. In this discussion, we'll review the anatomy of hearing, starting with a basic functional sketch and then filling in anatomical details as needed, and then discuss how the brain processes auditory input. We'll then return to the topic of the ear to talk about how it also contributes to vestibular sense, or our orientation in three-dimensional space.

To review, on a physical level sound waves are longitudinal waves that manifest as regularly repeating changes in pressure as air molecules move back and forth. The simplest way to think about the ear, then, is as a funnel that gathers together such waves and converts them into neural signals that travel to the brain. Now let's worry about how this happens.

> **MCAT STRATEGY > > >**
>
> "Hear" and "hair" sound very similar, which can help you remember that hair cells are responsible for hearing.

The cells responsible for this amazing feat are known as **hair cells**, because they have cute little stereocilia that poke out into a fluid called the endolymph that surrounds them. Sound waves cause hair cells to move around in the endolymph, and that swaying movement of the stereocilia opens up **ion channels** that let small positively-charged ions (cations) flow into the cell. This, in turn, triggers an influx of calcium ions through voltage-gated calcium channels, and this calcium influx then causes the release of neurotransmitters at the other end of the cell, to cells of the **vestibulocochlear nerve**, at which point neural signals encoding sound are transmitted. This is the **transduction** of sound.

Anatomically, the ear is divided into the outer, middle, and inner ear, and the hair cells are located in the **inner ear**, within a structure called the **organ of Corti**. The organ of Corti looks like a layer cake, with a flexible structure called the basilar membrane on the bottom, hair cells suspended in endolymph in the middle, and at the top lays a more rigid structure known as the tectorial membrane.

To summarize, sound waves enter the ear and cause the endolymph that surrounds the hair cells in the inner ear to vibrate. This ultimately causes the hair cells in the organ of Corti to release neurotransmitters that trigger nerve signals that move into the brain, towards the auditory cortex. This is the basic framework of how hearing works. Now we need to take a more detailed look at the anatomy of the ear and expand our understanding of the intermediate steps.

CHAPTER 3: SENSATION AND PERCEPTION

As we mentioned before, the ear is divided into outer, middle, and inner segments. The **outer ear** consists of the external structures of the ear. The fleshy bottom part of the ear is called the **earlobe**, and the cartilaginous, curly part on top is referred to as the **pinna**, or **auricle**. These structures funnel incoming sound waves into the external auditory canal, which is basically a tube that extends inward to the **eardrum**. The eardrum, known as the **tympanic membrane**, is the dividing point between the outer ear and the middle ear. As the name eardrum suggests, the tympanic membrane vibrates in response to sound waves. High-frequency sound waves cause it to vibrate at a high frequency, and vice-versa for low-frequency sound waves. The intensity of sound manifests as the amplitude of the sound waves, and straightforwardly enough, louder (higher-amplitude) sounds cause higher-amplitude vibrations of the eardrum. Imagine somebody playing a drum or any similar percussion instrument, but with sound waves, instead of hands or sticks, hitting the membrane.

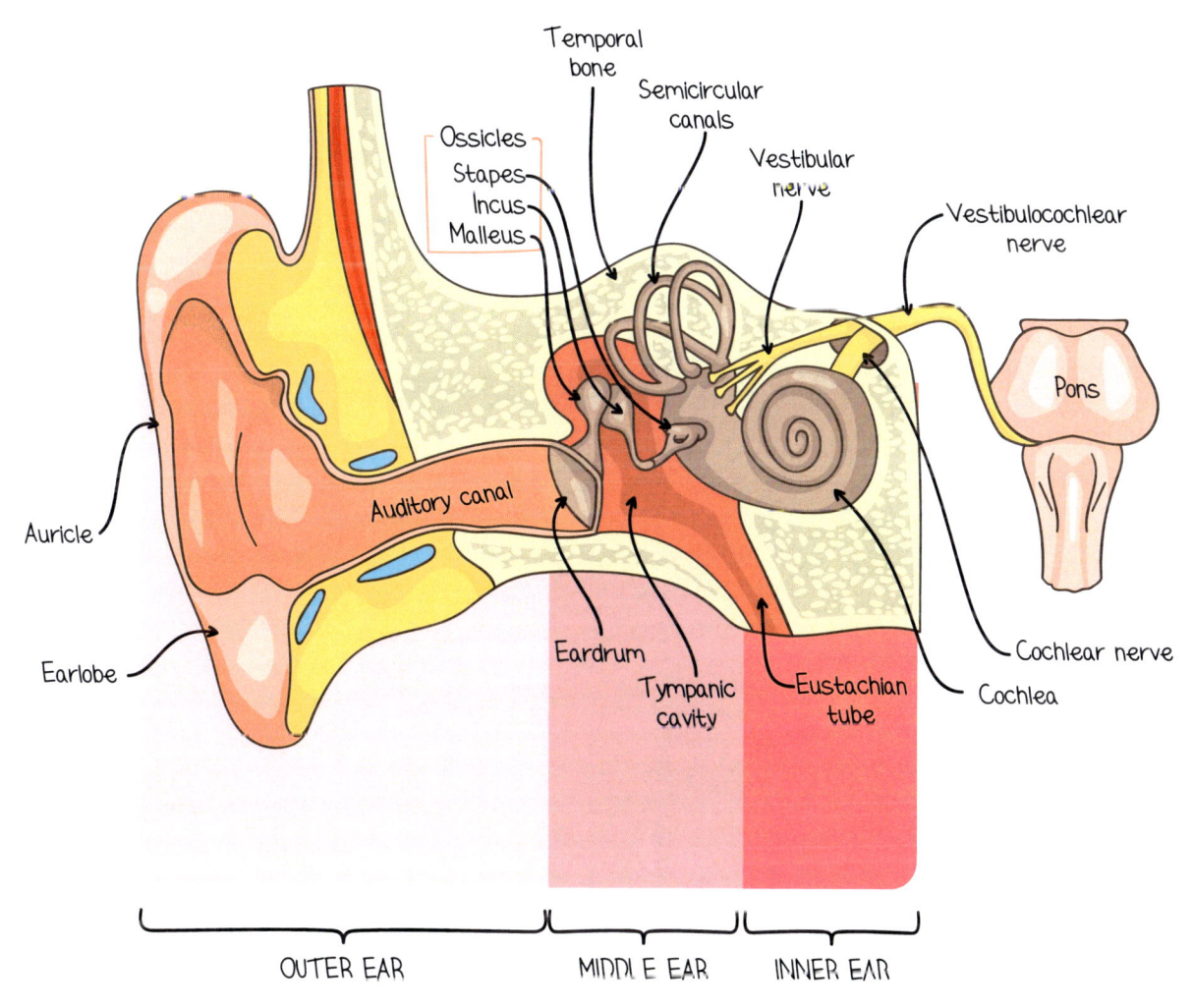

Figure 8. The anatomy of the ear

Next we've got the **middle ear**, which contains the charmingly named **ossicles**—think popsicles, except they're tiny bones—which are a set of three intricately-shaped bones that fit together to amplify the vibrations of the tympanic membrane. First, the **malleus**, or hammer, is connected to the tympanic membrane. It sends vibrations to the **incus**, or anvil, which then connects to the **stapes**, or stirrup. These are the smallest bones in the body. The stapes then connects to a membrane known as the oval window, which is the boundary between the middle ear and the inner ear, much like how the tympanic membrane is the boundary between the outer ear and the middle ear. In addition to the ossicles, the middle ear contains a connection to the nasal cavity known as the **Eustachian tube**, which is basically a valve that equalizes the pressure between the middle ear and the environment. If you've ever felt your ears "pop" in an an airplane, or in any other situation where you rapidly ascend or descend and therefore experience sudden changes in air pressure, that's the Eustachian tube at work.

So, as we've said, the oval window connects to the inner ear. The ossicles of the middle ear are able to amplify the vibrations from the eardrum by as much as ten times, so the oval window transmits much higher-amplitude oscillations to the inner ear. The structure of the inner ear is complicated. It's a multi-functional space, but a key aspect is that it contains fluid-bathed hair cells that can translate vibrations into nerve signals. The basic framework of the inner ear is known as the bony labyrinth, which contains the **membranous labyrinth**, which makes up the sub-structures of the inner ear. The membranous labyrinth contains **endolymph**, while the area between the bony labyrinth and the membranous labyrinth contains a similar fluid called **perilymph**.

The **cochlea** is the structure within the inner ear that is responsible for hearing. It's spiral-shaped and is divided into three layers, sometimes referred to as **scalae**. The inner and outer scalae are filled with perilymph, while the middle layer is suspended between two membranes and contains, as we discussed earlier, the organ of Corti. Hair cells protrude from the basilar membrane into the organ of Corti, and are bathed in endolymph. The layer below the basilar membrane is filled with perilymph, which vibrates in response to sound waves, and those vibrations are transmitted to the basilar membrane. The thickness of the basilar membrane isn't constant, and different thicknesses respond to different frequencies of vibrations. The basilar membrane responds to high-frequency vibrations close to the oval window that connects the middle and inner ears, and to low-frequency vibrations at locations further from the oval window. This phenomenon, sometimes referred to as **place theory**, allows the brain to infer information about the pitch of a sound based on which hair cells send signals.

MCAT STRATEGY > > >

Remember the basic logic of how the ear helps us perceive sound: the outer ear gathers up sound waves, the middle ear is our amplification system, and the inner ear does the actual job of hearing by converting mechanical signals into neural signals.

The nerve signals generated by the hair cells in the organ of Corti are transmitted through the **vestibulocochlear nerve**, a cranial nerve sometimes referred to as the **auditory nerve**. The medial geniculate nucleus in the thalamus is an important structure, through which which auditory signals pass on their way to the **auditory cortex** in the temporal lobe. The left hemisphere specializes in processing speech, while the right hemisphere specializes in processing background noise and instrumental music.

The function of the inner ear isn't just limited to sound. Hair cells in the inner ear are also responsible for the **vestibular sense**, which accounts for balance and contributes to our ability to orient ourselves in three-dimensional space. Within the inner ear, three endolymph-containing structures called the **semicircular canals** are responsible for sensing **rotational acceleration**. As their name implies, each of them looks like about half of a circle or an oval, and each ends in a bulge called an **ampulla**, which contains hair cells. When the head rotates, the endolymph in the semicircular canals moves, and the hair cells resist that acceleration. This mechanical stimulation of the hair cells causes a signal to be sent to the brain in much the same way that we saw for the cochlea, which is responsible for detecting sound. An interesting fact about the semicircular canals is that they're arranged perpendicularly to each other, like x-, y-, and z-axes on a graph, which helps relate to how they help us keep track of our movement in three-dimensional space.

Additionally, the inner ear contains yet another structure, called the **vestibule**. The basic job of the vestibule is to sense linear acceleration. In turn, it contains two sub-structures: The **utricle**, which detects acceleration in the horizontal plane, and the **saccule**, which detects acceleration in the vertical plane. These structures contain tiny little calcium carbonate specks called **otoliths**, which help stimulate the hair cells.

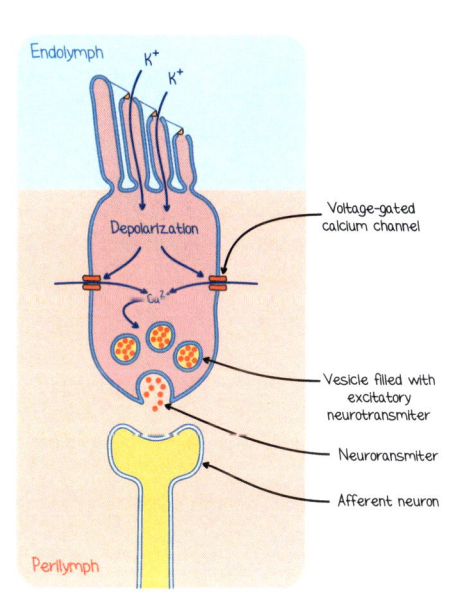

Figure 9. A hair cell

To review, the basic mechanism through which sound and vestibular sense work is that hair cells have the ability to convert a swaying motion in the endolymph into neural signals. The anatomy that supports this is complicated, but we can organize the basic structures into two groups of three: the ear is divided into the outer, middle, and inner ears, which respectively gather up sound information, amplify it, and convert it into signals. The inner ear is divided into the cochlea, which deals with sound, the semicircular canals, which sense rotational acceleration, and the vestibule, which detects linear acceleration. Logically grouping structures like this will help you make sense of what can otherwise be an overwhelming amount of information.

8. Other Senses

The category of "touch" is kind of an oversimplification; as we mentioned elsewhere, our bodies contain a variety of receptors that respond to specialized stimuli, such as light touch versus deep pressure versus stretching, and it also makes sense to group the perception of pain together with touch in a broader category known as **somatosensation**. *Soma* is the Greek word for body; the entire word therefore means sensation of the body.

Nerves in the skin are not distributed evenly. Some areas of the body that are highly sensitive have a very dense distribution of somatosensory nerves in the skin. Your hands are a perfect example: The tips of your fingers are exquisitely sensitive to small changes in stimulation. This makes sense, because we use our hands every day to carry out delicate and important motions, like writing textbooks. The skin on the back of your head, for example, though, doesn't have a very high density of nerves, because that isn't a part of the body that gets much use.

What do we mean by saying that one body part is more sensitive than another? Psychologists operationalize the concept of sensitivity using the **two-point threshold**, which refers to the minimum distance between two points that are stimulated at the same time on the skin such that we can perceive the two points as distinct from each other. The denser the distribution of nerves, the smaller the two-point threshold will be, and the more sensitive we say a certain area is. There's an interesting visualization called the homunculus, or "little man" in Latin, that was developed to help visualize this concept. It's a drawing of a person where the scale of each body part is proportional to the nerve density and the relative amount of space dedicated to processing the corresponding input in the somatosensory cortex of the parietal lobe.

Motor homunculus proportional somatotopical representation

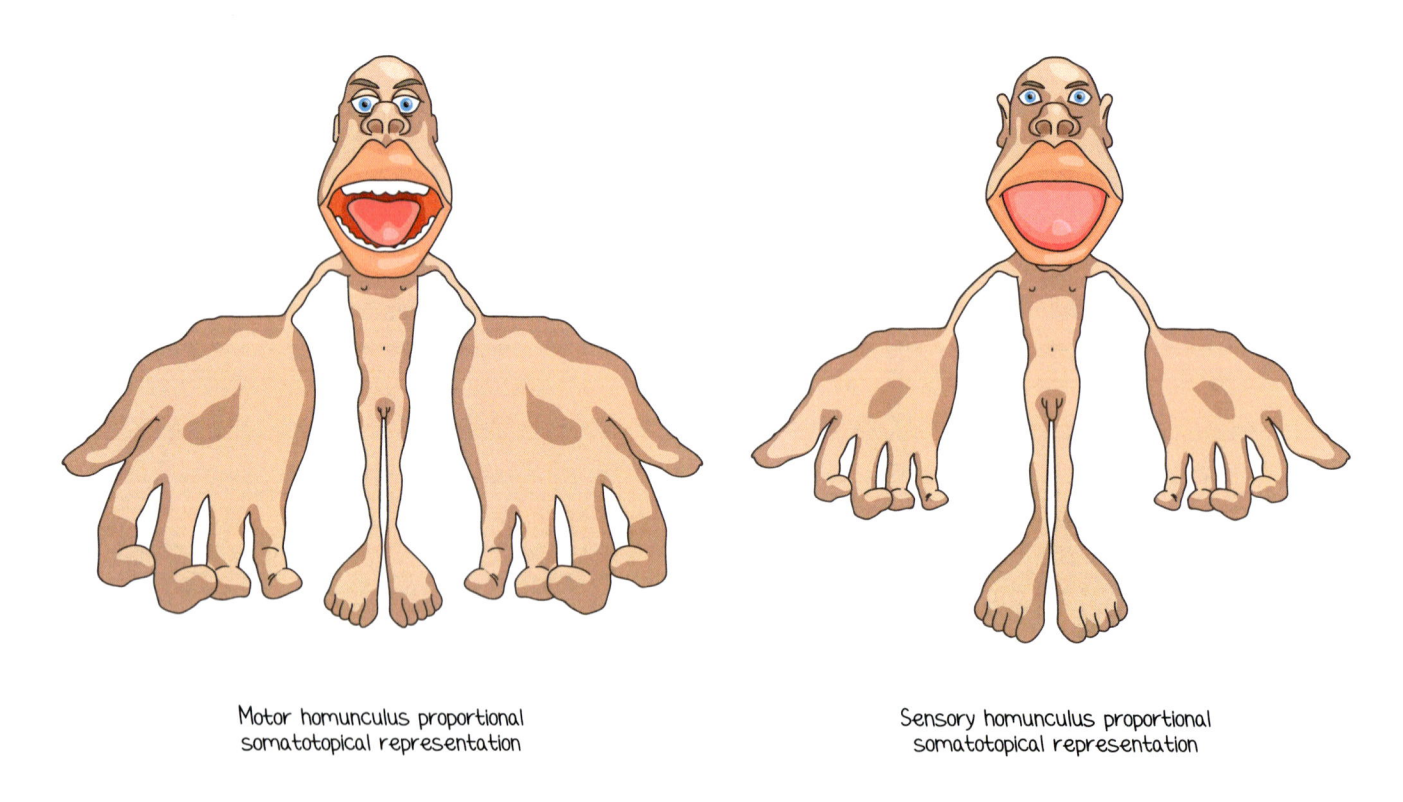

Sensory homunculus proportional somatotopical representation

Figure 10. Sensory and motor homunculi

Another noteworthy fact about somatosensation is that it's relative in some ways. For example, we tend to perceive temperatures as either warmer or cooler than the reference point of our skin, known as **physiological zero**, which usually ranges somewhere between 85°-90° Fahrenheit (29°-32°C)—that is, our skin is usually somewhat cooler than our core body temperature. Pain is also relative in the sense that some stimuli are more painful than others, to the point that an intensely painful stimulus can override a slightly painful stimulus, and in the sense that different people have different pain thresholds. These observations have been explained by the gate theory of pain, which suggests that the body can turn pain signals on or off in the spinal cord depending on the overall pattern of sensory input. This theory is not quite at the cutting edge of modern research—as you'll find out more about in med school, pain is the subject of a lot of intensive research right now—but it's still an influential idea that is worth being aware of for the MCAT.

Let's turn now to something more appealing than pain - that is, taste and smell. The receptors involved in both of these senses are chemoreceptors, although as we discussed previously, olfactory receptors respond to a huge range of different stimuli that are dissolved in the air, whereas gustatory, or taste, receptors, pick up on a smaller range of tastes based on substances dissolved in fluids. The input of these senses is also processed differently. Information about taste is processed first in the **taste center** of the thalamus, and then sent to the **gustatory cortex** elsewhere in the brain. Smells, on the other hand, are first processed in the **olfactory bulb**, which is located in the front of the brain, and are then passed along to the **olfactory tract**. From there, information on smells is processed by other parts of the brain, including the limbic system, which is involved in emotion. This helps explain why certain smells can be powerfully evocative of certain places, people, and times in our lives, even if we struggle to express that experience in words.

As a final note regarding our senses, the way that we've been talking about them in isolation is also a bit divorced from our lived experiences of the world: Real senses interact constantly. A simple example is how our perception of flavor reflects a combination of taste and smell. When we eat spicy food, we also add the sensation of pain to the mix - we might even enjoy that pain! If you take a second in the midst of your daily activities to stop and reflect on all the sensory input that you're processing in a given moment, it's actually astonishing! Sensation and perception are critical topics in psychology because they form the foundation for behavior, and while they may be very mechanically complex, keeping a high-level overview of these processes in mind should help you navigate their discussion on the MCAT.

9. Must-Knows

> Stimulus → transduction (stimulus converted to action potential) → sensation → perception
> Sensory receptors give information on location, type/modality, intensity, and duration of input.
> Types of receptors: photoreceptors (light); mechanoreceptors (sound, acceleration, touch); chemoreceptors (taste, smell); baroceptors (pressure); proprioceptors (body position); nociceptors (pain); osmoceptors (concentration)
> Absolute threshold: minimum signal to be detected (≠ threshold of conscious perception); just-noticeable difference (JND) = amount stimulus must change to be noticed
> Signal detection theory: ability to pick up true/false presence/absence of stimulus from environment
> Top-down vs. bottom-up processing: using expectations to structure perception vs. taking in info first
> Gestalt laws: principles describing how we integrate stimuli into consciously perceived shapes
> Visible light: EM waves with wavelengths between 380 nm and 740 nm (violet to red)
> Rods contain rhodopsin and are extremely sensitive to light, but do not detect color. They help us see in low light conditions, such as at night. Rods need to undergo dark adaptation when moving from light to dark.
> Cones: found in the macula and the fovea, near the center of the visual field and in the back of the eye. They are responsible for seeing color and seeing detail (acuity).
  – Three different types: short (blue, S), medium (green, M) and long (red, L)
> Cornea: a small, curved and translucent portion of epithelium that light must pass through to enter eye
> Lens: boundary between anterior and posterior chambers; changing its shape changes focus of light entering the eye (flattening = helps see farther-away objects, rounding = helps see nearer objects)
> Iris: structure in front of lens that controls amount of light entering (dilation = widening due to sympathetic NS stimulation or low light; constriction = narrowing due to parasympathetic stimulation or bright light).
> Retina: innermost layer; sclera: outermost layer (white color of eyes); choroid: vascular structure between retina and sclera
> Basic pathway of light: outside > cornea > anterior chamber > lens > posterior chamber > retina (sensing)
> Phototransduction starts in retina (rods and cones). Retina has three vertical layers: photoreceptors (rods/cones), bipolar cells (connect to ganglion cells), ganglion cells (comprise optic nerve); horizontal cells laterally connect photorecptors and bipolar cells, amacrine cells laterally connect bipolar and ganglion cells.
> Visual input: sent towards visual cortex by optic nerve; at optic chiasm, nasal sides of optic nerve cross over so that right visual field → right visual cortex and vice versa
  – After chiasm, optic pathway synapses at lateral geniculate nucleus (LGN; contains magnocellular neurons [motion] and parvocellular neurons [detail]), and sends input to visual cortex and superior colliculi
> Motion parallax: monocular depth clue based on relative motion of near vs. far objects
> Feature detection: ability to detect motion, color, shape, timing, and size
> Parallel processing: integrate simultaneous input; serial processing: sort incoming input to find specific info
> Sound waves (longitudinal) are detected by hair cells in ear.
  – Outer ear: catches sound waves w/ shape; middle ear: amplifies sound waves (malleus, incus, stapes); inner ear: turns vibrations into action potential via endolymph-bathed hair cells with stereocilia detectors
  – Organ of Corti: in inner ear; hosts endolymph-bathed hair cells on basilar membrane
> Left temporal lobe: speech; right temporal lobe: sounds and music
> Somatosensation: all sensation about and within the body
> Two-point threshold: minimum distance two simultaneously-stimulated points must be apart to be perceived as two points of stimulation, not one
  – Denser innervation in skin area (e.g. fingers) = smaller two-point threshold
> Physiological zero is the temperature we perceive as neither hot nor cold. It is approximately 85°-90° Fahrenheit (29°-32°C).
> Gate theory of pain: we can turn certain signals on or off depending on the overall pattern of sensory input.
> Taste: processed in the taste center of the thalamus, then sent to the gustatory cortex.
> Smells: first processed in the olfactory bulb, then passed along olfactory tract to limbic system and elsewhere.

End of Chapter Practice

The best MCAT practice is **realistic**, with a focus on identifying steps for further improvement. For those reasons, we recommend completing practice questions in an online setting that simulates the real MCAT interface, and taking advantage of advanced analytic features to help you determine how best to move forward in your MCAT study journey.

With that in mind, **online end-of-chapter questions** are accessible through your Next Step account.

As a further supplement, given the importance of active learning for effective studying, we also suggest that you consult the Must-Knows as a basis for creating a study sheet, in which you list out key terms and test your ability to briefly summarize them.

This page left intentionally blank.

CHAPTER 4

Consciousness

0. Introduction

We've discussed how sensory stimuli are perceived, but the awareness that we have of ourselves and of stimuli that surround us—that is, consciousness and attention—are important next steps in linking perceptions to eventual behavior.

1. Consciousness and Alertness

Consciousness is the awareness that we have of our surroundings, our internal states, and ourselves. Consciousness is often a topic for wide-ranging debates about things like whether robots could develop real awareness, whether zombies are conscious and so on—but for better or worse, we're not going to resolve those questions in an MCAT textbook. Instead, we'll just be looking at how these things are medically defined.

From a medical point of view, consciousness is important because it's not a steady-state phenomenon; humans aren't conscious all the time, and what's more, consciousness can vary in terms of degree and quality. As you may have experienced if you've worked as an EMT, in an emergency department or in elderly care, an evaluation of consciousness is an important early step in assessing a patient in several medical circumstances, such as during a hypoglycemic episode or head trauma. Medical issues that involve consciousness, such as sleep disorders and substance abuse disorder, are also common parts of everyday medical practice.

Let's start thinking about consciousness by taking our regular, everyday level of awareness as a baseline, and then think about how that awareness might increase or decrease. Increased awareness, where we're paying especially close attention to the various forms of sensory input that we're receiving, is known as **alertness**. The structure in the brain that is most closely associated with alertness is known as the **reticular formation**, and one of its subcomponents, the **reticular activating system**, plays an especially important role in this context. The reticular formation is part of the brainstem, but it's hard to specify its position in any more detail than that, because it's actually a complex network of neuron clusters that all contribute to the same broad goals. Alertness has received extensive attention from researchers because it has direct implications for high-stakes jobs. For instance, pilots, surgeons, and others must maintain high levels of alertness for extended periods of time, which can be quite challenging.

Just like our level of awareness can increase, it can also decrease. A mild example would be how we might start daydreaming and stop paying attention to our surroundings in a boring lecture. If the lecture is really boring, we might even become drowsy. We can also lose consciousness, and in fact, we do so every day when we fall asleep. However, as we'll see when we cover sleep in more depth below, there's more to sleep than just being a temporary and fairly easily-reversible loss of consciousness. Deeper **unconsciousness**, when a person cannot be easily roused, can also occur for various reasons, including trauma, loss of oxygen to the brain, and drug use -- including both drugs used for medical purposes, like in anesthesia, and excessive quantities of drugs used recreationally. An even deeper form of unconsciousness is a **coma**, which refers to someone who has lost consciousness, does not react normally to stimuli like light, sound, or pain, does not make any voluntary motions, and (to exclude heavy sleepers from this definition) is not in a normal sleep/wake cycle.

Now that we've established a basic framework for thinking about consciousness in terms of alertness and awareness, our next step is to fill in some of the details by exploring how the experience of consciousness itself can vary or be altered.

2. Sleep, Hypnosis, and Meditation

It's not something we often think about in these terms, but we lose consciousness every day when we sleep. Not only is sleep the form of altered consciousness that we most often experience, but it's also absolutely crucial to our ability to live, just as much as food. In fact, with proper hydration, it's possible to go for more than a month without food, but the official world record for staying awake is only 11 days straight, although some people have reported pushing it up to 19 days. Regardless, staying awake that long is an extremely bad idea and things start to get deeply weird—to the point of hallucinations—after a few sleepless days. World records aside, chronic low-level sleep deprivation is also associated with a range of bad outcomes, from poor cognitive performance to negative effects on virtually every system of the body, including increased risks of obesity, heart disease, and diabetes. So as hard as it can be, prioritize adequate sleep as you're studying for the MCAT, because being well-rested will help set you up for success both when studying and test-taking.

I. Stages of Sleep

Much of what we know about sleep comes from recording brain activity during sleep, through a technique called **electroencephalography**, or **EEG** for short. As we'll see shortly, there exist different stages of sleep, and each stage of sleep has a characteristic set of EEG waveforms. Of course, sleep doesn't only involve the brain—it's a whole-body activity—so similar techniques have been developed to measure muscle activity and eye activity. These techniques are known as **electromyography**, or **EMG**, and **electrooculography**, or **EOG**, and can be included in part of a comprehensive sleep study. Now, it wouldn't be science unless we had a fancy Latin-based term for a simple concept like "comprehensive sleep study", so a sleep study measuring multiple physiological parameters is called a **polysomnographic study**, which contains the Latin roots for Latin for "measuring ("graphy") many things ("poly") about sleep ("somno")".

MCAT STRATEGY > > >

A mnemnonic for sleep stages is: BATS Drink Blood: beta waves for being awake, alpha waves for drowsiness, theta waves for stage 1 sleep, spindles and K-complexes for stage 2 sleep, delta waves for stage 3 sleep, and then back to beta waves!

When a person is fully awake, an EEG will pick up **beta waves**, which have a high frequency and a low amplitude, and are not very rhythmic. Once we start getting fatigued, less alert, and especially when we close our eyes and rest—without falling asleep, though—our brain starts showing **alpha waves**, which have a lower frequency. Keep these in mind for now, since the brain will show very different wave patterns as we enter the sleep cycle.

CHAPTER 4: CONSCIOUSNESS

The highest-level division of sleep is between **rapid eye movement (REM) sleep**, and **non-REM sleep**. As the name implies, REM sleep is characterized by quick bursts of eye movement, and it's also sometimes called paradoxical sleep, because EEG shows brain waves similar to those observed when a person is awake, but muscle movement is very low, almost to the point of being paralyzed. REM sleep is also unique because various other physiological changes take place, including a loosening of the otherwise tight regulation of homeostasis, leading to irregularities in respiration and heart rate. Furthermore, the majority of dreaming happens during REM sleep. REM sleep is interspersed throughout the sleep cycle, and stages of REM sleep become longer as the night progresses. REM sleep is also very necessary, as suggested by a phenomenon known as REM rebound. This term describes how if we miss REM sleep on one night, the next night we'll spend more time in REM sleep to catch up.

As important as REM sleep is, however, when we first drift off to sleep, we enter non-REM sleep. More specifically, we enter **stage 1** of non-REM sleep, which is characterized by **theta waves**, which have an even lower frequency than alpha waves and tend to have low amplitudes, although they're somewhat irregular. Slow eye movement occurs in stage 1 sleep, and overall, stage 1 sleep is quite light. As we move into deeper sleep, we enter **stage 2**, in which eye motion stops and heart rate and breathing rate slow down. In stage 2 sleep, we continue to see theta waves, as well as bursts of activity called K-complexes and sleep spindles. K-complexes are periodic high-amplitude bursts, and sleep spindles are occasional high-frequency bursts of activity that are thought to play a role in memory consolidation.

Next, we move into **stage 3**, which is **deep sleep**. Just as a note, this stage was previously subdivided into stages 3 and 4, but they were combined together in 2008. It's also known as slow-wave sleep, and the slow, or low-frequency, waves in question are referred to as **delta waves**. Delta waves are notable because they're fairly high-amplitude. Stage 3 sleep is thought to be important for memory processing, as well as being a stage of sleep where the brain, crudely speaking, recovers from its daily activities.

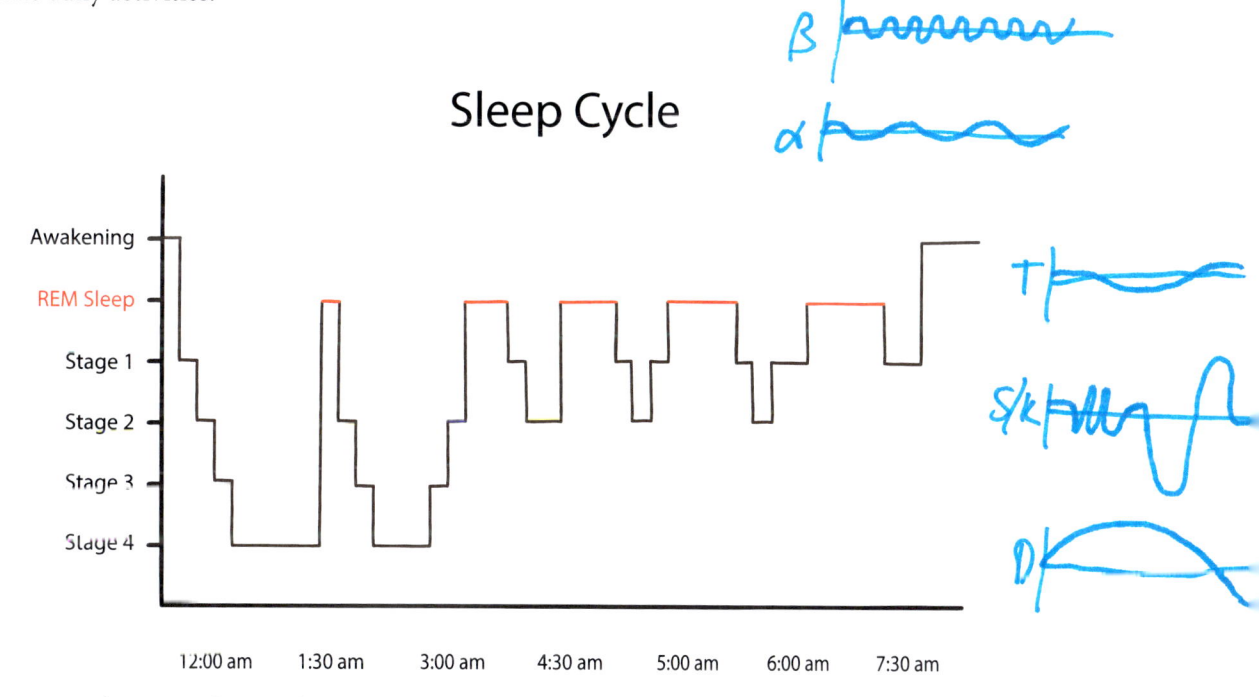

Figure 1. Hypnogram depicting sleep cycles

As we sleep, we successively move from stage 1 sleep through the various stages of non-REM sleep, then pop back up to REM sleep again, after which we repeat the process. Deep, slow-wave sleep tends to predominate towards the beginning of a night's sleep, while more time is spent in lighter REM sleep as the night progresses. In adults, each **sleep cycle** is about 90 minutes, although it is shorter in children, more along the lines of 50 minutes.

The body uses various signaling molecules to regulate our sleep-wake cycles, and if you've ever experienced jetlag, you know how disorienting it can be for that system to be disrupted. Our 24-hour sleep-wake cycle is known as our **circadian rhythm**, and it is mostly governed by **melatonin**, a hormone generated from the pineal gland that promotes drowsiness, and **cortisol**, which is best known for modulating the chronic stress response, but also contributes to wakefulness. You may have noticed that it can be difficult to fall asleep when you are stressed: Now you know why! Of course, not everybody sleeps at night. Hospitals, for instance, are staffed 24 hours a day. However, an increasing amount of research suggests that consistent night work may be linked to an increased risk of cardiovascular disease and cancer.

II. Sleep Disorders

As future doctors, whenever you learn about some sort of system that the body has, a natural follow-up question is to ask "How can it go wrong?". And indeed, there are several different sleep-wake disorders. For example, **insomnia**, the most common sleep disorder, makes it difficult to fall asleep. On the opposite end is **narcolepsy**, which involves excessive daytime sleepiness as well as abnormal REM sleep, cataplexy, or sudden loss of muscle control, sleep paralysis, and hypnagogic hallucinations, which are hallucinations that occur while going to sleep. Another disorder, **sleep apnea**, occurs when a person is unable to breathe while sleeping, either due to a physical obstruction or problems with neural signaling. Obese individuals are at an elevated risk for obstructive sleep apnea, which can cause significant health problems. Disorders like these, which interfere with whether or not sleep takes place, are collectively known as **dyssomnias**.

MCAT STRATEGY > > >

An important theme that emerges throughout this discussion is that consciousness—and as we'll see elsewhere in this chapter, attention—is not an all-or-nothing phenomenon. Therefore, be on the lookout for how passages and questions may test variations in consciousness!

Parasomnias are another category of sleep disorders that involve abnormal behavior during sleep. **Sleepwalking**, technically known as **somnambulism**, is a common example. During sleepwalking, a person can walk, talk, and engage in other activities while being fully asleep and not remember it the next day. Night terrors are another relatively common parasomnia, in which a sleeper is suddenly plunged into the fight-or-flight response. This often involves the sleeper sitting up and screaming. Such episodes only last for about 30 seconds to 3 minutes, and then the sleeper goes back to sleep and usually doesn't remember it the next day. **Nightmares** can also be considered parasomnias, since they occur during sleep.

III. Dreams, Hypnosis, and Meditation

That brings us to our final point about sleep -- what about the content of dreams? Especially for those of us who remember our dreams vividly, they can be highly-memorable and emotionally-significant experiences. **Dreams** are also often unrealistic, and even fantastic. So why do we dream, and what do our dreams mean? Not surprisingly for such a huge question, several ideas have been proposed. The famous early 20th-century psychiatrist, Sigmund Freud, who we'll be learning about elsewhere in this book, proposed dividing dreams into **manifest content** and **latent content**. The idea here is that manifest content refers to the surface-level plotline and details of a dream, while the latent content is the hidden meaning. An MCAT-relevant example is the fairly common experience that people have of dreaming that they show up to a final exam for a course, only to realize that they had never even taken the course, never mind studied for the test. That plotline would be the manifest content, and the latent content might be an underlying anxiety about tests, schooling, and professional success. Freud also identified the concept of wish fulfillment, which states that dreams provide a way to resolve a **repressed conflict** by allowing a person to visualize the satisfaction of a desire.

Modern theoretical approaches to dreaming include the more sober **activation-synthesis model**, which states that the activation of neurons in REM sleep results in a synthesis of that experiential input through dreaming; the problem-solving theory, which views dreams as a way that the brain unconsciously processes and works through problems encountered in one's day-to-day life; and the cognitive theory, which suggests that dreams reflect cognitive structures that play a role in our everyday lives, such as conceptions of self, others, and the world.

If you've been reading carefully, you might have observed that these theories aren't really mutually exclusive, because it could very well be true both that dreams are ways of unconsciously resolving problems and that they reflect important cognitive structures. Furthermore, none of these theories really refer to the underlying neurobiology of what's happening in the brain during dreaming. For a variety of reasons, that's a difficult research question to investigate, but scientists are continuing to chip away at this problem and to build more holistic and integrated frames for understanding dreaming on both neural and cognitive levels.

In addition to sleep, there are two other non-pharmacological forms of altered consciousness to be aware of: **hypnosis** and **meditation**. Hypnosis is a controversial subject, but at its core, it involves a practitioner, or hypnotist, inducing a hyper-suggestible state in a subject. In such a state, a subject may respond normally to most stimuli, but is extremely responsive to certain suggestions, with effects that may persist even after the hypnosis session. There is considerable skepticism as to whether hypnosis even exists as a well-definable state, beyond the parameters of ordinary suggestibility and motivation. That said, hypnotherapy is still practiced today.

Meditation, in contrast, has been a part of several religious traditions for millennia. Meditation is difficult to define precisely because there are many schools of practice, but a common theme is quieting one's mind to focus one's attention more deliberately. Meditation has been shown to alter brain wave patterns by promoting more alpha and theta waves, normally characteristic of drowsiness and sleep, and fMRI studies have shown that various specific brain areas are activated during meditation. In recent years, meditation has also been increasingly incorporated into non-religious approaches to counseling and wellness.

To summarize, there's a lot more to sleep than what meets the eye, to the point that sleep medicine is a subspeciality in its own right. Being aware of the basic architecture of sleep, in terms of its stages, the brain waves that appear in them, and the basic theories of dreaming, helps build a foundation for working with patients affected by sleep disorders. Furthermore, as a form of altered consciousness, sleep shares some parallels with other altered states like hypnosis and meditation.

3. Consciousness-Altering Drugs

Altering our consciousness through drugs is, for better or worse, a very common aspect of the human experience, as exemplified by the most common psychoactive drug in America: caffeine, found in coffee, tea, soda, energy drinks, and chocolate. In this section, we'll briefly review the numerous consciousness-altering drugs that the MCAT expects you to be aware of.

Since we already mentioned caffeine, let's start there. **Caffeine** is a member of a class of drugs broadly known as **stimulants**, which, as the name implies, increase activity in the central nervous system, have an energizing or invigorating effect, or mimic the effects of the sympathetic nervous system, simulating a fight-or-flight response.

Caffeine is a fairly mild central nervous system stimulant that primarily works by blocking receptors for adenosine, a compound in the brain that promotes drowsiness. Close to 85-90% of Americans consume at least some caffeine on a regular basis.

Partially for that reason, caffeine is a useful example of the distinction between **addiction** and **dependence**. Addiction is generally defined as a pattern of compulsive behavior that persists despite negative consequences. More specifically, it also involves repeatedly engaging in some sort of process that triggers the brain's reward pathway. So in this sense, at least in terms of negative consequences, caffeine has a very low potential for addiction. However, heavy daily caffeine users—like everyone involved in the writing and editing of this book—can develop dependence, which means that mild withdrawal symptoms, including headaches, drowsiness, and difficulty focusing, can develop upon discontinuing caffeine. This might sound confusing: how can someone be physically dependent, but not addicted? The idea is that even people who are dependent on caffeine don't show patterns of compulsive, reward pathway-driven caffeine use that persists despite negative consequences. Caffeine is also a great example of the phenomenon of **tolerance**, in which heavy users get accustomed to the effects of a drug, and need higher doses to get the same effect. **Nicotine** is another stimulant with relatively moderate consciousness-altering effects. Nicotine is most commonly consumed through cigarettes, which also contain many other harmful compounds, but it can also be administered through gum, patches, and in vapor cartridges, all of which have been used as ways to help people quit smoking. In contrast to caffeine, nicotine is highly addictive. It's unfortunately quite common for people to keep smoking even when they have been diagnosed with serious diseases caused by smoking. Currently, about 15% of adults in the United States smoke. This percentage used to be much higher—in the mid-1950s, about half of adult men were active smokers—and has been driven down through extensive public health initiatives focused on the close connection of smoking with dozens of health problems, including lung cancer, cardiovascular disease, and respiratory diseases.

Amphetamines are another important class of stimulants that are derived from amphetamine. For example, methamphetamine is formed by adding a methyl group to the amine in amphetamine. Amphetamines tend to increase energy and alertness, promote concentration and focus, and reduce appetite. However, they also have negative effects; for instance, chronic methamphetamine use can cause intense mood swings, hallucinations, and even psychosis. However, the specific effects of amphetamines, both positive and negative, vary across members of this class as well as the individual physiology of the user. In addition to recreational use and abuse, amphetamines are often prescribed as medications. For example, one of the trade names for amphetamine is Adderall, which may be familiar to you as a commonly-prescribed medication for attention deficit hyperactivity disorder, or ADHD. Thus, when it's prescribed to someone with ADHD, and taken to alleviate the symptoms of that condition, amphetamine is considered a therapeutic drug. But if someone without ADHD takes it either for fun or for a possible performance boost, it's considered a recreational drug, or drug of abuse.

MDMA, also known as **ecstasy** or **molly**, is another well-known member of the class of amphetamines. MDMA promotes a powerful sense of empathy and pleasure, along with the typical amphetamine-related effects of increased energy, focus, and appetite reduction. MDMA is mostly used recreationally, and there are no disorders for which it is prescribed, but several research groups in psychology have investigated whether MDMA can be incorporated into therapy. MDMA promotes the release of serotonin, norepinephrine, and dopamine; by doing so, it depletes the brain of its serotonin reserves, causing users to experience depression after use.

Finally, **cocaine** is a strong stimulant that works by blocking the reuptake of serotonin, dopamine, and norepinephrine. The vast majority of cocaine use is recreational and illicit, although it does have some limited medical uses as a local numbing agent for nose and mouth procedures. It is derived from the coca plant, which has for millennia been used traditionally in the Andes mountains of South America. As a powder, cocaine is generally snorted—or, technically, insufflated—although it can also be dissolved and injected. Processing cocaine with sodium bicarbonate and water results in a more readily smokable, rapid-onset form commonly known as crack.

CHAPTER 4: CONSCIOUSNESS

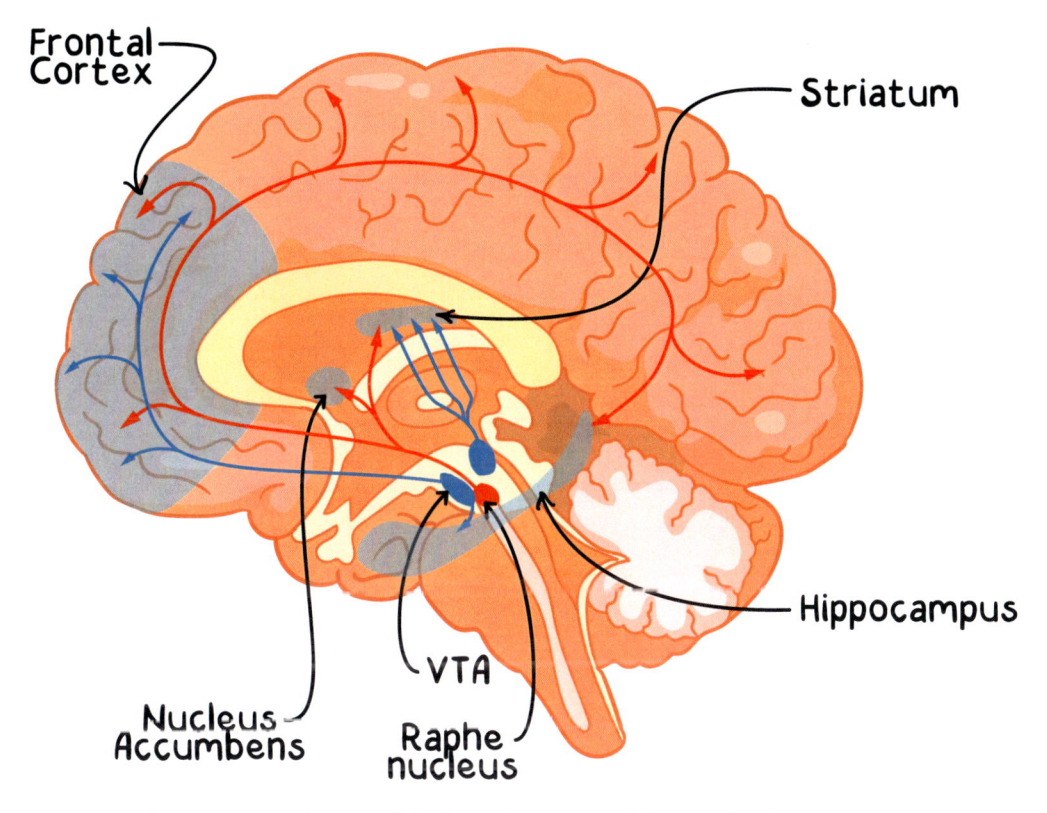

Figure 2. Dopamine and serotonin pathways of the brain (one part of the mesolimbic pathway, the medial forebrain bundle, is not pictured, but is between the nucleus accumbens and the VTA).

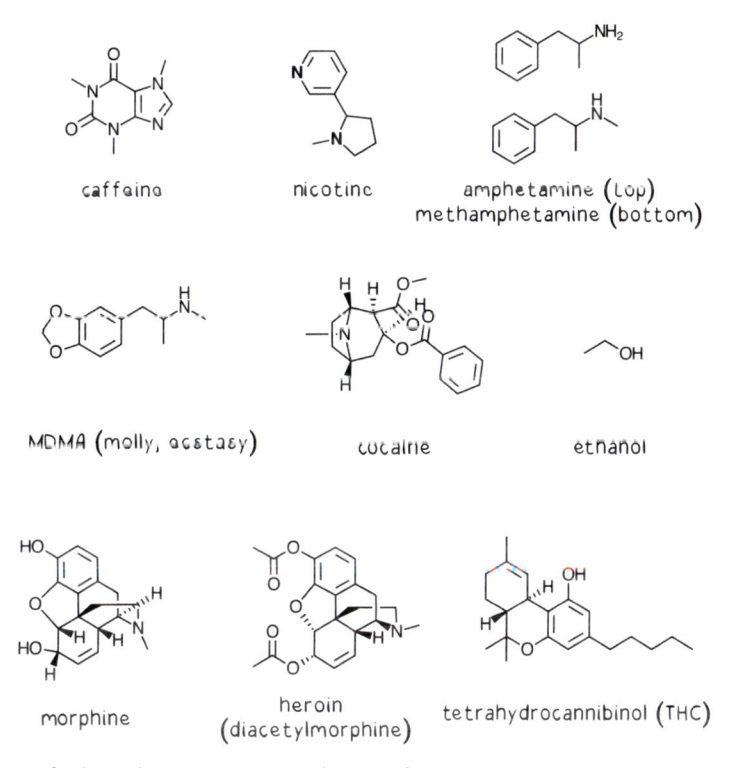

Figure 3. Chemical structures of selected consciousness-altering drugs

73

Well, what goes up must come down, so after stimulants, we need to move on to **depressants**, which work by reducing activity in the central nervous system. This has both psychological and physiological effects, because after all, many physiological processes depend on neural signaling for coordination. So we'd expect stimulants to raise your heart rate, and depressants to lower it. The same pattern holds for processes like the respiratory rate and blood pressure.

Alcohol, or more technically, **ethanol**, is a depressant found in beer, wine, and spirits. Its primary mode of action is enhancing the action of **GABA receptors**. Recall that GABA is the main inhibitory neurotransmitter in our brains. Therefore, ethanol basically makes the brain act as if it's receiving more GABA input than it actually is. That is, it makes neurons fire less often, slowing the brain down. Now this might come as a surprise if you've ever dealt with drunk people who get excited. But the idea here is that relatively low doses of alcohol dial down a drinker's conscious inhibitions and planning ability, as mediated through the frontal lobe, but higher doses more directly affect speech, motor function, cognition, memory, and so on. Regarding memory in particular, high doses of alcohol can cause anterograde amnesia, or blackouts, by interfering with the consolidation of short-term memory into long-term memory. Extremely high doses of alcohol can repress respiratory control to the point that an individual stops breathing, potentially resulting in death.

As that last point implies, alcohol is dangerous. In any given year in the US, on the order of 80,000 to 90,000 alcohol-attributable deaths occur. This includes deaths from acute alcohol intoxication and deaths caused by injuries and risky behavior under the influence of alcohol, but also deaths due to chronic conditions that alcohol either causes or contributes to, like liver disease. Long-term alcohol use also elevates the risk of many cancers and of cardiovascular disease. **Korsakoff syndrome** is a psychiatric condition associated with chronic alcoholism that involves amnesia—both anterograde, or for events starting after the syndrome develops, and retrograde, or for events before the onset of the condition—and a tendency for confabulation, or invented memories. More specifically, Korsakoff syndrome is associated with a lack of vitamin B1, or thiamine, which can be depleted in heavy drinkers, especially in those who also do not have an adequate nutritional intake.

A final important fact about alcohol is that for people who are physically dependent on alcohol, suddenly discontinuing drinking can lead to very unpleasant, and even fatal, withdrawal symptoms that include hallucinations, excruciating anxiety, and seizures. This tendency for withdrawal to be dangerous is shared by other depressants that increase GABA receptor activity. **Benzodiazepines** and **barbiturates** are two such classes of depressants. Barbiturates were developed first, and were used for a while to treat anxiety and insomnia, but are super-risky in terms of overdose risk, propensity for addiction, and the danger of withdrawal. Benzodiazepines are used for similar purposes, and, interestingly, to treat ethanol dependence, but still have some dangers, including a high risk of addiction. Barbiturates and benzodiazepines should not be combined with alcohol, as doing so greatly increases the risk of an overdose.

Next, let's discuss **opioids**, which are derived from and named for the opium poppy. Opioids cause sedation, sleepiness, and respiratory depression, as well as pain relief and euphoria. They exert their effects by binding opioid receptors on neurons. **Morphine** is a naturally occurring opioid, while **heroin** is a more potent, and highly addictive, version of morphine that was developed by pharmaceutical researchers in the late 19th century. Its name comes from the idea that it might make you feel like a hero. It was initially marketed as a non-addictive substitute for morphine in cough syrup. Both morphine and heroin are however highly addictive, as are the majority of opioids. Since then, many different opioids have been developed, with varying levels of potency, length of effect, and so on. Some relatively well-known examples include codeine, hydrocodone, oxycodone, and fentanyl.

Now, you might wonder about what it means that we have opioid receptors in our neurons; why would they have developed in the first place? The answer is that our body produces compounds that interact with those receptors. The most commonly known are **endorphins**, which block pain and can induce feelings of euphoria. Endorphins in particular are also released after intense exercise and are commonly associated with the so-called runner's high. As such, opioids such as morphine and heroin can be thought of as extremely potent endorphin agonists.

Next, **hallucinogens** distort perceptions, enhance sensory experiences, and promote introspection. Their physiological effects usually mimic sympathetic nervous system activation. **LSD** is probably the most famous hallucinogen, while other examples include ketamine, peyote, psilocybin, which is present in hallucinogenic mushrooms, and PCP. Their mechanisms are complex and go beyond our scope.

Finally, **marijuana** is a drug derived from the plant species *Cannabis sativa* and *Cannabis indica*. A major psychoactive constituent of marijuana is **tetrahydrocannabinol**, usually abbreviated as **THC**. However, THC is just one of over a hundred cannabinoids in marijuana. These compounds bind with cannabinoid receptors in the brain. Just as we saw with opioids, the presence of cannabinoid receptors implies that we may have some kind of related internal system. And we do, in fact—compounds produced by the body known as endocannabinoids are involved in a wide range of processes that include appetite, mood, and pain sensation. Some non-psychoactive cannabinoids in marijuana, such as cannabidiol or CBD, have received attention due to possible therapeutic effects on pain and seizure activity. The legal status of marijuana has been changing rapidly in recent decades, and it continues to be a focus of intense research. The effects of marijuana include stimulant, depressant, and hallucinogenic properties, so it doesn't really fit into the classification we presented above.

As we've mentioned, addiction is defined as compulsive behavior that triggers the **reward pathway** and is repeated pathologically despite negative consequences. What we've called the reward pathway is more technically known as the **mesolimbic pathway**, which is made up of a set of structures containing dopaminergic neurons. It consists of the nucleus accumbens, the ventral tegmental area, the olfactory tubule, and the medial forebrain bundle. It is powerfully associated with motivation and reinforcement learning, and any activity that produces psychological dependence—including drug use and gambling—activates this pathway. Other brain structures involved in emotion, like the **amygdala**, may also contribute to addiction. Addiction is associated with intense cravings for the high given by a drug or other addictive activity. Furthermore, it is thought that the concepts of positive and negative reinforcement might be helpful for understanding addiction.

> **MCAT STRATEGY > > >**
>
> Dependence, tolerance, habituation, and addiction are classic examples of a situation where we use words interchangeably in everyday life, but need to make a careful distinction in the Psych/Soc section of the MCAT.

Likewise, **tolerance** refers to the phenomenon of a user needing an increasing dose of a substance to get the same effect. If someone requires a drug to function normally, they are said to be **habituated** to that drug and **dependent** on it. As we discussed with caffeine, dependence is not quite the same as addiction, because it may be a more stable state, without the compulsivity associated with addiction. When someone who is dependent on a drug discontinues it, they may undergo withdrawal. Although withdrawal can be deadly for ethanol and other depressants that modulate GABA signaling, for other drugs, withdrawal is generally safe (in the sense that it won't kill you), but can range from being mildly unpleasant for a drug like caffeine to miserable or even unbearable for opiates. Withdrawal is often accompanied by especially intense cravings for a drug.

4. Attention

If you reflect on all the years you've spent in school, you may notice that attention is one of the major themes that comes up in the classroom: on the one hand, teachers might tell students to pay attention, and in particular to put away their phones, but on the other hand, students might complain about how hard it is to pay attention in a certain set of lectures.

Attention sits right at the intersection of several other major psychology topics, serving as a crucial link between perception and higher-level cognitive processes involving learning and memory. Now, we all probably know what attention is, if for no other reason than how often we get told in our early lives that we need to pay more attention to things, but let's be accurate and stipulate that attention is the ability to direct our awareness to a single aspect of stimuli from the external environment.

I. Selective Attention

It follows from the above definition of attention that paying attention to something means not paying attention to other things. For that reason, attention is often viewed as a spotlight; imagine your mind's focus zooming around from here to there, picking out various things you need to notice or want to think about. This idea is rooted in the work of **William James**, a pioneer of psychology who worked in the late 19th century and described attention as having a **focus**, a **fringe** area we aren't paying attention to, and a **margin**, which lies in between the focus and the fringe. This isn't technically a theory, since it's not specific and testable, but it's a nice metaphor for us to use as a jumping-off point.

Paying attention to something means being able to think about it, remember it, learn it, and so on—but what about those things we're not paying attention to? Figuring this out is at the core of understanding **selective attention**. Scientists have tried to answer two major, closely related questions about selective attention: How does it work, and what happens to the information we're not paying attention to?

One of the first psychologists to focus on selective attention was Donald Broadbent, who conceptualized the mind as working like a filter. The **Broadbent model of selective attention** posits that the dozens of input streams of sensory information undergo basic processing for things like color, shape, and so on, and then enter a **sensory buffer**. From that sensory buffer, the mind picks something to focus on, process, and assign meaning to, and then the rest of the information in the buffer decays.

This sounds reasonable enough, and some experimental evidence supports it. In particular, this model was tested using the dichotic listening task, in which experimental subjects are given headphones and are told to focus on audio input coming into one ear, but not another. If listeners are then asked to recall information about what they heard, they tend to only remember the information that came into the ear they were told to pay attention to, but not vice versa. This experimental setup can also be applied to a task known as **shadowing**, in which subjects are asked to repeat words as soon as they hear them. This tests attention a bit more directly, whereas asking subjects to recall information shifts the focus towards memory. In any case, it's pretty clear that we process the information stream that we're focusing on much more than the one we're not focusing on.

However, the question of what happens to unattended input isn't quite as simple as the Broadbent model would suggest. In particular, it seems fairly clear that we must be processing unattended input on some level. An intuitive example of this is what's known as the **cocktail party effect**, which describes how if you're in a room with a lot of different groups talking, like at a party, you can be focused on the conversation you're having with your group of friends, but if someone across the room mentions you by name, you'll immediately notice. So on some level, we must be processing input that we're not directly paying attention to, so that we can immediately notice if something important happens, like someone talking about us. We might also use that ability to react in an emergency situation, such as if someone in the background collapses.

To account for the cocktail party effect, a psychologist named **Anne Treisman** proposed a modification of the Broadbent model according to which, instead of passing through an all-or-nothing buffer, unattended-to information is attenuated, or reduced in intensity. After attenuation, particularly intense or important information might come to our attention. An advantage of the attenuation theory is that the degree to which input is attenuated can depend on various factors, including context and coherence. So if we're primed to be on the lookout for our names in a social setting, either through an experimental setup or a deep sense of insecurity, audio input containing our name is more likely to make it through the buffer. Strong evidence exists that we process unattended-to input at least to some extent, while not fully interpreting it. As such, **Treisman's attenuation model** has proven to be quite influential in research on memory.

That said, when we're working on a focused task, we can definitely miss things happening in the background. This is known as **inattentional blindness**, which was brought to researchers' attention by the fantastically named invisible gorilla experiment. In this experiment, subjects were shown a video of people passing a basketball around and asked to analyze it, by counting either the number of passes or the different types of passes made by each team. In the meantime, a woman walks straight through the scene, either carrying an umbrella or dressed up in a full-body gorilla suit. After the study participants finish watching the video, they were asked whether they saw anything unusual. About half of the people who watched the video with the woman in the gorilla suit didn't notice anything out of the ordinary. This wasn't a fluke; inattentional blindness has been robustly replicated. In fact, it's what magicians rely on to perform their tricks.

The related concept of **change blindness** refers to failure to notice changes that take place between two stimuli. A classic everyday example is when someone fails to notice your new haircut, or that you've changed into a different-color shirt, or something like that. Change blindness is related to inattentional blindness, in that our expectations and level of focus clearly play a role in whether we notice differences between two stimuli, but it's a more specific phenomenon.

Unattended stimuli might also affect us in interesting ways. For example, we rarely pay specific attention to the color of the rooms that we're in, or other aspects of the interior decor and architecture, but the sum total of those factors can affect our mood, and maybe even our behavior, although research is very much still out on the degree to which blue, for instance, is actually a calming color in any measurable sense. Along similar lines, urban planners have often wondered about the degree to which our behavior and mood are shaped by aspects of our environment that we may not consciously notice.

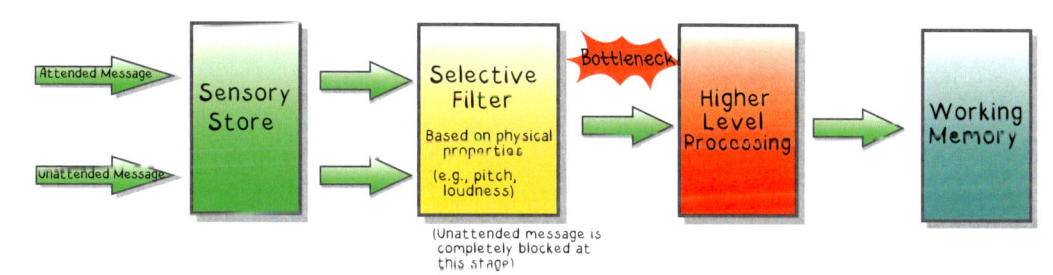

Figure 4. Broadbent's filter model.

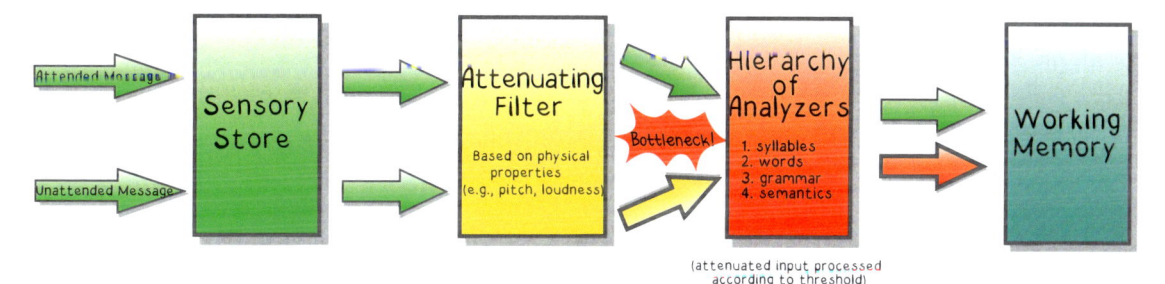

Figure 5. Treisman's attenuation model.

II. Divided Attention

For a variety of reasons, **multitasking** is a common temptation; being able to reliably do multiple things at the same time would certainly be a huge productivity boost, and would also help alleviate tedious or otherwise unpleasant obligations. However, even anecdotal experience suffices to confirm that beyond a certain point, trying to multitask can be counterproductive. As such, psychologists have invested considerable efforts into figuring out to what extent we can multitask and what actually happens in our brain when we do.

One basic question has to do with whether or not we can actually pay attention to multiple things at the same time, or whether what we think of as multitasking is actually just rapidly switching back and forth between tasks. These possibilities are referred to as **simultaneous attention** and **sequential attention**, respectively. While it would be going too far to say that simultaneous attention is a myth, compelling evidence suggests that multitasking generally involves sequential attention, or switching back and forth between tasks. This might even be true in circumstances where we consciously perceive ourselves as genuinely engaging in simultaneous attention, because of how quickly we can switch back and forth. As an analogy, when we watch an animation, we consciously process visual input too slowly to be able to see the individual still images.

The evidence is fairly clear that multitasking—regardless of whether it involves simultaneous attention or rapid shifts of sequential attention—degrades one's ability to perform cognitively complex tasks in comparison to doing those tasks in isolation. This should be fairly intuitive: Try playing chess while having a thoughtful conversation with a friend. Odds are decent you'll play a bad game of chess and be a bad conversationalist. It's as if we have a finite amount of attention that we can allocate among various tasks, and the more demanding one of those tasks becomes, the less attention we can pay to the others. This insight was formalized by a psychologist named **Daniel Kahneman**, who proposed a model of attention in which we have a certain capacity for attention that we allocate among tasks, with the attention required for each task depending on our expertise, the difficulty of the task, our level of psychological arousal, and so on.

Based on some interesting experimental findings, in which experienced piano players were able to shadow speech while reading and playing sheet music, **Allport's module resource theory** posits that instead of a central structure in the brain that allocates attention among all competing demands, we have distinct, specialized modules. This means that we can multitask reasonably well as long as the tasks draw from different modules, but will run into trouble if we try to do two similar tasks at the same time.

In this context, it's helpful to make a distinction between **controlled processing**, which takes place when we consciously focus on exactly how to carry out a task, and **automatic processing**, which takes place when we can more or less do something on autopilot. For example, if you've ever learned to play a musical instrument, the first steps of learning require exhaustive, careful attention to be able to produce even the most basic sounds, but after you become skillful enough, you can play familiar pieces of music without breaking stride. In fact, you may even be able to sustain a conversation with someone while you do so. Learning a foreign language and driving are other common examples of skills that start off with controlled processing and then proceed to automatic processing. In general, automatic processing places fewer demands upon our attention, facilitating multitasking. Nonetheless, mistakes are possible in both processing modes, so don't assume that one is inherently better than the other.

The most common attention-related psychological disorder is **attention-deficit/hyperactivity disorder**, or **ADHD**. ADHD has three subtypes: a predominantly inattentive type, a predominantly hyperactive-impulsive type, and a combined type. The symptoms associated with the predominantly inattentive type relate to difficulties in sustaining attention. These symptoms include not paying close attention to details, having trouble sustaining attention on tasks, and being easily distracted. These key symptoms exemplify the degree to which theories about attention in general, and divided attention in particular, give us a toolkit with which to think about the impact of ADHD.

5. Must-Knows

- Consciousness is awareness of our surroundings and ourselves and can be split into at least 4 broad states: alertness, daydreaming, drowsiness and sleep.
- Sleep stages: alertness (beta waves), drowsiness (alpha waves), stage 1 (theta waves, light sleep), stage 2 (theta waves, sleep spindles and K-complexes, memory consolidation), stage 3 (delta waves, deep sleep/slow-wave sleep, memory processing), REM sleep (rapid eye movement, dreaming, irregular respiration and heart rate)
- Sleep cycles repeat throughout night; about 90 min in adults
- The body's 24-hour clock is called the circadian rhythm and is regulated by melatonin and cortisol.
- Sleep-wake disorders are called dyssomnias and include insomnia, narcolepsy, cataplexy, sleep paralysis, hypnagogic hallucinations and sleep apnea.
- Sleep disorders (disorders that occur during sleep only) are called parasomnias and include sleepwalking (somnambulism), night terrors, and even nightmares.
- Theories about the content of dreams: Freud's idea of manifest and latent content of dreams and wish fulfillment; the activation-synthesis model; problem-solving theory; cognitive theory
- Addiction: a pattern of compulsive behavior despite negative consequences; dependence: the onset of withdrawal symptoms on cessation; habituation: requiring larger doses to experience an effect
  – The mesolimbic pathway is the reward pathway often active in addiction. It consists of the nucleus accumbens, ventral tegmental area, olfactory tubule and medial forebrain bundle.
- Stimulants increase CNS activity and include caffeine, nicotine, amphetamines, cocaine and MDMA
  – Amphetamines increase energy and reduce appetite; MDMA increases energy and empathy and works by stimulating the release of serotonin, dopamine and epinephrine.
  – Cocaine works by blocking the reuptake of serotonin, dopamine and norepinephrine.
- Depressants decrease CNS activity and include alcohol, benzodiazepines and barbiturates
  – Alcohol is a major health problem in many countries, including the US.
  – Benzodiazepines and barbiturates are both most commonly used to treat anxiety, and are very dangerous in combination with alcohol.
  – Korsakoff syndrome is most frequently caused by chronic alcohol use. Its symptoms include memory loss, confusion and confabulation.
- Opioids are a group defined as opioid-receptor agonists and include morphine, heroin, codeine, hydrocodone, oxycodone, and fentanyl; are effective for pain relief but tend to be highly addictive and also constitute a major health crisis in the US.
- Hallucinogens distort perceptions and enhance sensory experiences and this group includes LSD, ketamine, psilocybin and PCP.
- Marijuana is usually not put into strictly any one category. It acts on endocannabinoid receptors and has a wide range of effects and medical uses.
- Selective attention: ability to pay attention to just a few things in our environment and pay less or no attention to others
- Broadbent filter model: unimportant and background information is filtered out of the sensory buffer and lost
- Treismann attenutation model: unimportant and background information is attenuated, but if something important happens we can notice. Explains cocktail party effect.
- Inattentional blindness: we miss things if we're focusing elsewhere; gorilla party experiment.
- Change blindness: we miss things that have gradually or subtly changed in our environment.
- Multitasking may happen sequentially or in parallel; often impairs performance in both tasks.
- Simultaneous attention: processing two tasks at the same time to multitask.
- Sequential attention refers to switching between tasks rapidly to multitask.
- Allport's module resource theory: Attention isn't regulated by a single center, but divided among modules in the brain according to task. Multitasking using different modules works well, but using similar ones does not.
- Attention-deficit/hyperactivity disorder: inattentive type, hyperactive impulsive type and combined type

End of Chapter Practice

The best MCAT practice is **realistic**, with a focus on identifying steps for further improvement. For those reasons, we recommend completing practice questions in an online setting that simulates the real MCAT interface, and taking advantage of advanced analytic features to help you determine how best to move forward in your MCAT study journey.

With that in mind, **online end-of-chapter questions** are accessible through your Next Step account.

As a further supplement, given the importance of active learning for effective studying, we also suggest that you consult the Must-Knows as a basis for creating a study sheet, in which you list out key terms and test your ability to briefly summarize them.

CHAPTER 4: CONSCIOUSNESS

This page left intentionally blank.

This page left intentionally blank.

Cognition and Language

CHAPTER 5

0. Introduction

Cognition is a very broad topic, and in this section we're going to approach it from multiple angles. To organize our thinking on the topic, though, it's helpful to have an overarching model in mind for what the mind does, broadly speaking, abstracting away from concrete details like the organization of brain tissues and how axons send action potentials. An influential framework in the last 50 years has been the **information processing model** of cognition. In simple terms, this perspective views the mind as being like a computer that receives data, processes it, stores some of it, and makes decisions based on how it's processed. To some extent, this might seem like a pretty obvious idea—especially since our society is saturated by computers—but it forms an important contrast with the previously dominant psychological paradigm of behaviorism, which asserted that only behavior could be studied scientifically and avoided any speculation about internal states. This point of view was also influential in developing the framework of memory that we'll be reviewing elsewhere.

1. Cognitive Development

The topic of cognitive development is often associated with the work of a psychologist named **Jean Piaget**, whose decades of research output, from the 1920s until his death in 1980, had a profound impact on developmental psychology. Piaget is perhaps most famous for proposing a set of developmental stages that every child passes through on their way to adulthood. For the MCAT, you need to recognize these stages and their associated cognitive passages, as well as know their age ranges. We'll start by reviewing them and then step back to analyze how Piaget thought about learning in general.

The first stage proposed by Piaget is the **sensorimotor stage**, which extends from **birth until about 2 years old**, the point at which a child really starts to acquire language in earnest. As the name implies, during this period, infants primarily interact with the world through processing sensory input and by engaging in motor activities. For instance, a curious baby might crawl around and put various things in her mouth as a way of exploring, or might repeatedly knock food down from her highchair both as a way of getting rid of unwanted food and as a way of exploring, and confirming, her caregivers' reactions to this behavior. The most important aspect of this stage is the acquisition of **object permanence**, which means understanding that objects exist outside of one's perception—in other words, that things don't go away when you stop seeing them. A conventional example of how this manifests is through the game of peek-a-boo. The idea is that babies find this game so funny because they haven't fully acquired the principle of object permanence, meaning that on some level they think the person playing peek-a-boo with them is emerging from nowhere in every round of the game. You can think of children in the sensorimotor stage as not having object permanence yet. So-called **circular reactions** are another major feature of this developmental stage; this concept refers to the intentional repetition of something that either happened accidentally, like dropping a toy, or had an interesting effect, like flipping a light switch. A further important phenomenon in this stage is **stranger anxiety**, which describes a transition that usually occurs at around 8 or 9 months, from a previous pattern in which infants are generally open to strangers to a new one in which strangers provoke intense worry.

The next three stages all have operational in their name: the preoperational stage lasts from about age 2 to age 7, the concrete operational stage lasts from about age 7 to age 11, and the formal operational stage comes later. Before we get into the details, let's identify what Piaget meant by **operational**. Given the context of a theory of cognitive development, Piaget was interested in aspects of rational thought and cognition. In particular, he was interested in how children develop the ability to reason logically about the world, which, according to Piaget, manifests in the ability to engage in operations—that is, mental manipulation of objects of thought. Logical and mathematical reasoning was a particular concern of Piaget, as was the ability to recognize phenomena such as **conservation**, which is the idea that the same amount of a substance is preserved even as it is transferred between containers with different shapes. That is, a taller bottle doesn't necessarily contain more water.

In the **preoperational stage,** which more or less corresponds to early childhood, from about **age 2 to age 7**, children represent objects symbolically, using words and images, and often take part in very vivid imaginative play based on those representations, but can only engage in very minimal logical thinking. Instead, children at this stage are characterized by **egocentrism**, or difficulty imagining the world from the perspective of others, and have not yet developed an understanding of conservation. Children's understanding of conservation at this stage is dominated instead by **centration**, or a tendency to focus on a single property or parameter of an object to the exclusion of others. In other words, a child who observes water being poured from a short, wide container to a tall, narrow container, and concludes that the tall container has more water, is focusing just on the property of height. Another example is that a child in this stage might be very happy to receive two pieces of chocolate, in contrast to an older sibling who only receives one, even if the two pieces of chocolate are smaller and both children are getting the same actual amount of chocolatey goodness. To summarize, though, the four key features of this stage are: egocentrism, lack of conservation, centration, and symbolic thought. While children in this stage may use abstract reason, their abilities tend to be minimal and flawed.

The **concrete operational** stage lasts from the ages of **about 7 to about 11**. To a nontrivial extent, the name of this stage captures what it's about — that is, children make dramatic steps forward in abstract reasoning, but only as applied to concrete objects. For example, they develop an understanding of conservation—a prototypically concrete cognitive task. They lose egocentrism and become more skilled at solving problems that involve taking others' perspectives into account. Children at this stage also develop logical reasoning skills, but again, they tend to do better when logical problems are posed in terms of concrete objects. Interestingly, they also tend to perform better with inductive tasks—or generalizing logical conclusions based on empirically observed phenomena—than with deductive tasks, which involve applying logical principles to make predictions in a top-down way.

Finally, the **formal operational stage**, which starts at **about age 11 and goes until age 16**—and then persists into adulthood—is where the ability to fully engage in abstract logic kicks in. At this point, adolescents become able to handle hypotheticals, reason abstractly, and make nuanced moral judgments.

As we've mentioned, Piaget's stages are mostly concerned with the development of logical, abstract reasoning skills, and therefore do not directly apply to phenomena such as emotional development. Another concept crucial for understanding Piaget's research is that of a **schema**. In psychology, a schema refers to a cognitive framework that organizes information about things that one perceives in the outside world, with implications for the actions that can be taken in response. A very simple example would be understanding cows as animals with black-and-white splotches that produce milk. If you then encounter an animal that otherwise looks and functions like a cow, but is brown, then you have two options: either you can preserve your schema by concluding that that animal must not be a cow, or you could expand your schema by acknowledging that cows can have additional colors. Piaget would label these two options as **assimilation** and **accommodation**, respectively, and posit that these processes are at work from early childhood to adulthood.

Although Piaget's stages end at late adolescence or early adulthood, life obviously continues thereafter. Changes in cognition do take place in adulthood as well, in particular involving the relative balance between fluid and crystallized intelligence. **Fluid intelligence** essentially refers to problem-solving skills that can be applied to new situations, without any reliance on previously existing knowledge, while **crystallized intelligence** reflects the ability to deploy one's knowledge and skills to solve problems.

It's also a familiar, but unfortunate, reality that cognitive performance can decline with age, especially after 65 years of age. In its more extreme manifestations, when cognitive decline and memory impediments interfere with a person's ability to function in the world, this is known as **dementia**. Dementia isn't a specific condition, in the medical sense; instead, it's a constellation of symptoms that may have multiple causes. The most famous cause is Alzheimer's disease, which involves the formation of beta-amyloid plaques in the brain, but dementia can also occur as a result of accumulated tiny brain bleeds, or micro-strokes, or in response to other conditions that affect the brain. For example, a condition called hepatic encephalopathy occurs when a damaged liver can no longer effectively remove toxins from the body, and those toxins impact brain function.

> **MCAT STRATEGY > > >**
>
> Piaget's stages are an excellent example of pure memorization for the Psych/Soc section of the MCAT, but also illustrate how investing the effort needed to understand what a psychologist was trying to accomplish can help foster more solid long-term learning.

Circling back to Piaget, it's also important to note that his proposed stages were intended as universal statements about human development, regardless of culture. Not surprisingly, this point of view has been critiqued. For instance, the Soviet psychologist **Lev Vygotsky** emphasized the role played in cognitive development by feedback, input, and assistance from people surrounding a child -- with clear implications for cultural factors in development.

Hereditary and environmental factors—some biological, some cultural—also impact cognitive development. As we'll discuss in more depth later, it's highly likely that intelligence is heritable to a meaningful extent, and genetic conditions can also impact cognition. Down's syndrome, which involves trisomy of chromosome 21 and cognitive deficits, is a familiar example. Exposure to toxic chemicals in the womb or in early childhood can also impact cognitive ability, as often exemplified by fetal alcohol syndrome. As alluded to earlier, different cultures can also place different emphases on how cognitive skills are developed and fostered. For the purposes of the MCAT, you're certainly not expected to be able to rattle off a comprehensive list of examples of these phenomena; instead, the key goal when it comes to cognitive development is to understand Piaget's stages thoroughly, but also have a general sense that they aren't the whole story.

2. Problem-Solving

One of the simplest, most observable, and most practically relevant applications of cognition is **problem-solving**; however, it shouldn't come as a surprise to anyone who has lived in the world that we're not always successful at solving problems, which means that problem-solving has attracted significant attention from psychologists.

Let's explore some ways of solving problems. One of the most elementary options available to us is **trial and error**, where we more or less just try different options and see what works. This approach is clearly not the most sophisticated, but it's sometimes a viable option when we have the time or resources to explore many possible solutions and when we lack a conceptual understanding of the problem that would allow a more sophisticated approach. We readily associate trial and error with how animals and children learn, but it also has an interesting pedigree in more sophisticated domains too. For instance, the world-famous inventor Thomas Edison, who made groundbreaking discoveries in fields ranging from electricity to motion picture recording in the late 1800s and early 1900s, was well known for extensively using trial and error. To a certain extent, even today, screening various molecules for potential use as medications involves trial and error. Both in Edison's experiments and in modern drug design, trial and error can be useful when we understand the problem we're trying to solve enough to come up with a workable space of possible solutions, but not enough to predict the exact solution.

Moving up a level of sophistication, an **algorithm** is a problem-solving technique that involves applying a fixed set of steps. Algorithms are unlike trial and error, in that a lot of thought and insight can go into designing an algorithm, but they're similar to trial and error in that actually applying an algorithm doesn't require a conceptual understanding of the problem. Algorithms are perhaps most famous as how computers work, which illustrates the point precisely, since software engineers have the job of understanding a problem and breaking it down into very specific instructions, or an algorithm, that a computer can apply without any conceptual insight whatsoever. Algorithms are also used in medicine, as ways to codify the various "if-then" decisions that need to be made when treating a patient with a certain condition.

Importantly for the MCAT, though, many students use algorithms when solving chemistry or physics problems that involve equations. Doing so can be a double-edged sword: On the one hand, it can be comforting to have a routine to apply to a certain kind of problem, but on the other hand, relying too much on algorithms can cover up a lack of understanding of the material, which becomes problematic when a question asks about, say, acid-base chemistry in a new or unexpected way. Therefore, it's often the case for students that a major part of studying for the MCAT is reducing reliance on less than fully adaptive algorithms, and transitioning to a problem-solving approach that more closely reflects how the MCAT presents things.

Moving to a more conceptual approach to problem-solving, we can apply either deductive or inductive reasoning to solve problems. **Deductive reasoning** is **top-down**; it involves applying general principles to a specific situation. For example, if we're trying to find a drug that will interact with a certain receptor, we might notice that the its active site is rich in positively-charged residues, and apply the general principle that opposite charges attract to predict that a negatively-charged molecule would interact with that receptor. In contrast, inductive reasoning is a **bottom-up** process, where successive observations are extrapolated to identify general principles. In our example of drug design, we might test various compounds for interactions with the receptor and gradually notice that compounds richer in negatively-charged atoms interact more closely with the positively-charged active site, based on which we might formulate the principle that oppositely-charged amino acids are attracted to each other. Both inductive and deductive reasoning are common strategies that can produce good results. However, inductive reasoning is vulnerable to overgeneralizations, and deductive reasoning is profoundly dependent on the validity of the general principles.

We also routinely use **analogies** as a problem-solving tool. This means recognizing that a new problem is similar to a problem that we've seen before, and then solving the new problem in the same way that we solved the old one. A closely related problem-solving technique is **intuition**, which happens when we just have a gut sense of how to solve a problem. Often, intuition corresponds to analogies that we aren't consciously aware of. Interestingly, analogies and intuition are commonly applied in clinical settings in medicine, where experienced clinicians can draw upon years or even decades of experience to rapidly assess a new situation and react accordingly. Pushing this idea even further, occasionally we just get flashes of insight about how to solve problems that are facing us. This is why the advice is sometimes given to "sleep on" a problem, with the idea that our brains can work on it subconsciously. **Insight** as a problem-solving tool is probably most familiar in relation to problems we encounter in our daily lives, but it actually does have an interesting history in science too. For instance, August Kekulé, a pioneering chemist who worked in the 19th century, explained that he saw the cyclic structure of benzene in a daydream about the mythological figure of the ouroboros, which is a snake that eats its own tail. Polymerase chain reaction, or PCR, is also often described as having occurred to its inventor in the form of a sudden insight. These moments are sometimes known as "Eureka" moments, based on the historical tale according to which Archimedes, the ancient Greek philosopher and scientist, discovered what is now known as Archimedes' principle in a bath, and then jumped out yelling "Eureka!", which means "I have found it!" in ancient Greek.

A common barrier to problem-solving occurs when we have difficulty seeing a novel approach for solving a problem because we find ourselves trapped in certain ways of looking for solutions. A **mental set** is a framework that we use for conceptualizing a problem and trying to solve it, and **fixation** refers to getting stuck in our old ways of thinking about things. More particularly, **functional fixedness** describes a tendency to see objects as only having a certain function—usually the functions they were designed for—and having difficulties applying objects in novel, or untraditional ways. A classic illustration of this was proposed by a psychologist named Karl Duncker. In **Duncker's candle problem**, a participant is given a candle, a book of matches, and a box of thumbtacks, and is asked to figure out how to attach the candle to a wall in such a way that the candle wax won't drip down onto the floor. The solution to this problem is to remove the thumbtacks from the box, and then to tack the box to the wall to use as a candle-holder. However, many people have trouble seeing this solution because they only perceive the box as something that contains thumbtacks, not as an object that could be utilized for other purposes.

Building on this general theme of difficulties in seeing or incorporating new perspectives, **belief perseverance** refers to people's tendency to maintain their beliefs—or sometimes even strengthen them—in the face of contradictory evidence. Belief perseverance is a major concern in public health, especially with regard to the rising tide of anti-vaccination beliefs in the United States and Europe in recent years. Physicians and public health advocates have found that directly challenging patients, or their parents, about the efficacy of vaccines can backfire and even generate more resistance, and are therefore brainstorming ways to communicate effectively with patients about this issue. Inaccurate assumptions about one's own level of skill or expertise can also get in the way of problem-solving. Being too sure of oneself is known as **overconfidence**, which can interfere with solving problems effectively by making one less likely to even perceive a problem in the first place, and if a problem is perceived, by making one more likely to jump in with a hasty, inappropriate solution. Overconfidence may also be linked to belief perseverance, although it's certainly not the only explanation for it. Underconfidence can also be an impediment to problem solving, though, since someone who does not consider themselves capable of solving a problem is unlikely to put much effort into doing so, especially when initial attempts don't succeed.

3. Biases and Heuristics

Our cognitive processes, including but not limited to attempts to solve problems, can also be impeded by **cognitive biases**, which are systematic, generally subconscious patterns of thought that skew our reasoning. Everyone is vulnerable to cognitive biases, although with careful attention and training it might be possible to minimize their effects. **Confirmation bias** occurs when we reason in a way that favors information that supports conclusions that we have already made, or beliefs that we already have. For example, we might be more likely to notice a news story or opinion piece that supports an argument that we feel passionate about, and when reading such a story, we might pay particular attention to specific pieces of data that help support our perspectives. That's not to say that we're consciously trying to ignore other information, or that we wouldn't respond rationally to information that challenges our viewpoints if we are forced to confront it, just that we're naturally attracted to information that fits into how we already see things.

> **MCAT STRATEGY > > >**
>
> Biases and heuristics can be very easy to get confused; we present some illustrative scenarios here, but it can also help (1) to relate these concepts to personal experiences of yours, and (2) to focus on contextual clues that can unambiguously distinguish one term from another.

Hindsight bias, in contrast, refers to our tendency to retrospectively view events as having been highly predictable even if it wasn't so simple in the moment. History is a classic example of this, since we construct explanations for various historical events that imply that it was obvious whether a given candidate would win or lose a presidential election, or a certain army would win or lose a battle, even if things were actually much more fluid and difficult to assess at the time. Hindsight bias is also relevant in medicine, especially at morbidity and mortality reviews, in which clinicians debrief on cases where patients had negative outcomes, up to and including death. When reviewing a case with a negative final outcome, every error may seem like a logical foreshadowing of the end point, although in reality it can be quite difficult to figure out exactly how much suboptimal charting or mistakes in other aspects of patient care contributed to the poor result.

Next, **causation bias** refers to our tendency to infer cause-and-effect relationships incorrectly, either because one event follows another—which is technically known in logic as the "post hoc ergo propter hoc" fallacy, which is Latin for the "after this, therefore because of this" fallacy—or because two events tend to co-occur. The latter refers to the all-too-common tendency to mistake correlation for causation. This bias can be surprisingly persistent, even in physicians and other professionals who are trained in how to infer causality. For example, if a patient stops experiencing symptom A after taking medication B, it might be tempting to conclude that medication B caused symptom A to vanish. That might or might not be the case. After all, symptom A could have been an inherently self-limiting problem, like a stuffy nose caused by a cold, which would have gone away anyway, regardless of any medications. Clinical trials are designed to address this concern, but it's a pattern of thought that recurs with surprising frequency in real life.

In making assessments of situations and solving problems, we also use **heuristics**, which are commonly defined as mental shortcuts: that is, more or less fixed cognitive processes that we use to solve problems rapidly and/or in situations where we have incomplete information. Conceptually, heuristics are similar to biases, but the difference is that heuristics are themselves problem-solving methods—that is, they may be somewhat fuzzy or flawed, but they're ways of solving problems that often work at least well enough for practical purposes—whereas biases are more general cognitive patterns that affect our decision-making processes. Furthermore, the examples of heuristics that you'll encounter on the MCAT specifically refer to ways that we assess the probability of certain outcomes.

The **representativeness heuristic** is used when we make decisions based on what we consider to be the prototypical example of a category. In particular, the representativeness heuristic occurs in contexts where we need to make judgments about how probable something is. In one of the first experiments that established the concept of the representativeness heuristic, one set of participants was asked to estimate the proportion of college students who were majoring in certain topics. Another group of participants was given a personality sketch of a hypothetical student named Tom, who basically fit a set of stereotypes about nerdy, antisocial engineering majors, and was asked to estimate the probability of Tom majoring in various subjects. The participants who were given the personality sketch of Tom considered it much more probable that he was an engineering major than would be implied by the other participants' assessments, even though they were given no specific information suggesting anything about his major. Significant concerns have been raised about the impact of the representativeness heuristic on various higher-level social phenomena, like the criminal justice system, because it implies that people involved in various stages of the process, ranging from police officers to jurors, will conclude that someone is more likely to be a criminal if he or she fits the profile of a typical criminal—a concept that is itself deeply vulnerable to stereotypes. Correspondingly, people who don't fit the profile of being a criminal, such as police officers, might benefit from more favorable assumptions made by jurors, judges, other police officers, or prosecutors.

The logic of the **availability heuristic** is similar to that of the representativeness heuristic in that it also involves reasoning about the probability or likelihood of a certain event, but it's different in that it involves being influenced by examples of a certain phenomenon that come to mind quickly. A classic example is how sensationalistic news stories about certain types of crimes lead people to think that they're at risk every time they step outside, even if objectively those crimes are very rare and more mundane dangers are not. Another vivid example is something informally known as **medical students' disease** or second-year syndrome, which refers to how medical students who are learning about a wide range of unusual, diverse, and often gruesome illnesses begin to interpret every slight symptom or physical oddity they experience as signs of a rare and serious illness.

The representativeness and availability heuristics are often confused, and medical students' disease is actually a fantastic example in terms of telling these two apart. The driving motivation behind medical students' disease is that students are exposed day in and day out to descriptions of these diseases, meaning that these conditions are very directly available in their consciousness and easy to recall, but that doesn't mean that they think it's typical for otherwise healthy people be diagnosed with rare diseases.

This example makes a good rule of thumb that will help you distinguish these terms on the MCAT: The representativeness heuristic must refer to some assessment of what's typical, or a certain stereotype, while the availability heuristic must refer to something in recent memory or that immediately comes to mind. In reality, of course, something could be both representative and available in the sense we've been discussing, but for testing purposes, any scenario will clearly be one or the other.

4. Intelligence

Intelligence is the parameter that comes to mind perhaps most immediately when we think about cognition, and it might seem a little surprising that we've reserved this topic for the end of our broader discussion of cognition. However, there's a reason for this: Exploring topics like Piaget's stages of cognitive development, various aspects of problem-solving, and factors such as biases and heuristics that can impede our ability to reason effectively give us at least some sense of how multifaceted intellectual function is, with corresponding implications for how we view intelligence.

The first aspect of intelligence that we need to consider is how we can define intelligence in the first place. This turns out to be a complex question; even though we've all had the experience of recognizing that some people are smarter than others, it turns out to still be very tricky to pin the concept down in a precise and scientifically legitimate way. Luckily, the MCAT will never expect you to define intelligence. So we can use a working definition of intelligence as the ability to detect patterns, process and store information, understand ideas, and problem-solve. What the MCAT does expect you to be familiar with are some of the various ways that researchers have analyzed intelligence over the years, and how those conclusions have been applied for practical purposes.

One of the most influential ways of thinking about intelligence was developed by a psychologist named **Charles Spearman** in the early 1900s. He noticed that children's performance in various subjects in school tended to show correlations—that is, even though history and math test different cognitive skills, students who do well in history tend to do well in math, and vice versa. One logical possibility for this observation would be that some underlying capacity drives performance across multiple, seemingly-unrelated subjects. That underlying capacity is **general intelligence**, which was then labeled the ***g* factor**. It might not seem stunning that doing well on cognitive tasks is associated with being smart, but Spearman's real contribution was to give a more formal mathematical and empirical basis for this fairly obvious statement. Perhaps more surprisingly, the *g* factor has had a long and persistent life in psychological research, and tests that measure it—or purport to measure it—have shown correlations with a wide range of outcomes. Interestingly, the *g* factor can be inherited, with a heritability of roughly 50%. This certainly leaves some room for environmental factors, but points to an important role for genetics.

> **MCAT STRATEGY > > >**
>
> Highlights about intelligence for the MCAT include the concept of general intelligence, the distinction between fluid and crystallized intelligence, and the idea that IQ has a normal distribution like many physiological parameters. Being aware of potential pitfalls in IQ testing is also a good idea.

Most modern approaches to general intelligence recognize fluid and crystallized intelligence as distinct components of the *g* factor. **Fluid intelligence**, as mentioned above, refers to one's ability to reason on the fly, or to solve novel problems, while **crystallized intelligence** describes one's ability to bring knowledge and skills to bear on problem-solving. A key point here is that crystallized intelligence doesn't just reflect memorization; instead, it has to do with how one can apply what one knows.

Spearman was not the first person to think about intelligence, though. An earlier pioneer in this field, Francis Galton, is worth noting. Galton was a thought-provoking figure historically. He made important advances in several fields, inspired by the work of Charles Darwin—who, believe it or not, was his cousin—on evolution. However, much of his intellectual career was devoted to laying the foundations for **eugenics**, a paradigm that espoused selective breeding programs for humans, endorsed extremely racist ideas about differences between populations, and provided a framework for horrifically unethical practices like the forced sterilization of poor people. Eugenics is now regarded as a disastrous wrong turn in the history of biology and anthropology, and it's impossible to view Galton's career outside of that context, but Galton's idea of **hereditary genius**, articulated in an 1869 book by the same, is worth being aware of for the MCAT.

At almost exactly the same time that Spearman was formulating the idea of the *g* factor, in 1904, a French psychologist named **Alfred Binet** was tasked by the French government with finding a way to determine which students had cognitive deficiencies so that they could be educated accordingly. After conducting extensive research to identify the levels of performance in various cognitive domains that were typical for children at certain ages, Binet was able to calculate a given child's "mental age" relative to his or her chronological age. That is, a high-performing child at the age of 10 might be able to function on the level of a 12-year-old. With a little bit of mathematical tweaking, this idea developed into the **intelligence quotient**, or **IQ**, which was initially defined as a child's mental age divided by his or her chronological age, multiplied by 100. So in our example, a child with a mental age of 12 and a chronological age of 10 would have an IQ of 120. However, extending this concept to adults can be problematic. It wouldn't make sense to say that a 40-year-old functioning at the level of a 60-year-old would have an IQ of 150! Nonetheless, IQ tests for adults have been developed, in which IQ reflects an estimate of general intelligence, including both fluid and crystallized intelligence.

Another interesting aspect of IQ is that it has a **normal distribution**. We don't have to be too precise statistically here, but this basically means that IQ shows a standard bell curve distribution, with most people having scores clustered around the mean and fewer and fewer people having more extreme scores. Normal distributions are commonly seen for physiological features, like height. For a variable with a normal distribution, 68% of the population is captured within plus or minus one standard deviation of the mean, and 95% of the population is captured within two standard deviations. The standard deviation of IQ is generally defined as plus or minus 15 points, so 68% of the population has an IQ between 85 and 115, and 95% of the population has an IQ between 70 and 130. These values correspond to the 2.5th and 97.5th percentiles, respectively.

IQ tests and the applications thereof would be a strong contender for the most controversial topic in psychology in the last 80 years, for several reasons. One reason for this is that IQ tests are high-stakes. They can influence the educational resources that a child receives, and **standardized tests** like the SAT, which is not technically an IQ test but purports to measure many of the same qualities of general aptitude, have a huge impact on the opportunities that people have after high school. Differences across racial and cultural groups in terms of IQ scores have been observed, and extremely intense debates have taken place about whether those observed differences reflect actual population-level differences in cognitive ability, or instead may be due to factors such as cognitive biases in testing, differences in exposure to education or the broader effects of poverty and class. The latter points are extraordinarily important factors to consider when approaching the concept of intelligence testing. Verbally-based questions, for instance, may wind up testing vocabulary, which can be strongly impacted by environmental exposure and formal schooling, instead of intelligence. Attempts have been made to address this point by using visual questions that require pattern recognition and extrapolation, but the counterpoint has been made that even those ostensibly neutral questions might be affected by cultural bias, since our educational system gives students extensive training from early years in arranging information in rows and columns and looking for patterns to extrapolate. Other societies (e.g. hunter-gatherer societies) may tend to highlight other ways of organizing information.

As we mentioned earlier, intelligence is somewhat hereditary—that is, within the context of family-level inheritance patterns—and somewhat influenced by environment. A notable finding in this regard is the **Flynn effect**, which describes how IQ scores steadily increased in many developed countries throughout the 20th century, before possibly peaking in the 1990s. Possible explanations for this effect include improvements in nutrition, general education, overall health, and environmental stimulation. No complete consensus exists regarding this point, but it's a powerful example of the impact of environment on the achievement of intellectual potential at the level of entire populations.

> **MCAT STRATEGY > > >**
>
> Intelligence can serve as the basis of questions about the nature vs. nurture debate, and the plethora of terms and theories related to intelligence can also serve as fodder for related passages and questions on the MCAT.

Although cognitive-based measures of intelligence, like IQ, are predictive of academic achievement, it's also clear that IQ alone is no guarantee of happiness or success. Thus, IQ cannot be the whole story of human ability. In the 1980s, the psychologist Howard Gardner proposed the **theory of multiple intelligences**. Originally, Gardner proposed seven intelligences: musical, visual-spatial, verbal-linguistic, logical-mathematical, bodily-kinesthetic, interpersonal, and intrapersonal. Some of these domains are pretty self-explanatory based on their names, but a few are worth commenting on in a bit more depth. Three of Gardner's categories—visual-spatial, verbal-linguistic, and logical-mathematical—correspond to subcomponents of the g factor, or general intelligence, that are also addressed in IQ-based approaches to intelligence. So in that sense, Gardner's project isn't about replacing previous ideas about intelligence, but rather about refining and extending them. Musical and bodily-kinesthetic intelligence are not traditionally included under the rubric of general intelligence, but it's pretty straightforward to understand what those concepts get at. Since "inter" and "intra" can be tricky prefixes to remember, it's worth highlighting that interpersonal intelligence has to do with how we relate to one another. In other words, it's basically social intelligence. Intrapersonal intelligence, on the other hand, has to do with how we relate to ourselves and our emotions. In the 1990s, Gardner suggested adding an eighth form of intelligence, naturalistic intelligence, that would describe the ability to relate to and pick up important patterns in the natural world.

A common misconception is that Gardner's theory of multiple intelligences includes emotional intelligence. This isn't quite true, although Gardner's intrapersonal intelligence does involve recognition of one's emotions. Instead, the term **emotional intelligence** was popularized by Daniel Goleman. Emotional intelligence in this sense involves recognition of both one's own emotions and those of others, as well as emotional self-regulation. Goleman proposed that emotional intelligence be viewed as an equal counterpart of traditional intelligence, and even suggested that an emotional intelligence quotient, or EQ, be used alongside IQ. Further extensions of the concept of multiple intelligences have been put forward; for instance, a pop-psychology book in 2013 argued for creative intelligence as a distinct capacity. As these examples show, the concept of multiple intelligences has struck a chord with many people, both in the field of psychology and in the general public. As with just about everything relating to the topic of intelligence in psychology, some controversy exists around the concept of multiple intelligences, mostly regarding whether it's preferable to use intelligence in a strict sense and to call everything else an aptitude, or to extend the definition of intelligence to cover a broader range of domains. Food for thought, but the MCAT will not expect you to take a side in this debate.

To summarize, intelligence is a deep and non-obvious topic, and we've covered various ways of thinking about the topic. For the MCAT, the key point is to be aware of the major ways that researchers have conceptualized intelligence, with the most important landmarks being Spearman's g factor, Binet's concept of mental age versus chronological age, and Gardner's theory of multiple intelligences. It's also worth having a general awareness of the pitfalls and controversies associated with intelligence testing, since those topics could be addressed in passages.

5. Language: Components and Theories

Communication is one of the most basic parts of being human, and language is at the heart of our ability to communicate with each other. Interestingly, language is thought to be uniquely human. But anyone who's had a pet knows that animals absolutely do communicate. The difference is that human language has a unique degree of structural complexity and ability to use arbitrary symbols to refer to both concrete objects and abstract ideas. For instance, what relationship does the concept of physiology, for example, have to do with the literal sounds in the word "physiology?" In contrast, the range of meaning that a cat's meow or a dog's bark can express is possibly broad, but way less than what we can do with language. Some thought-provoking research has shown surprisingly sophisticated communication strategies in birds, bees, and other animals, but human language still stands out.

It's important to clarify what psychologists and linguists mean by **language**. In particular, there's a difference between studying languages—that is, the thousands of different linguistic systems that people use to communicate, the most widespread of which include Chinese, English, Spanish and Hindi—and studying language, which means focusing on the structure of language, the underlying similarities shared by all human languages and/or the cognitive aspects of learning and using linguistic systems. Language as studied by psychologists and linguists is also distinct from how language is understood in the context of literature; that is, our current discussion of language is not going to yield a direct payoff for the CARS section.

Human language consists of multiple components that operate in parallel whenever we speak, or when we listen to and understand someone else speaking. **Phonetics** deals with the speech sounds that we produce, often on a level that doesn't consciously register with us as speakers or contribute directly to meaning. So, for example, a phonetician might be concerned with the precise articulatory details of how we produce sounds in our vocal cavity, or with exactly how long we continue to pronounce vowel sounds depending on the context, or with intonation patterns that don't directly affect meaning. Moving up a level of complexity, **phonology** deals with how we structure and organize speech sounds in ways that do affect meaning, as well as processes that affect such sounds. For instance, phonologists are interested in defining phonemes, or the units of sound that distinguish meaning in each language. As an example, the English words "deep" and "dip" mean two different things, and are only differentiated by the vowel sounds "ee" and "i" -- but many other languages don't distinguish those two sounds. Another example is how the plural marker in English, which we write with an "s", is pronounced as either an "s" or a "z" depending on its environment -- so we say it as "s" in cats, but as "z" in dogs. It'd be really hard to actually pronounce it as an "s" in dogs (go ahead, try!), because English has an automatic process that causes consonants in a cluster to be similar to each other.

Our reference to a plural marker brings us to **morphology**, which in the field of linguistics refers to the study of how words are formed. This can include ways that various words are derived from underlying roots, like how we can add an "-er" or "-or" suffix to a verb and create a noun that describes someone who engages in that action; thus, a baker is someone who bakes, an investigator is someone who investigates, and so on. Morphology can also include ways that words change to indicate grammatical relationships, like how to indicate past tense, we change "jump" to "jumped" or "eat" to "ate". As indicated by how "eat" changes to "ate," morphology isn't always regular, and the acquisition of irregular forms is a milestone in a child's language development. Languages also show tremendous variation in the kinds of grammatical relationships they encode through morphology and the ways that they do so.

The field of **semantics** specializes in meaning, either on the level of words or sentences. On the word level, it may take some time for children to learn the precise definition of various words. For example, kinship terms can be difficult. As an example of a semantic puzzle on the sentence level, consider the sentence "Every student at this school speaks two languages." There are two possible ways we could interpret this sentence. Without any other context, the most likely interpretation would be that each student speaks two languages that may or may not overlap, so that one student might speak English and Spanish, another might speak English and Punjabi, and so on. Another interpretation might be that there are two specific languages that each student speaks. For instance, in a bilingual English-French school, every student might speak two languages (English and French) and maybe other languages too.

> **MCAT STRATEGY > > >**
>
> Much more could be said about the components of language that we've reviewed, but for the MCAT, it suffices to have a rough understanding of these domains (phonetics, phonology, morphology, syntax, semantics, and pragmatics), because they can be given as answer choices.

This example points to the importance of context, which brings us to **pragmatics**. In everyday speech, we use "pragmatic" to mean practical, down-to-earth, and real-world, but in linguistics it has a completely different meaning. The study of pragmatics is basically the analysis of non-literal meaning, which, when you think about it, is a basic component of how we interact with each other. After all, if you ask someone "Could you pass the hot sauce?", you're not literally asking about their ability to do so. We can choose to interact with each other informatively, non-informatively, or share too much information, we can decide to tell the truth or lie or tell half-truths that lie somewhere in between, we can choose how polite or rude to be to other people, and so on, and all of those aspects of language use that give texture to our lives fall under the rubric of pragmatics.

Although we've been focusing on spoken language, **sign languages** are also full-fledged linguistic systems, with all of the above components. The only structural difference is that phonetics and phonology, which correspond to sounds in spoken language, refer to physical motion of the hands in sign language, but in both cases, these systems deal with how words are physically articulated. Just like spoken languages, there are many different sign languages that are not mutually intelligible, and there's no relationship between a sign language and the spoken language spoken in the vicinity. That is, American Sign Language is not a version of English that's just "translated" into physical motion. It's a distinct system with a grammar and structure of its own.

People have been interested in language for centuries, but the scientific study of language only really took off in the 19th century, when linguists focused on establishing relationships between languages based on descent from a shared ancestor and sketching out the basic structural features of human language. In the 20th century, psychologists and linguists turned a closer eye to language acquisition on the individual level, trying to answer the question of how children learn languages as they grow.

The psychological school of **behaviorism**, pioneered by **B. F. Skinner**, dominated American psychology in the mid-20th century. Broadly speaking, this approach focused exclusively on observable behavior, and thought of learning strictly in terms of concrete behavior that emerged in response to rewards or punishments. In 1957, Skinner published a book called *Verbal Behavior* that applied this framework to language. This theory, sometimes also called the **learning theory of language**, states that language is a learned behavior that develops in response to environmental stimuli and responses, ranging from direct coaching to how a verbal request for a cookie may be rewarded with a tasty baked snack. Importantly, Skinner denied the existence of any specialized capacity for language learning in the brain, seeing language as just another example of behavior that emerges from training.

Two years later, Noam Chomsky, probably the most well-known American linguist of the late 20th century, published a scathing 30-page review of *Verbal Behavior*, tearing down the learning theory of language in particular and Skinner's behaviorist theories of psychology in general. This review, in some ways, launched Chomsky's career, and the research program that he spent the next decades developing is often referred to as the **nativist theory of language acquisition**, because it places a strong emphasis on the idea that humans have a hard-wired neural capacity for learning language. In other words, our ability to learn language is native, or in-born. This theory was articulated before modern brain imaging, so it doesn't point to specific brain structures, but instead views the so-called **language acquisition device** as a general capacity distributed throughout the brain.

Another central aspect of Chomsky's approach to language is that it posits deep, underlying, and somewhat abstract linguistic structures that undergo transformations to generate the structures that we produce when we speak. Because these transformations generate the sentences we speak, this framework is called **generative linguistics**. The goal of this framework is to explain patterns we've already mentioned, like how "The doctor examined the patient" and "The patient was examined by the doctor" describe the same action, as well as some interesting asymmetries, like how you can ask "What did Jane buy?", but if you know she bought a coffee and something else, it would be really weird to ask "What did Jane buy a coffee and?"

The nativist theory doesn't exclude the importance of environmental stimuli -- after all, the specific language we learn as children is obviously based on our environment, and as we mentioned previously in our discussion of nature versus nurture, children who are deprived of language in their early lives are at an ongoing deficit. However, it treats the environment as only a secondary influence. The **interactionist theory** places a greater emphasis on how children interact with their environment. It differs from Skinner's language approach in that the interactionist school doesn't deny that we have an inborn capacity for language, and it views environmental input less as a dry system of rewards and punishments, and more as a rich, interactive process.

6. Language, Cognition, and the Brain

Many people experience their own thoughts as words, and even if you perceive your thoughts as images or some other sensory representation, words are necessary to convey our thoughts to others (or at least to do so in more depth than what can be done in a game of charades). For that reason, it's no surprise that people have long thought about the relationship between language and cognition.

That said, precisely because we need language to articulate our thoughts about the relationship between language and thought, this is a notoriously tricky topic, and it's easy to get caught up in logical circles. In the late 1800s and early 1900s, linguists in the Americas started studying indigenous languages in more depth than they had previously. These studies yielded novel insights into linguistic structure, because many of these languages have dramatically different grammatical structures from those in European languages, and this spurred intense thought into all sorts of issues related to grammar.

This brings us **Benjamin Lee Whorf**, who was an engineer by profession. He had a lifelong passion for Native American languages, and wound up auditing classes and working with a Yale linguistics professor named **Edward Sapir**. Whorf studied a Native American language known as Hopi, which is spoken in Arizona, and concluded that Hopi grammar contained no linguistic forms for expressing time, at least as generally understood by Europeans and European-Americans, and that Hopi speakers therefore don't have a concept of time passing continuously, with huge philosophical ramifications for their worldview in general. Whorf was probably wrong about a lot of things involving Hopi, but the idea that the grammatical categories —like present, past, and future tenses of verbs, and things like conditional and subjunctive moods—and vocabulary of the language that we speak can shape our cognition turned out to be quite influential. Sometimes this concept is known as the **Sapir-Whorf hypothesis**, and sometimes as **linguistic relativity**. A particularly strong version, which claims that language actually dictates thought, is known as **linguistic determinism**. You should be prepared to recognize any of these terms on the MCAT.

> **MCAT STRATEGY > > >**
>
> Be wary of trick questions related to linguistic relativity! This topic provides the test writers with an opportunity to test a topic that is interesting, but often misunderstood, using analogical situations that are perfect for skill 2 (Scientific Reasoning and Problem-Solving) questions in the Psych/Soc section.

Let's be very clear about some things that linguistic relativity does not refer to: It is not just a simple statement that languages are different. The fact that different languages have different grammar and vocabulary is pretty obvious to anyone who's ever studied another language. Sometimes those differences might be unexpected—for instance, it can definitely be surprising to learn that some languages only have three or four basic color terms—but that's still not linguistic relativity. Instead, linguistic relativity always involves some link to cognition. For instance, we might wonder how speakers of languages with different color systems perform on color characterization tasks; perhaps, someone whose native language has a word for pink might be quicker to distinguish color stimuli involving pink than a speaker of a language that only has basic words for red and white. In fact, psycholinguists have spent a lot of time and energy investigating possibilities like that. The evidence is not especially conclusive one way or the other, but in general, the strongest pieces of evidence tend to relate to narrowly-defined questions instead of broad statements about language and thought. Regardless, linguistic relativity is one of those ideas that consistently draw the interest of both researchers and members of the general public.

A natural follow-up question when thinking about language and cognition would be to try to correlate human linguistic ability with specific brain structures. This turns out to be both easy and hard: Easy in the sense that there's just a few structures you should be aware of for the MCAT, but hard in the sense that the problem becomes more complicated the more that researchers dig into it. Two particular brain areas associated with language were identified well over a hundred years ago—that is, way before imaging techniques like MRI—on the basis of studies of patients with aphasia. **Aphasia** is a blanket term that refers to an impaired ability to communicate, and depending on the specific pattern of dysfunction, several different types of aphasia have been identified.

In **Wernicke's aphasia**, named after the psychologist who identified it, affected individuals can speak fluently, but what they say doesn't typically make sense, and they have great difficulty with language comprehension. The brain area linked to this type of aphasia, **Wernicke's area**, is located in the superior temporal lobe of the dominant hemisphere, which is generally the left hemisphere, and is thought to be involved in language comprehension. Therefore, a stroke or lesion affecting this area will knock out a person's ability to understand language or make sense, but they can still produce sentences with ease. This type of aphasia is also known as **fluent aphasia**, because affected individuals can produce sentences easily, and **receptive aphasia**, because this disorder involves problems understanding.

Broca's aphasia, likewise named after Pierre Paul Broca who characterized this disorder, shows the opposite pattern. That is, affected individuals can understand spoken language with no major problems, but they have extreme difficulty producing language. Some of the patients who Broca worked with could produce fewer than five words. This disorder corresponds to **Broca's area**, which is in the frontal lobe of the dominant hemisphere. This type of aphasia is sometimes also known as **non-fluent aphasia**.

This information paints a really nice picture: Wernicke's area handles comprehension, while Broca's area handles production. We can even link this distinction to the location of these areas, since language production takes conscious thought and judgment, so it makes sense for it to be localized to the frontal lobe, whereas comprehension happens more or less automatically. Information gets from Wernicke's area to Broca's area through the **arcuate fasciculus**, and damage to that structure results in a condition known as **conduction aphasia**, which involves severe difficulty repeating words. This is exactly what you'd expect if the structure responsible for transferring information from the comprehension center to the production center is damaged.

Of course, things are never quite that simple when it comes to the human brain. It turns out that multiple other areas in the brain play various roles in language. However, the most important point to be aware of for the MCAT is that, generally speaking, regions in the temporal lobe tend to handle language-related processing functions, and this includes the **auditory cortices**.

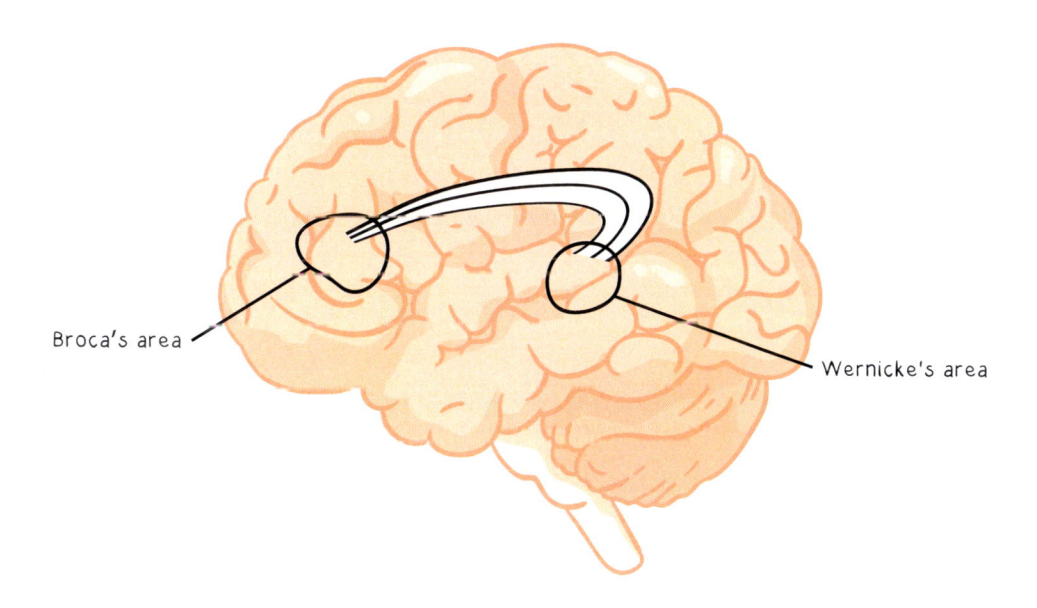

Figure 1. Areas of the brain primarily responsible for speech

6. Must-Knows

- Information processing model treats the brain somewhat like a computer, handling input and creating output
- Behaviorism focus on measurable external outcomes, no attempt to directly determine internal states
- Jean Piaget introduced the idea of cognitive stages:
  – Sensorimotor (0-2 years): lacking object permanence, circular reactions, stranger anxiety.
  – Preoperational (2-7 years): symbolic thought, egocentrism, centration, lack of conservation.
  – Concrete operational (7-11 years): understand conservation, logical reasoning.
  – Formal operational (11-16 years): abstract logic, handle hypotheticals, reason abstractly.
- Fluid intelligence: problem-solving skills; crystallized intelligence: knowledge and its application
- Cognitive performance declines with age. Dementia is defined as severe cognitive decline. It is often caused by Alzheimer's disease, but can have a multitude of causes.
- Down's syndrome is caused by trisomy 21 (having 3 copies of chromosome 21 instead of 2) and fetal alcohol syndrome is caused by prenatal alcohol exposure. Both impact cognitive functioning.
- Problem-solving strategies: trial and error, algorithms, deductive and inductive reasoning, and analogies.
- Mental set: framework for solving a problem. Functional fixedness: seeing only a prescribed set of uses for a particular object or property
- Belief perseverance: people's tendency to maintain beliefs in the face of contradictory evidence
- Overconfidence and underconfidence can both get in the way of problem-solving.
- Biases and heuristics: patterns we use to quickly make judgements, heuristics used to problem-solve
  – Confirmation bias: disregard of evidence contrary to one's beliefs, favorable interpretation of ambiguous evidence and selective recall of only supporting evidence
  – Hindsight bias is the phenomenon that all events in retrospect seem significantly more predictable than they were at the time, and the actual outcome appears as the only likely outcome.
  – Causation bias is our tendency to infer cause-and-effect to almost any set of events occurring in close proximity or that we expect to be causally related.
  – Representativeness heuristic: Using prototypical categories to misestimate the likelihood of a certain behavior, outcome, or property
  – Availability heuristic: Finding events that immediately come to mind more likely (medical students' disease)
- Components of language, from lowest to highest level: phonetics (direct sounds that we produce), phonology (sound structures affecting meaning), morphology (word formation/construction), syntax (phrases/sentences), semantics (literal meaning), pragmatics (real-world language use, nonliteral meaning)
- Sign languages share all components of language and are full-fledged linguistic systems.
- Three conflicting theories of language acquisition are tested on the MCAT.
  – Learning theory of language: all language is learned behavior (environmental stimuli, conditioning)
  – Nativist theory of language acquisition: humans have an innate, hard-wired capacity for learning language
  – Interactionist theory: emphasizes interactions with the environment, without denying inborn capacity
- Linguistic relativity (Sapir-Whorf hypothesis): the language we speak shapes our cognition.
- Linguistic determinism (strong Sapir-Whorf hypothesis): language simply dictates thought.
- Aphasia: impairment of the ability to communicate
  – Wernicke's aphasia: fluent speech that doesn't make sense; difficulty with language comprehension. It is caused by damage to Wernicke's area in the superior temporal lobe of the dominant hemisphere and is classified as both a fluent aphasia and receptive aphasia.
  – Broca's aphasia: extreme difficulty producing language, without significant difficulties understanding spoken language. It is caused by damage to Broca's area in the frontal lobe of the dominant hemisphere.
  – Conduction aphasia: severe difficulty repeating words and is caused by damage to the arcuate fasciculus, a structure connecting Broca's and Wernicke's areas.

End of Chapter Practice

The best MCAT practice is **realistic**, with a focus on identifying steps for further improvement. For those reasons, we recommend completing practice questions in an online setting that simulates the real MCAT interface, and taking advantage of advanced analytic features to help you determine how best to move forward in your MCAT study journey.

With that in mind, **online end-of-chapter questions** are accessible through your Next Step account.

As a further supplement, given the importance of active learning for effective studying, we also suggest that you consult the Must-Knows as a basis for creating a study sheet, in which you list out key terms and test your ability to briefly summarize them.

This page left intentionally blank.

Emotion, Stress, Memory, and Learning

CHAPTER 6

0. Introduction

Perceptions and cognition set the stage for more complex psychological phenomena, such as emotion, stress, memory, and learning, which will form the core of this chapter.

1. Emotions: Components, Culture, and Biology

Emotion is a basic element of the texture of our inner lives -- just as fundamental to human existence as other aspects of psychology like cognition and learning. In fact, evolutionary psychologists have pointed out that emotions, and the ability to sense and act upon them, have been highly adaptive in the evolutionary trajectory of humankind, insofar as humans are deeply social creatures and emotions are fundamental to how people perceive and express their needs, wants, and desires in a group setting.

Although the existence of emotion in general is a basic property of human psychology, a question of perennial interest in the study of emotion is the degree to which emotions are culturally specific or universal. Cultural variations certainly do exist with regard to the expression and perception of emotions; for example, cultures may have very different expectations with regard to under what circumstances it's considered acceptable to express negative emotions like anger and sadness. Some emotions may also be specific to a certain culture; for instance, the Portuguese word *saudade* refers to a type of sweetly sad longing that is felt to be unique to Portuguese and Brazilian culture.

In contrast, though, the psychologist Paul Ekman proposed that certain basic emotions are universal -- by which he meant both that they have essentially the same meaning no matter where someone grows up in the world and that they correspond to predictable, hard-wired facial expressions. The first pair of **Ekman's universal emotions** is, unsurprisingly enough, happiness and sadness. The expression for happiness includes smiling and wrinkling one's brow. In the expression for sadness, the corners of the mouth are lowered and the inner side of the brows

> **MCAT STRATEGY > > >**
>
> Ekman's universal emotions provide an excellent opportunity to put kinesthetic, or physical, learning into practice - that is, make the faces to help solidify your knowledge of the terms!

are raised. Next, surprise is expressed by opening one's eyes wide, thereby raising the eyebrows, and optionally by opening one's mouth slightly. Fear also involves widening the eyes and raising one's eyebrows, but with the lips retracted backwards towards the ears. Anger is expressed by lowering one's eyebrows, pressing one's lips together, and glaring. Disgust is shown by wrinkling one's nose and possibly lifting up one's upper lip. Ekman originally proposed these six, but then argued that a seventh emotion should be included: contempt, which is expressed by pulling a corner of the mouth upwards.

Ekman's proposal has stirred up an entire subfield of research, with thousands of articles written on the topic, and not everyone necessarily agrees with Ekman's classification. An important point is that Ekman did not say that these are the only emotions, or the only emotions that matter, or even that these are like the basic building blocks of emotions from which more complicated emotions like anxiety, jealousy, and ecstasy are constructed. Instead, Ekman's proposal is that these core emotions are present and recognizable across all cultures, and therefore in some sense represent part of our common psychological heritage as humans.

Emotion is rooted in the brain. In particular, the **limbic system** is associated with emotion. This is a tricky point of terminology, because the limbic system isn't a single structure, and it's arguably not even a coherent system. Instead, it's a grouping of structures, mostly in the midbrain, in the vicinity of the thalamus, in the medial part of the temporal lobe, that are involved in emotion, memory, and motivation. The limbic system contains many structures. In particular, extensive evidence exists that the **amygdala** is implicated in processing emotional stimuli, and several disorders involving emotional processing are correlated with abnormalities or changes in the amygdala. The amygdala has neurons that project to the **hypothalamus**, which is an important link between the nervous system and the endocrine system. Thus, the amygdala and the hypothalamus both play important roles in translating between stimuli, conscious perceptions, and the physiological manifestations of emotion.

Emotion can be a very physical phenomenon. For example, emotions like anxiety and fear are associated with activation of the sympathetic nervous system, which is the component of the autonomic motor system that is responsible for the "fight-or-flight response." To review, increased activity of the sympathetic nervous system has effects including dilation of the pupils, increased conductivity of the skin, reduced peristalsis and less blood flow to the muscles responsible for digestion, and increased blood sugar levels. Other manifestations of emotion can include blushing in response to embarrassment, breaking into a sweat as a sign of nervousness, and so on.

Furthermore, emotions have three components: cognitive, physiological, and behavioral. The **cognitive component** of emotions is what's most likely to come to mind when we think of emotions: it's what's going on in our heads, so to speak, when we feel a certain way. The **physiological component** refers to how emotions manifest physically in our body. The **behavioral component** is a little bit slipperier. As the name suggests, it refers to the way in which we behave when we feel a certain emotion. Joy might be associated with jumping up and down, and intense fear might be associated with running away. However, freezing up and not responding at all can also be a response to fear. This brings up an important point, which is that people's behavioral response to emotions can be quite variable. Nonetheless, for all that we're not dealing with one-to-one relationships, the behavioral component of emotion is important not least because we interpret other people's emotions through behavioral cues.

CHAPTER 6: EMOTION, STRESS, MEMORY, AND LEARNING

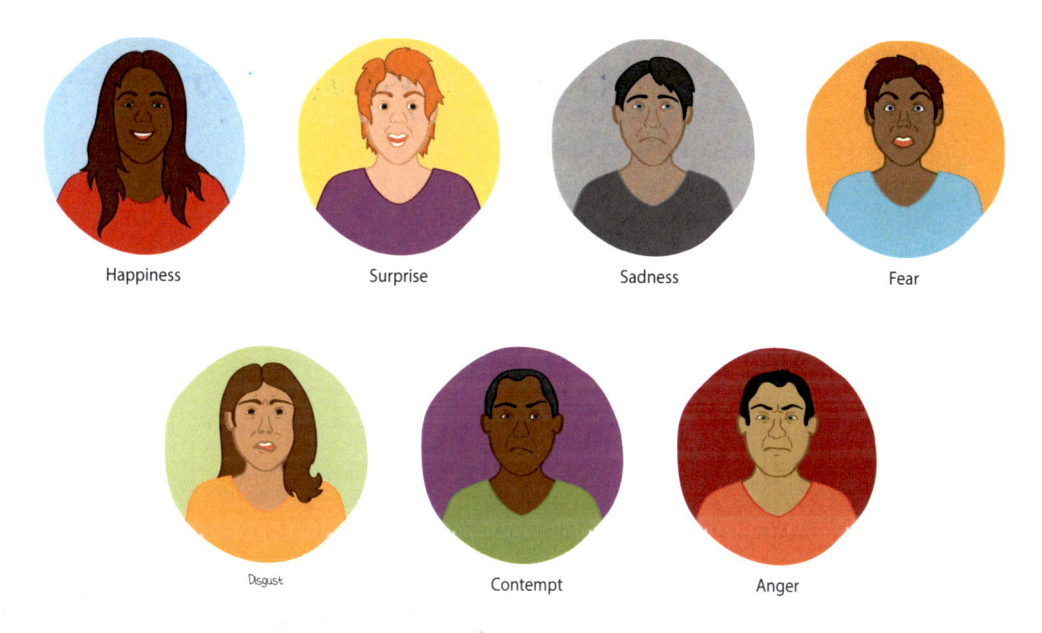

Figure 1. Ekman's seven universal emotions

2. Theories of Emotion

I. Background

The three main theories that have been proposed to account for links among the cognitive, physiological, and behavioral components are the James-Lange, Cannon-Bard, and Schachter-Singer theories of emotion, although a fourth theory known as the Lazarus theory is also worth being aware of.

These theories are a perennial source of confusion for students, largely because the names of the theories don't provide much of a "hook" for understanding the differences between them. Stepping back, it's useful to take a quick look at the historical background of these theories. In particular, some of these theories are relatively old: the James-Lange theory was developed in the late 1800s, the Cannon-Bard theory was developed in the 1920s, the Schachter-Singer theory was developed in the 1960s, and Richard Lazarus was most active from the 1970s to the 1990s. As such, it's not particularly productive to worry about how much these theories agree with modern neuropsychological research. Instead, the goal is to understand the basic proposals of these theories and how they can be applied to various situations.

With that in mind, let's work through these in a scenario where you see a bear, get scared, and run away. Physiologically, of course, getting scared involves a response from the sympathetic nervous system, including elevated heart rate and blood pressure. Naively, we might imagine the following sequence of events: we encounter a stimulus, or the bear, then have an emotional response, or fear, which triggers a physiological response, leading to a

103

behavior like running away. The thing is, though, that this intuitive account is almost certainly wrong, and we can make sense of the MCAT-relevant theories of emotion as a set of improvements on our naive explanation.

II. The James-Lange Theory

[handwritten: stimulus → physiological response → emotion]

The **James-Lange theory** involves a simple modification of the intuitive explanation that we suggested above. Namely, according to the James-Lange theory, the physiological response occurs immediately after the stimulus, causing the emotional response. In other words, we see a bear, then our heart starts racing, and then we perceive that physiological response as fear. The main historical contribution of the James-Lange theory is that it called attention to the central role of physiology in shaping our psychological perceptions, which is an insight that continues to be relevant in modern psychology. However, the James-Lange theory is not adequate as a complete theory of emotion. Among the various critiques that have been raised, an issue to notice is that different people can have different emotional responses to similar or identical stimuli, and even to the physiological responses to those stimuli. For instance, some people love watching horror movies and getting scared, and other people don't. Moreover, our emotional response to a stimulus might depend on the context: sympathetic nervous system activation (elevated heart rate, etc.) might be enjoyable in the context of a horror film but frightening in the case of what appears to be a real threat.

III. The Schachter-Singer Theory

[handwritten: stimulus → physiological response → context → emotion]

The **Schachter-Singer theory** addresses this problem by adding another stage to the James-Lange theory: cognitive appraisal of the context. So we'd see the bear, have a physiological response, appraise that response in context, and then have a conscious emotion and/or behavior. The 1962 experiment that Schachter and Singer conducted is an example of the surprisingly large category of influential but highly unethical psychology experiments from the 1950s and 1960s.

In this experiment, the researchers injected subjects with either epinephrine, also known as adrenaline, or a placebo, telling them that they would receive a shot of a made-up vitamin called "suproxin." Some of the participants who received epinephrine were informed that the shot would trigger effects characteristic of sympathetic arousal, others were misinformed about the effects and were told that they'd have side effects like foot numbness, and others were told nothing at all. After the injection, they were told to wait with a research confederate who would act either really euphoric or really angry. During this time, their reactions were observed, and they were also asked to reflect on the experiment. The people who were not informed at all about the epinephrine experiment showed the strongest emotional reactions to the odd behavior of the research confederates, whereas those who were warned about experiencing symptoms of sympathetic arousal showed the lowest level of emotional reactions to the confederates, and those who were misinformed fell somewhere in between. From this finding, Schachter and Singer concluded that having an appropriate conceptual frame for physiological effects—that is, appraising them as having resulted from an injection—allowed subjects to handle their emotions more appropriately, whereas the subjects who were experiencing physiological effects without an appropriate conceptual frame had to find some cognitive context within which to work through those sensations, and this cognitive context was provided by the research confederates' unusual behavior.

The Schachter-Singer theory shares a deep commonality with the James-Lange theory in that both prioritize the physiological response relative to the conscious experience or labeling of an emotion. However, in the

> **MCAT STRATEGY > > >**
>
> The James-Lange theory is the simplest of the four theories tested on the MCAT, and is a reversal of our common-sense ideas. The Schachter-Singer theory adds contextual appraisal, and the Cannon-Bard theory is signaled by key terms like "simultaneous." The Lazarus theory includes "labeling."

Schachter-Singer theory, the contextual appraisal step is inherently linked to the physiological response. Recall the logic of the Schachter-Singer experiment: the epinephrine injection induced a certain physiological response, and then the researchers manipulated the conditions that influenced how subjects handled it. So in that sense, we can view the Schachter-Singer theory as being like the James-Lange theory, but with the extra baggage of contextual appraisal, and we can remember that idea through the fact that J comes before S, which reminds us that the James-Lange theory was modified by the Schachter-Singer theory.

IV. The Cannon-Bard Theory

The **Cannon-Bard theory** of emotion takes a different approach, and proposes that after a stimulus, the physiological response (elevated heart rate, etc.) and emotional response in the brain happen simultaneously and separately, and jointly lead to a cognitive response. The key words here are *simultaneous* and *separate*. If you encounter a question on the MCAT for which the Cannon-Bard theory is the correct answer, it's very likely that the question will use the word "simultaneous" or a synonymous phrase like "at the same time." So keep an eye out for that.

V. The Lazarus Theory

In contrast to the other theories, the **Lazarus theory** privileges a cognitive assessment of the entire situation. The idea is that we first label the situation that we're in as good or bad, and then experience a physiological response and a conscious emotion. The Lazarus theory is similar to the Schachter-Singer theory in that it emphasizes the active role of our cognition, and attempts to explain why different people have different emotional responses to things. The key difference is that in the Lazarus theory, the cognitive labeling comes first, whereas in the Schachter-Singer theory, contextual appraisal is tightly linked to the physiological response. Also, from a purely practical point of view, the MCAT tends to emphasize the Schachter-Singer theory more.

The key to successfully answering questions on theories of emotion is to be able to recognize the distinctive features of each theory that can be presented directly in a question stem. So let's quickly review with that in mind. James-Lange is the simplest of our theories, and it states that we experience emotions in the following order: stimulus, then physiological reaction, then emotion. The Schachter-Singer theory says that we have to add a contextual appraisal of the physiological response, and the Cannon-Bard theory says that the physiological reaction and conscious psychological experience of emotion happen separately and simultaneously. The Lazarus theory, finally, puts a cognitive labeling stage first. Carefully watching out for these diagnostic clues is the key to succeeding on questions dealing with this subject.

3. Stress

For many of us, stress in one form or another is a constant companion - and that generally does not stop being the case in medical school, residency, or even in clinical practice. The potential sources of stress, or stressors, in the world are myriad. On one hand, cataclysmic events, which are typically external and broad-scale, such as natural disasters, wars, epidemics, and the like, can be a massive source of stress for thousands, if not millions of people at a time. On the other hand, events in daily life can be stressors, including tasks like doing homework if you're a student, or commuting to and from work and school. Events and transitions in one's personal life can also be sources of stress. Examples might include starting or ending a relationship, or a new job, or graduating from college and figuring out what comes next, and so on. Broad categories like those can be useful for organizing our thinking about stressors, but another important distinction can be drawn between **independent stressors** and **dependent stressors**. Independent stressors are outside of our control. Cataclysmic events would be an example, as would things like unexpected illnesses, random-seeming layoffs from work, and getting into a car accident through no fault of one's own. Dependent stressors, in contrast, are those that are impacted by our own behaviors and to some extent are therefore within our control. Although control is a pretty vague concept, and one that can be extensively and productively debated in the context of psychological and behavioral disorders, but the distinction between dependent and independent stressors is of interest in terms of assessing people's motivation and coping strategies.

Making choices can also be a source of stress, often because choices involve a conflict. The terms avoidance and approach have been used to describe such conflicts. This choice of terminology can seem a little bit random, but basically the idea is that we want to avoid bad options and we want to approach good ones. Therefore, an **avoidance-avoidance conflict** is one where we have to choose between two bad options. So, depending on where you wind up going to med school, an example from your future might be the choice between going to a boring mandatory wellness seminar at 8 am or having the school's administration yell at you about professionalism violations. An **approach-approach conflict** involves choosing between two good options. An **approach-avoidance conflict** is one where you're dealing with a decision that has both upsides and downsides, and a **double approach-avoidance conflict** is one where you're choosing between two options that each have upsides and downsides.

Now, in order for a stressor to be a stressor, we have to perceive it as such. However, discrepancies exist in the degree to which certain things stress people out. This points us to a process known as **stress appraisal**. A distinction is made between **primary appraisal**, which refers to the process through which a person sees a certain event as a threat or a stressor, and **secondary appraisal**, which refers to a person's assessment of his or her ability to deal with that stressor.

Stress has a surprisingly broad range of psychological, emotional, behavioral, and even physical impacts. When thinking about the effects of stress, it's helpful to distinguish between distress, eustress, and neustress. **Distress** is basically a form of stress that has a negative effect on you; it's the default way we tend to think about stress, but it's worth distinguishing distress as a specific concept in contrast to **eustress**, which refers to positive stress. Positive stress might initially seem like sort of a surprising concept, but there are some situations where stress brings out the best in us. Think, for example, of an athlete playing in a big game. That's definitely stressful, but if all goes well, it's still ultimately a positive and productive experience. Furthermore, since stress can refer very broadly to any kind of life transition, eustress is also sometimes defined as including major changes like employment, graduating school, or marriage. Finally, sometimes a third type of stress is defined: **neustress**, or neutral stress. This refers to stressors that don't have much of an impact on you one way or the other, or that you perceive as neutral or inconsequential.

General adaptation syndrome is a concept developed around 1950 to integrate the various findings that were being discovered at that time regarding how the body responds to stress. According to this framework, the initial response to stress is alarm, a stage in which the sympathetic nervous system becomes activated to marshal the fight-or-flight response needed to deal with an acute stressor. As stress persists, the body shifts over to resistance, a stage mediated by the steroid hormone cortisol, which is responsible for the chronic stress response. Eventually, the body's resources will be drained, resulting in exhaustion, at which point the body becomes more vulnerable to the long-term negative side effects of stress, such as an increased susceptibility to illness, fatigue, and other medical conditions. The most well-known negative impacts of chronic stress on the body include elevated blood glucose and blood sugar levels, with a concomitant higher risk of cardiovascular disease, as well as impairment of the immune system. Additional impacts include reduced fertility and a greater risk of developing psychological conditions such as depression. Of note, the wide-ranging effects of chronic stress have caused stress to emerge as a topic of particular interest among researchers investigating socioeconomic disparities in health, since chronic stress may serve as a mediating variable for observed relationships between lower socioeconomic status and higher rates of negative health outcomes.

Repeated exposure to stressors that one is unable to change or avoid can lead to a phenomenon known as **learned helplessness**. A common example from animal experiments is that if an animal continually receives an electric shock upon trying to escape its enclosure, it will eventually stop even trying. Learned helplessness is also a highly relevant response pattern in human beings, and it has received attention for potential links to psychiatric conditions such as depression.

CHAPTER 6: EMOTION, STRESS, MEMORY, AND LEARNING

There are a wide range of coping strategies that people can employ to manage stress. Some are healthier and more productive than others. Maladaptive strategies can include substance abuse; verbal, emotional, and even physical aggression; self-harm; and status-seeking as a way to compensate for stressors. We should be clear that maladaptive stress responses aren't necessarily a conscious choice on people's behalf; instead, the persistence of maladaptive stress responses both within an individual and across generations is a thought-provoking example of the complex ways in which conditioned and observational learning can shape people's habits both in good ways and in bad. In contrast, practices such as meditation and exercise are more adaptive responses to stress, both because they have positive psychological and physical outcomes in general, and because the impacts of meditation and exercise include increased resilience towards stress. Of course, whether we assess a stress management technique as adaptive or maladaptive depends on a more holistic understanding of a person's psychological context. For example, although we generally would consider exercise to be an adaptive response to stress, it can also be the case that unhealthy amounts of exercise can be incorporated into an eating disorder. As always, context matters.

> **MCAT STRATEGY > > >**
>
> Because patterns in the assessment and response to stress can vary considerably across people and even within a person depending on the circumstances, whenever stress is tested on the MCAT, be sure to pay close attention to context clues! Also, hopefully the terms we discuss here will broaden your conceptual toolkit for understanding what you're going through in terms of MCAT stress.

4. Memory: Encoding and Storage

The ability to remember information about our surroundings is a prerequisite for being able to apply cognitive processes to reason about that information. There are multiple stages of how memories are processed in our mind, starting with encoding and storage.

I. Encoding

Before we can store a memory, we have to have something to store. This is where **encoding** comes in. As we mentioned in our discussion of attention, we can process environmental input either automatically or in a controlled, more deliberate way. Regardless, the perceptual processes of our nervous system mediate that processing, so that sensory input is transformed into an object of sorts that we can store or perform cognitive operations on. This latter process is encoding. For instance, we can use visual encoding to generate an image of an object, auditory encoding to store information about how something sounds, semantic encoding to encapsulate meaningful information about a stimulus, and so on.

Several techniques, some that we deploy consciously and some that we deploy unconsciously, can affect the ease with which information is encoded. For example, **priming**—which can be either positive or negative—refers to the effects of context on our ability to perceive subsequent stimuli. In a word-recognition task, previous exposure to stimuli related to medicine might increase the speed with which a participant recognizes words like "doctor" or "nurse" relative to words related to other topics. **Negative priming** occurs when a stimulus inhibits the processing of subsequent stimuli. For instance, consider the **Stroop task**, in which the task is to identify the color that is used to write a word depicting another color, so that if you see the word "yellow" written in red text, your task is to say "red." This is obviously a challenging task. But now consider a variation where the word "yellow" written in red is followed by the word "black" written in yellow, followed by "blue" written in black, and so on, such that the color stimulus that is ignored in one stage is the one that has to be produced in the next step. Many people find this to be even more difficult, because in any given step you have to produce the color stimulus that was suppressed just beforehand. This is an example of negative priming.

Chunking is another technique that can be used to promote encoding. In this process, a complex stimulus is broken down into multiple small, more meaningful components that are easier to encode. For instance, this technique is often used with phone numbers: a linear sequence of ten numbers—say, 5, 1, 0, 8, 6, 7, 5, 3, 0, 9—is much easier to remember if you break it down into 510-867-5309. Chunking can be deliberately used as a study technique, which brings to the topic of mnemonics in general.

Mnemonics, like the phrase "SNoW DRoP" for Southern, northern, and western blotting involving DNA, RNA, and protein respectively, are most fundamentally tricks to help with encoding. Relatedly, the **method of loci** can be used as a way to encode information by mentally mapping it onto an imagined space, with multiple rooms, hallways, and so on. The method of loci is used by professional memorizers, like people who compete to see who can memorize the most digits of pi. Regarding the deliberate use of various techniques to assist in encoding information, it's also worth noting that psychological arousal restricts our focus of attention. This can be a good thing or a bad thing; it's something we can leverage by using the sense of urgency of an upcoming exam to focus on the material we need to study and tune out other distractors, but it can be a bad thing if negative forms of arousal cause us to procrastinate unproductively, or if we're so focused on something that we miss a stimulus that would really be useful. This hypothesis is particularly associated with the work of a psychologist named **J. A. Easterbrook**.

II. Storage

Once we've encoded input, it can be stored in memory. There are multiple different types of memory, and the blizzard of associated terminology can be a challenge for students. So much like we've done with other complex topics with detailed terminology, let's start by focusing on the main divisions of memory, and then fill in the rest of the picture with narrower divisions and terminological distinctions.

The highest-level classification of memory separates it into three categories according to duration: sensory memory, short-term memory or working memory, and long-term memory. **Sensory memory** is virtually instantaneous; the idea here is that in any given moment in time, we're taking in and temporarily storing a vast amount of information that will decay very quickly, on the order of seconds, without **rehearsal**, or a conscious decision to pay attention or to reinforce the memory. **Long-term memory** is, as the name suggests, long-term -- on a scale ranging from hours to years. Of note, there's not thought to be any particular limit on the number of items that we can store in long-term memory. Short-term and working memory are two separate concepts that are a little bit trickier to define, both in terms of their exact duration and what they involve. However, we can roughly think of them as operating on a scale of tens of seconds to minutes. **Short-term memory** describes our ability to store information on that time scale, and it's generally thought to have a relatively small capacity. The traditional guideline to describe the limits of short-term memory storage is the 7 ± 2 rule, which states that we can generally hold roughly 5 to 9 items in our short-term memory. **Working memory**, instead, focuses more on the cognitive and attentional processes that we use to perform mental operations on information that we're holding in our short-term memory. Working memory is thought to draw on a capacity known as the visuospatial sketchpad, which describes a buffer of sorts that is used to hold onto visual and spatial information as it is processed by working memory.

Within this basic framework, psychologists have identified several distinct subtypes of memory. The following main types of long-term memory can be distinguished: semantic memory or explicit memory, procedural memory or implicit memory, and episodic memory. **Semantic memory**, also known as **explicit and declarative memory,** refers to memory of specific pieces of information. The presence of several distinct names for this concept can be frustrating, but the key idea here is that this is the kind of memory that would pay dividends on a trivia night. Again, the focus is information. In contrast, **procedural memory**, also known as **implicit memory**, refers to the memory of how to do something. Riding a bicycle is a great example of this contrast, in that memories of how to ride a bicycle may be very persistent, but it might be difficult or outright impossible to state in explicit terms how to do so.

Episodic memory, instead, relates to our memory of experiences. Distinguishing among these types of memory is both useful from a broad conceptual perspective and for interpreting symptoms in patients with memory disorders.

A couple other types of memory are worth noting, although they don't quite rise to the same level of conceptual significance as the ones we've previously discussed. A so-called **flashbulb memory** refers to the phenomenon that many of us have experienced of having an extremely vivid and detailed memory of important moments in our lives, either positive or negative ones. The metaphor here is from photography; it's like the flash of a camera goes off and imprints all the details of a consequential moment in our mind. **Eidetic memory** (also called photographic memory) is a somewhat similar idea, but it's more focused on information recall and less associated with strong emotional experiences. It refers to the ability to remember a stimulus in great detail after a relatively short exposure. Claims regarding eidetic memory are quite common, and strong evidence supporting it is highly elusive, although individual variation certainly does exist in terms of memory storage. In any case, it's mostly worth being aware of for our purposes just so that you're not taken aback if you encounter it as a term. **Iconic memory** refers to how a highly-detailed visual image can remain in our perception for a brief period of time—on the order of a second or so—after the stimulus itself is removed or changed. Finally, **prospective memory** refers to memories related to plans to do something in the future.

Even leaving the biological aspect of memory storage aside for the time being, our memory doesn't just work by storing an unstructured blob of random facts, procedures, and experiences. Instead, our memories and knowledge are thought to be organized in semantic networks. For example, a rocking chair (or any other type of chair) might be linked back to the more general category of "chair," which itself can be linked back to the even more general category of "furniture," which would also contain things like beds and couches, and furniture could in turn be related back to the general category of "stuff." Such a network is hierarchical, in that we proceed from most specific to most general, and there does exist some evidence suggesting that hierarchical networks are a good model for at least some aspects of knowledge storage. However, a sort of linear, top-down approach doesn't capture everything, because we also have to account for metaphorical or emotional associations, like how a rat is an example of a mammal, but also has negative connotations, and can even be used as a slang term for someone who provides incriminating information to authorities. As such, we might imagine that the concept of "rat" is present in, or at least adjacent to, multiple overlapping conceptual networks. The concept of **spreading activation** suggests that when a concept is brought to mind, activation spreads across adjacent nodes of a conceptual network. For instance, activating the concept of a bright yellow school bus might prime us to think about categories like yellow things, vehicles, children, and schools. The semantic content of these conceptual networks is sometimes referred to as **schemas**, a general term used for ways in which we organize our knowledge and perceptions about the world.

This concept can also help explain the phenomenon of **source monitoring errors**, which occur when we have a memory or piece of knowledge that is, in and of itself, perfectly correct, but for which we misattribute the source. For instance, we might remember that we heard a piece of news from a friend, when we in fact heard it from a family member, or we might incorrectly assume that a familiar name is a figure from history, whereas in fact it refers to a character in a famous novel.

6. Memory Retrieval and Loss

I. Retrieval

Once we have memories and knowledge stored in our head, they're not of much value to us unless we use them. The process of calling upon our memories and stored knowledge is known as **retrieval**. An important distinction needs to be made here between **recall**, which is an active process, and **recognition**, which is a passive process. That is, being asked to name the enzyme that catalyzes the rate-limiting step of glycolysis would require recall, whereas being able to recognize that phosphofructokinase is that enzyme would require recognition. Generally speaking, recognition is thought to be easier than recall, in that it requires shallower knowledge and less active mastery. As we discussed earlier, our memories are stored in semantic networks or schemas. Interestingly, speed and accuracy in recall and recognition tasks can be used to probe those schemas, as **semantic activation** primes us to more quickly retrieve concepts that are adjacent to already-activated concepts.

Several factors can favor or disfavor the recall of various items. Numerous experiments have investigated the recall of items on a list, and it's been found that people are more likely to recall items at the beginning of a list than they are to recall items in the middle of the list. This phenomenon is known as the **primacy effect**. Likewise, items at the end of a list are more likely to be remembered than those in the middle, which is known as the **recency effect**. The term **serial position effect** unites these two observations by pointing out that, in general, the extreme ends of a list are more favorable than the middle of a list in terms of promoting recall. The **spacing effect** describes how we are more effective at recalling information when our learning process is spaced out than when we try to learn everything in one big rush. This is why cram sessions are ineffective, and why spaced repetition is built into your study plan for the MCAT. Another principle at the heart of effective studying is the **dual-coding effect**, which proposes that studying multiple modalities—like visual learning and text-based learning—is more effective than using a single modality because our brain codes visual, auditory, and semantic representations separately.

Somewhat surprisingly, emotions can also affect memory retrieval. To some extent, this is linked to the effect of strong emotions on memory storage, in that emotionally intense memories are generally more likely to be stored. However, this effect can also take place on the retrieval level, in two ways. First, being in a certain mood might favor the recollection of memories with similar emotional overtone; for instance, being in a happy mood might favor the recall of good times, and being in a depressed or anxious state might promote the recall of negatively tinged memories. Second, interestingly, a state-dependent effect can exist in which being in a certain mood might promote the recall of memories—even those that are neutral in and of themselves—that were encoded when you were in a similar mood. To make this more intuitive, imagine getting angry and remembering events that happened, or information you learned, a previous time you were angry. Interestingly, the more general phenomenon of **state-dependent memory** can also apply to states of consciousness induced by psychoactive substances. The evidence for state-dependent learning in rodent models is quite strong. Similarly, recall can be context-dependent, in that being in the same physical setting where a memory was encoded and stored can promote its recall.

An effect specific to episodic memory is the **misinformation effect**, in which information that we subsequently obtain can affect how we remember an event. For instance, if you learn something really bad about someone who you previously had a decent relationship with, you might then recollect interactions with them through that light; as an example, you might remember those interactions as being more tense and emotionally negative than they actually were at the time. More seriously, from the point of view of the criminal justice system, the misinformation effect helps explain ways in which witnesses can be biased. After learning that someone is a criminal, or even that someone has been arrested, a victim of a crime might be more likely to remember the event as involving that specific person.

This brings us to an important insight: memory is an active process. **Reproductive memory**—or a model in which we encode information and then reproduce it as needed, much like how we might look something up on a computer's hard drive—is an insufficient model that is at best an oversimplification of how memory works. Instead, to a great extent, memory is **reconstructive**; that is, we build our memories based on our perceptions of ourselves and others, information that we have about the context of events, and so on. This is a factor that can drive the formation of false memories, and is a reason why care is needed when debriefing witnesses about sensitive acts or potential crimes. The essence of the insight here, as disturbing as it may be, is that false memories are often not acts of deliberate deception; instead, even our most sincerely held memories may be, to a non-trivial extent, the product of **cognitive reconstruction** rather than a simple recording or reproduction.

CHAPTER 6: EMOTION, STRESS, MEMORY, AND LEARNING

II. Memory Loss

Another fact about memories is that they can be lost. In fact, forgetting things that we learn is inevitable. However, research has found that the process of re-learning things is faster than learning them the first time, and that each successive round of re-learning leads to less forgetting. This dynamic is familiar to anyone who's struggled through glycolysis and the citric acid multiple times -- but hopefully, learning it for the MCAT will go more quickly than learning it for, say, high school biology classes. The **Ebbinghaus forgetting curve** formalizes the insight that forgetting is a fact of life, but repeated rounds of learning cause the forgetting process to slow down and for more information to be consolidated into longer-term memory.

What's more, memories and pieces of knowledge can enter into conflict with each other. This process is known as **interference**, and it can be either proactive or retroactive. In **proactive interference**, older memories inhibit the consolidation or retrieval of new memories. That is, if you're set in your ways about how to perform a certain task, those old memories might get in the way of learning how to do things a different way. In other words, this is the "you can't teach an old dog new tricks" syndrome. In contrast, in **retroactive interference**, new memories or knowledge interfere with older knowledge. For example, if you become skilled at playing a new version of a video game, with a new interface and new controls, it might be difficult to play the old version, even though you were once good at it. In a nutshell, proactive amnesia is forward-looking, and retrograde amnesia is backward-looking.

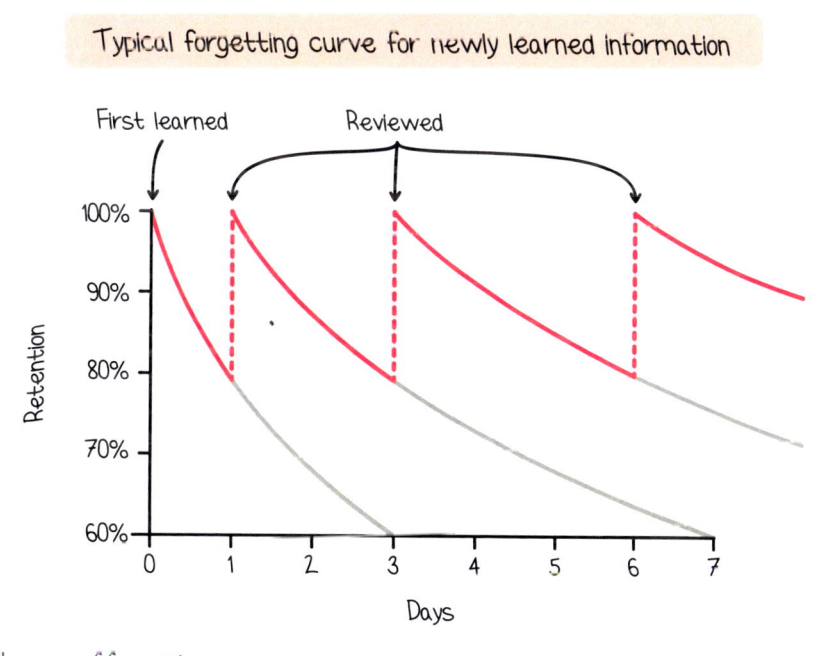

Figure 2. Ebbinghaus' curve of forgetting.

Amnesia refers to more generalized processes of memory loss: not losing isolated bits of information, but losing memories of entire experiences, periods of time, and/or broad swaths of information. Much like with interference, we can distinguish between backward-facing and forward-facing types of amnesia. **Retrograde amnesia** describes the inability to remember previous events, and **anterograde amnesia** refers to the inability to form new memories.

There are two disorders related to amnesia that are important for the MCAT: **Alzheimer's disease** and **Korsakoff's syndrome**. Alzheimer's disease is more familiar, so we can start there. Alzheimer's disease is thought to be responsible for a majority of long-term cases of dementia in the United States, although its definitive diagnosis can only be established by examining brain tissue, which is not always performed. Its underlying causes have not been fully elucidated, but neurofibrillary tangles involving tau proteins and plaques formed of beta-amyloid proteins are characteristic of the disease. The early manifestations of Alzheimer's disease involve forgetfulness and short-term memory loss, but the disease progresses to involve more severe anterograde and retrograde amnesia, as well as cognitive deficits, difficulties thinking and speaking, and emotional disturbances. Patients with late-stage Alzheimer's disease require around-the-clock care and experience extreme limitations in interacting with other people, as well as intense physical deterioration. There is no known cure for Alzheimer's, and no established preventive measures. Alzheimer's disease remains among the top focuses of ongoing scientific and clinical research.

Korsakoff's syndrome is a distinct disease that also causes anterograde and retrograde amnesia, but is also marked by a tendency for confabulation, or elaborate fictional stories. In contrast to Alzheimer's disease, which remains largely mysterious in terms of underlying causes, prevention, and treatment strategies, the biochemical basis of Korsakoff's syndrome is simple: it is caused by a deficiency of thiamine, or vitamin B1. As such, Korsakoff's syndrome is caused by nutritional deficiencies; it was first discovered in severe alcoholics, and has also been observed in people with eating disorders or who are malnourished for any other reason. Since Korsakoff's syndrome is caused by a vitamin deficiency, it is considered to be a preventable disease, and intense administration of large amounts of thiamine is the primary treatment strategy.

> **MCAT STRATEGY > > >**
>
> Make a careful note of diseases and clinical conditions that are mentioned here; they are common fodder for MCAT questions.

Perhaps partially due to the prevalence of Alzheimer's disease, the perception exists that memory loss is an inherent part of aging. That's not quite true. Aging does tend to reduce fluid intelligence, as we discuss elsewhere, and it likewise does reduce the pace of acquiring new declarative knowledge. However, aging in and of itself does not cause the loss of previously-acquired semantic knowledge, or impair the ability to deploy crystallized intelligence.

As a final point, it's worth noting and reflecting upon the fact that so far we've been treating memory as a purely psychological phenomenon, with minimal to no reference to its biological basis. Yet, after all, the brain is a biological machine. To a great extent, that's because the biological underpinnings of memory are quite complicated and incompletely understood. That said, there are a few general points about the biology of memory that we should make. Perhaps the most crucial principle is that the mechanism underlying memory and learning is thought to be the development and evolution of synaptic connections. This can involve the formation of such connections, but also the strengthening and reinforcement of connections, and even the pruning or loss of those connections. Losing synaptic connections may sound like a bad thing, but it's not necessarily that simple. Synaptic pruning is an important stage in early childhood development, and it has been proposed that insufficient synaptic pruning may be a factor implicated in the development of conditions such as autism.

The changeability of synaptic connections is the primary driver of **neuroplasticity**, or the ability of the brain to rewire itself in response to learning new information or to compensate for disease or injury. Increasingly, findings are supporting the importance of neuroplasticity of a contributor to lifelong learning and as a source of functional resilience in individuals affected by brain injuries or pathologies. However, it's worth noting that what we termed lifelong learning can manifest both in the formation of new connections and in the solidification of previously existing patterns through the long-term potentiation, which is the strengthening and reinforcement of synaptic connections. Much remains to be learned about neuroplasticity, but it's undeniable that the biological basis of memory is remarkably intricate.

7. Classical Conditioning

"Learning" on the MCAT tends to focus on ways that animals and humans can be trained to exhibit certain behaviors, namely **associative learning**. In this discussion, we'll focus on a learning paradigm that psychologists started exploring around the end of the 1800s and beginning of the 1900s. This paradigm is known as **classical conditioning**, basically because it's the "classic version", so to speak, of psychological research into conditioning.

Classical conditioning was launched by a Russian psychologist named **Ivan Pavlov**, who had some dogs. You may have learned about Pavlov's dogs before, but even if that's the case, hang tight and don't skip ahead; it's worth reviewing, both because misconceptions about this experiment are common and because it provides a fantastic illustration of these ideas. Pavlov was primarily a physiologist, and his main area of research was gastrointestinal physiology. He was researching salivation in dogs, and noticed that they started salivating before food hit their mouths. That spurred him to look into the behavior of salivation more closely. Now, unsurprisingly, it turned out that the dogs salivated in response to the smell of meat. But Pavlov's genius is that he didn't stop there: he also wondered about what other stimuli could trigger the salivary response.

Pavlov paired the stimulus of tasty-smelling meat with a metronome, a device that produces a rhythmic beat. Sometimes you might hear about Pavlov using bells instead; that's historically less accurate, but it doesn't really matter from our point of view. In any case, the dogs would smell the meat and hear the metronome, and would salivate. Eventually, just the sound of the metronome would be enough to induce salivation. That is, the dogs had learned to associate the metronome with delicious meat, and therefore salivated in response to the metronome. This experiment is so familiar that it's easy to take it for granted, so let's pause, recognize what's so important about this experiment, and then use it to introduce some important terminology.

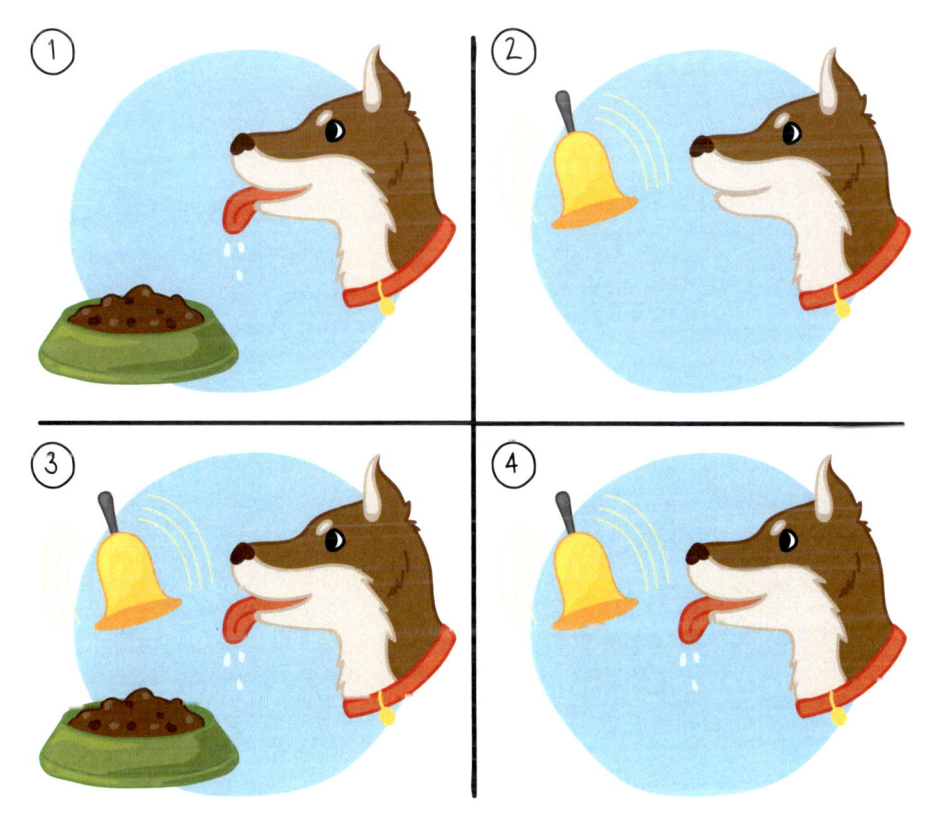

Figure 3. Classical conditioning of Pavlov's dogs.

Broadly speaking, you can divide the great experiments in science into two categories: those that discover a new fact or phenomenon, and those that shed light onto previously unknown mechanisms that underlie familiar behavior. Pavlov's experiment falls firmly into the second category. People have known for literally thousands of years that dogs can like food and get excited for it -- put Pavlov nailed down the mechanism, or at least a mechanism, through which the learning around this process happens.

The baseline response of a dog is to salivate when it smells meat. That's just something dogs do. It is the natural state of a dog. For this reason, in Pavlov's experiment, the smell of meat is an example of an **unconditioned stimulus**, and the initial response of salivating is an **unconditioned response**. The term unconditioned means that it just sort of *is*, like a reflex. At the start of Pavlov's experiment, the metronome—or bell, if you prefer that version—is termed a **neutral stimulus**, because it's just some random thing that the dogs don't care about and doesn't elicit any particular response. Through repeated pairing with the smell of meat, though, conditioning happens. The term **acquisition** is used to refer to successful conditioning. Once the dogs have learned to associate the sound of the metronome with meat, the metronome becomes a **conditioned stimulus**, and salivation becomes a **conditioned response**.

MCAT STRATEGY > > >

Variable ratio is how slot machines pay out at casinos. Casino owners want people to keep playing as long as possible.

Now, here's a question: what term would we apply to salivation in Pavlov's experiment? Think about this for a second. It's a tricky question, because we used salivation as an example of an unconditioned response, when paired with the smell of meat, and as an example of a conditioned response, when paired with the metronome after the conditioning process. Therefore, framing the question that way isn't really the right way to look at it. Instead, we need to look at pairings of a stimulus and response. In other words, determining whether a response is conditioned or unconditioned requires looking at the context of what provokes the response. Another way to understand the process of acquisition is that the whole point of classical conditioning is to transform an unconditioned response into a conditioned response.

Now, nothing is forever, right? And learning *definitely* isn't forever. If you keep stimulating the dogs with the metronome without providing any meat, they'll eventually stop salivating in response. This is known as **extinction** in the framework of classical learning, and it's linked to the broader phenomenon of **habituation**, which refers to the fact that repeated stimuli elicit a diminished response over time. For example, you know how if you walk into a kitchen where someone's cooking some tasty food, it'll smell really good, but you'll stop noticing the smell after a few minutes? That's habituation in action. Then if you step away for a second to get some fresh air and enter the kitchen again, you'll probably notice the smell again, although not necessarily quite as intensely as you did at first. This process, in which an intervening stimulus causes you to become re-sensitized to the original stimulus, is called **dishabituation**.

This covers the core concepts of classical conditioning, but there are a few other terms that we should add to our toolkit to prepare for any questions on this topic. First off, extinction of a conditioned response isn't necessarily the end of the story. Under some circumstances, the conditioned response can re-emerge without requiring a separate conditioning process; this phenomenon is known, reasonably enough, as **spontaneous recovery**. That said, when spontaneous recovery occurs, the conditioned response tends to be less strong, an effect that gets amplified as more cycles of extinction and recovery repeat.

Another interesting fact about classical conditioning is that under some circumstances, a conditioned stimulus similar to—but not exactly the same as—the original conditioned stimulus can also elicit a conditioned response. For example, if Pavlov's dogs were trained with a metronome that produced a steady beat, maybe they would also salivate in response to rhythmic, regular ringing of a bell or tapping of fingers. This phenomenon is known as **stimulus generalization**, because, it involves generalizing the properties of a specific stimulus to include other,

CHAPTER 6: EMOTION, STRESS, MEMORY, AND LEARNING

similar ones. The opposite of stimulus generalization is responding selectively to only one or a very limited range of stimuli, which is known as **discrimination**.

Classical conditioning is often somewhat challenging for students, both because of the relatively large amount of specific terminology, and because—as we'll see below—it's necessary to keep classical conditioning separate from the related, but crucially distinct, phenomenon of operant conditioning. One should always keep in mind that the defining purpose of classical conditioning is to shift an unconditioned response to a conditioned response, and that the learner has not learned to perform some specific behavior to get a reward.

8. Operant Conditioning

Classical conditioning is limited to specific stimulus-response relationships, and doesn't really give us a toolkit for incentivizing someone to do something more or less frequently or to even create a distinct, complex behavior. That's where **operant conditioning** comes in, which is strongly associated with the mid-20th century psychologist B. F. Skinner, who pioneered a paradigm known as behaviorism in which psychology is studied through the lens of observable behavior, rather than trying to guess at internal states.

The key concept of operant conditioning is **reward**, which sharply distinguishes it from classical conditioning. These rewards are known as **reinforcers**, and somewhat tautologically, reinforcement is defined as anything that increases the frequency of behavior. Conversely, **punishment** is defined as anything that decreases behavior. An additional set of adjectives we can put before either of these terms is **positive** or **negative**, where these words don't refer at all to the subjective quality of good or bad, but instead to whether something was added or removed.

MCAT STRATEGY > > >

The contrasts between reinforcement and punishment and between negative and positive make up a natural 2-by-2 conceptual matrix, so it's as if this topic was designed for multiple-choice questions. indeed, asking you to characterize a reinforcer in these terms is a classic MCAT question.

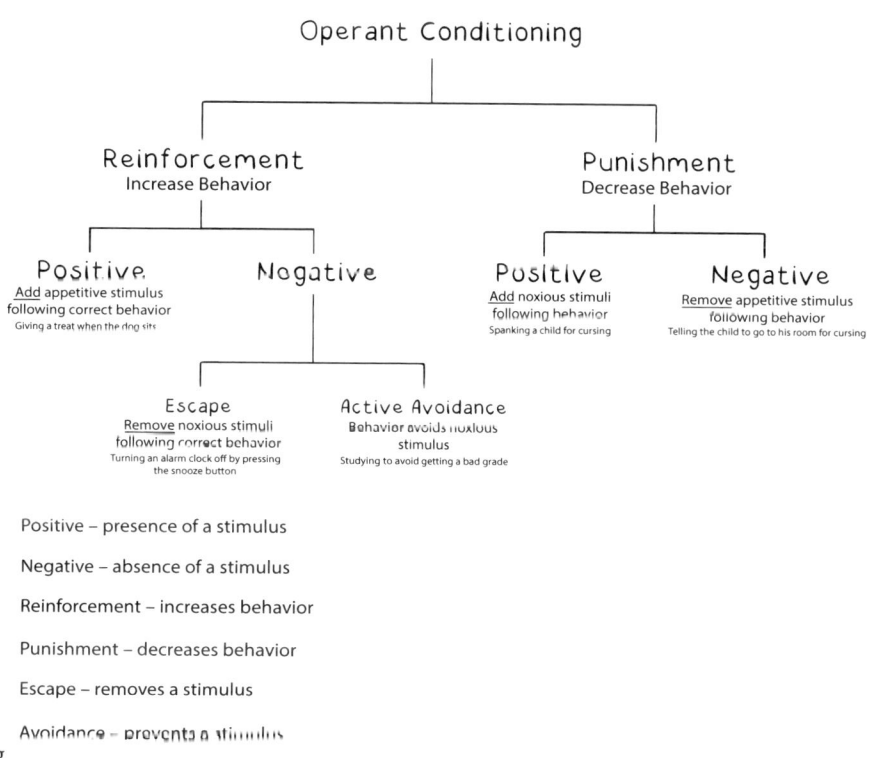

Operant Conditioning

- Reinforcement — Increase Behavior
  - Positive: Add appetitive stimulus following correct behavior. Giving a treat when the dog sits
  - Negative
    - Escape: Remove noxious stimuli following correct behavior. Turning an alarm clock off by pressing the snooze button
    - Active Avoidance: Behavior avoids noxious stimulus. Studying to avoid getting a bad grade
- Punishment — Decrease Behavior
  - Positive: Add noxious stimuli following behavior. Spanking a child for cursing
  - Negative: Remove appetitive stimulus following behavior. Telling the child to go to his room for cursing

Positive – presence of a stimulus
Negative – absence of a stimulus
Reinforcement – increases behavior
Punishment – decreases behavior
Escape – removes a stimulus
Avoidance – prevents a stimulus

Figure 4. Operant conditioning.

Let's dive into some examples: **Positive reinforcement** would mean administering a pleasant stimulus immediately after a behavior we would like to see increase, like giving an animal a treat as it exhibits a desired behavior, like touching the tip of your finger with its nose. **Positive punishment** means administering an aversive stimulus, or adding anything, that decreases behavior. For example, in the past, if children showed signs of nail-biting, their nails would be coated with a harmless but foul-tasting material so that biting their fingernails would immediately be followed by a highly unpleasant taste experience. Keep in mind that whether something is actually punishment depends entirely on the learner, and some children didn't mind the taste at all. Therefore, their behavior didn't decrease and they were by definition not punished. Conversely, intended rewards might not always be rewarding either, as some children might have disliked attention - and found attention from a teacher after solving a problem to be punishing, even if it was never intended to be. From a behaviorist perspective, intent is meaningless. **Negative punishment**, in contrast, would mean removing a pleasant stimulus right after a behavior occurs in order to decrease it, like how you might close your hand around a treat if a young puppy tries to nip at your hand instead of taking it gently. **Negative reinforcement** is taking away a stimulus in order to encourage a behavior; for this to make sense logically, the stimulus must be unpleasant, or aversive. A common example of this is hurrying to come out of the rain, or be done with math homework; in both cases, the aversive stimulus (being cold and wet, or having homework) encourages a behavior (running inside quickly, or sloppily hurrying through your homework).

> **MCAT STRATEGY > > >**
>
> It's really easy to mix up positive/negative reinforcement/punishment, especially in a stressful situation, like when taking the MCAT, mostly because we have a tendency to use "positive" and "negative" to mean "good" and "bad." Instead, try your best to think of "positive" and "negative" in this context as having a mathematical meaning, like plus and minus. That is, you add a stimulus or subtract one.

An important distinction is also made between escape learning and avoidance learning. **Escape learning** involves a behavior aimed to terminate an aversive or unpleasant stimulus. The example that we gave of physically getting out the rain to stop being wet, cold and uncomfortable and having your phone short out is one such case. **Avoidance learning**, instead, as the name implies, refers to a behavior that is intended to prevent an aversive stimulus from ever even happening. So, for instance, a child might clean his or her room to avoid getting in trouble, or a cat might avoid hot pavement.

We can also tweak the regularity with which we provide rewards. This is known as a **schedule of reinforcement**. One option would be to provide reinforcement every time the target behavior is performed. This is known as **continuous reinforcement**. Although continuous reinforcement is extremely effective, especially in the early stages of the acquisition process, but from a real-world point of view, it's not always practical in terms of resources. The other option is to pick one of many partial reinforcement strategies-- that is, reinforcement is applied in a subset of cases in which the target behavior occurs. **Partial reinforcement** can be structured according to ratios, depending on how many instances of the behavior have occurred, or on time intervals.

Fixed and variable schedules can also be used. Thus, we have another 2 x 2 structure that generates four options: **fixed ratio, variable ratio, fixed interval,** and **variable interval**. So, an example of a fixed ratio schedule would be if a rat was given a food pellet every four times that it pushed a lever. A variable ratio schedule would instead give the rat a food pellet somewhere between every two to eight times it pushed a lever. The precise upper and lower bounds don't really matter; the crucial point is that the ratio should vary unpredictably within a roughly similar range. A fixed interval schedule would involve giving a reinforcement for the behavior after a certain time elapses, and a variable interval schedule would provide reinforcement for the behavior after an unpredictable amount of time passes. Generally speaking, variable schedules tend to be more effective than fixed schedules, and ratios tend to be more effective than intervals, so a variable-ratio reinforcement schedule will lead to the largest increase in the frequency of the behavior and is most resistant to extinction. Not coincidentally, this is precisely the reinforcement schedule that casinos deploy with slot machines.

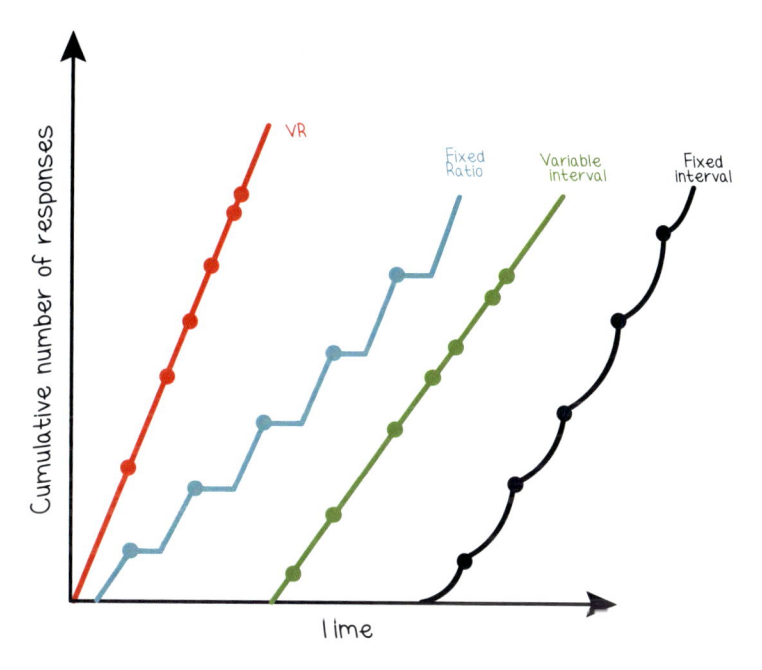

Figure 5. Types of reinforcement schedules (VR: variable-ratio; FR: fixed-ratio; VI: variable interval; FI: fixed-interval).

For the most part, you should try to keep classical conditioning and operant conditioning separate in your head. An interesting point of overlap occurs because classical conditioning can be used as a tool within operant conditioning. The idea here is to take a primary reinforcer—that is, something that an organism responds to naturally, like how an animal might respond to food or a person might respond to a small reward—and use the principles of classical conditioning to associate that primary reinforcer with another stimulus that is originally neutral, like a clicker in animal training or cute little tokens or points with humans. Once associated with a favorable response, this new stimulus is referred to as a conditioned stimulus. In humans, these systems can even be further developed into a structure known as a **token economy**, in which these tokens can be accumulated and exchanged for a reward that triggers a more direct response, to the point that it could be suitable as a primary reinforcer. So, for instance, imagine that an elementary student gets a point or a sticker every day he or she completes a task successfully, and then gets to exchange ten stickers for a lollipop. This example serves to convey the basic point, although of course, these systems can get more complicated -- to the point that you might wonder what the difference actually is between the token economy and the actual economy that uses currency. .

A few additional factors complicate the process of operant conditioning. Researchers quickly figured out that operant conditioning can be used to train subjects—including both animals and people—to perform pretty complex behaviors. But especially in the context of animal training, that doesn't happen immediately. For example, it's possible to do things like train dolphins to leap out of the water and go through a hoop. Now, how does that work? Dolphins either don't speak English, or any other human language (or if they do, they've kept it a secret!). So we can't just go up to a dolphin and ask them politely to jump through a hoop. The strategy of just waiting for a dolphin to spontaneously jump through a hoop and then rewarding it, a process called capturing, is also probably not going to pay off, unless you have ample time on your hands. The solution, then, is to use a technique called **shaping**, in which progressive approximations of a target behavior are rewarded.

What's more, it turns out that learning isn't necessarily limited to the specific behavior that is incentivized or disincentivized. **Latent learning** describes a form of non-associative learning in which a subject learns something that's kind of in the background of the experimental design. The key experiments on this topic had to do with rats in mazes; for instance, in one experiment, rats were divided into three groups. One group was placed into a maze with food at the end, one group was placed into a maze but never received food, and the final group was placed into a maze with no food ten times, but on the eleventh time, there was indeed food at the end of the maze. Those rats very quickly learned to run to the end of the maze once there was food, indicating that during their previous seemingly aimless wandering around the maze, they had been building a mental map that they could use .

Just like with classical conditioning, the patterns instilled by operant conditioning aren't permanent. Extinction is a concern, and in particular, there's a tendency for animals to revert back to their instinctive behavior unless reinforcement continues. This phenomenon is known as **instinctive drift**. It's of practical relevance for anyone seriously engaged in the practice of operant conditioning, and it also underscores the fact that operant conditioning is, to some extent, a set of cognitive mappings that is overlaid on the basic biological underpinnings of behavior. That fact can also be utilized productively by choosing high value reinforcers and target behaviors that correspond relatively closely to an organism's behavioral predispositions. For instance, it would be much easier to use operant conditioning to teach a tiger a specific set of behaviors related to stalking and capturing prey using meat as a reinforcer than it would to try to deploy highly valuable one-on-one time with a celebrity as a reward to train a tiger to make funny faces. It's a silly example, but it does serve to illustrate the point that relatively hard-wired cognitive and biological factors play a role in associative learning, or are even the basis of most associative learning.

9. Observational Learning

There was a period in the mid-20th century where psychologists—most famously B. F. Skinner and his colleagues in the behaviorist framework—sought to really push the boundaries in terms of trying to explain as much human behavior as possible in terms of conditioning. And indeed, as we've discussed, the power of conditioning to shape a wide range of behaviors is remarkable, but it's also not the whole story; in particular, considerable evidence exists that learning happens through observation.

One of the key experiments establishing the importance of observational learning was conducted by **Alfred Bandura** in 1961. The experiment involved using so-called **Bobo dolls**, which had a low center of mass and a dense, rounded bottom component. This combination allowed them to pop right up after being knocked down. And indeed, this is what happened. Bandura set up an experiment where children get the chance to play with the Bobo dolls after watching an adult act aggressively or non-aggressively with them. The aggressive behavior was pretty gruesome -- adults would hit the Bobo doll in the face, smack it with a hammer, even yell out things like "kick him!", and so on. It turned out that the children who observed the aggressive play were much more likely to engage in aggressive play with the Bobo dolls themselves.

CHAPTER 6: EMOTION, STRESS, MEMORY, AND LEARNING

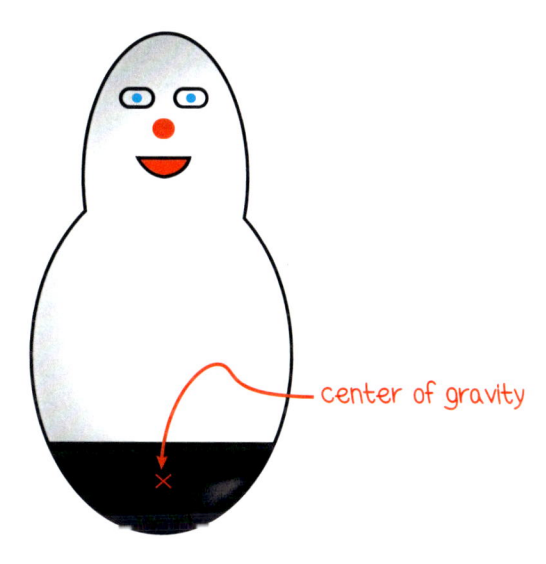

Figure 6. A diagram of the "Bobo Doll" used in Bandura's experiment.

Further experiments by Bandura, and other psychologists working in this field of research, have explored the difference between observational learning and the factors that influence someone to engage in a learned behavior. Carefully making this distinction is critical when attempting to apply the logic of observational learning to explain broader trends in society. For example, violence in television and video games has received a lot of attention in terms of its possible ability to normalize and even cultivate violent behavior. This suggested effect of violent media is rooted in the theories of observational learning—the parallels with Bandura's Bobo doll experiment are clear—but, at the same time, questions about the effects of media on their consumers are complicated by the general fact that society and human behavior are very complex phenomena and by findings indicating that whether someone engages in learned behavior is shaped by a variety of parameters, including motivation and socialization. Nonetheless, findings on observational learning support the importance of modeling as a way that behavior is transmitted, and the research literature increasingly indicates that observational learning and modeling take place at very young ages in infancy.

Imitation is a subtype of observational learning, but care should be taken not to view observational learning as simply imitative, for a couple of important reasons. First, the behaviors that someone picks up through observational learning don't have to match those of their model perfectly; instead, some variation is possible, reflecting the fact that people are independent agents capable of their own thoughts and of extrapolating their observations to their own specific context. Second, and more importantly, observational learning can be a source of lessons about what not to do. For instance, if you see your friend blow off studying for an exam, and then have negative consequences due to failing it, that can be a lesson for you not to make the same mistake. More broadly, our criminal justice system, in some sense, draws on this principle through the hope that legal penalties can serve as a deterrent. The effectiveness of this idea has been much debated, but for our purposes, it's worth noting the link between this big-picture social question and the psychological patterns explored in the Bobo doll experiment.

As researchers have accumulated evidence pointing to the critical role played by observational learning both in humans and in animals, increasing attention has been focused on the biological basis of observational learning. In the 1990s and early 2000s, scientists discovered a type of neuron that is activated both when an organism performs an action and when an organism observes an action being performed. These are known as **mirror neurons**, and they are strongly implicated as contributing to observational learning. Additionally, it's been proposed that mirror neurons contribute to empathy, or the ability to feel other people's emotions from their perspective. The ability to experience emotions vicariously (e.g., feeling sadness in response to another person's sadness) is also crucially linked to empathy. Nonetheless, a lot remains to be understood about the structural properties and functions of mirror neurons, so we can't quite consider them to be a closed case.

As we alluded to by mentioning that societal discussions about issues like whether exposure to violent media causes violent behavior draw on the principles of observational learning, it does seem to be the case that observational learning can have a powerful impact on individuals' behavior. A particularly relevant example for clinicians is how observational learning can lead to the replication of behavioral patterns within a family, with regard to both interpersonal relationships and health-related behaviors, such as patterns of diet, exercise, and self-care. As such, a basic understanding of the principles of observational learning will be a powerful element of your toolkit in your future career.

CHAPTER 6: EMOTION, STRESS, MEMORY, AND LEARNING

10. Must-Knows

- Jean Piaget introduced the idea of cognitive stages
  - Sensorimotor (0-2 years): lacking object permanence, circular reactions, stranger anxiety.
- Ekman's universal emotions: fear, anger, sadness, happiness, disgust, surprise, contempt (optional)
- Limbic system is associated with emotion (esp. amygdala [emotion processing] and hypothalamus [connects the CNS with the endocrine system]).
- Emotions have cognitive, physiological and behavioral components.
- Major theories of emotion:
  - James-Lange: stimulus > physiological response > emotion
  - Cannon-Bard: stimulus > simultaneous physiological and cognitive responses > emotion/behavior
  - Schachter-Singer: adds contextual appraisal to James-Lange
  - Lazarus: stimulus > labeling > physiological response > emotion
- Stressors: independent (we have no control over) vs. dependent (we have control over)
- Conflicts: avoidance-avoidance (two bad things), approach-approach (two good things), approach-avoidance conflict (one thing w/ pros and cons) and double approach-avoidance (two things w/ pros and cons)
- Stress can be divided into eustress (good), distress (bad), and neustress (neutral).
  - General adaptation syndrome: 3 stages of stress adaptation: alarm, resistance and exhaustion
  - Repeated exposure to unavoidable stressors causes learned helplessness
- Encoding (visual, auditory, semantic): transformation of sensory input into a cognitive object.
- Priming: in our response to subsequent stimuli based on prior ones; negative priming: prior stimulus inhibits the processing of a current one, such as in the Stroop task
- Chunking, mnemonics, and method of loci enhance learning.
- Memory systems can be ordered by the time spans which they retain information: instantaneous (sensory memory), brief (short-term memory and working memory) and life-long (long-term memory).
  - Visuospatial sketchpad is drawn on by working memory.
  - Memory can also be organized by content as semantic memory or explicit memory, procedural memory or implicit memory, and episodic memory (also cf. flashbulb, eidetic, iconic memory).
- Semantic networks store memory, retrieved through spreading activation.
- Source monitoring errors: accurate info, wrong source
- Non-associative learning encompasses habituation, dishabituation, sensitization, extinction, instinctual drift, imprinting, latent learning and observational learning; associative learning = conditioning
- Classical conditioning: unconditioned stimulus/response > conditioned stimulus/response (Pavlov's dogs)
- Operant conditioning: frequency of behavior is increased by reinforcement and decreased by punishment; positive = addition of a stimulus, negative = removal of a stimulus
- Reinforcement schedules: continuous, fixed ratio, fixed interval, variable ratio, and variable interval
- Conditioned stimulus = previously neutral stimulus paired with an unconditioned stimulus
- Shaping: rewarding progressive approximations of a target behavior; capturing: waiting around for a behavior to happen to reward
- Latent learning: background learning that happens and information gathered even when no rewards are present
- Extinction: the decrease in response over time in the absence of reinforcement, while instinctive drift refers to reversion to instinctive behavior
- Observational learning was famously studied in Alfred Bandura's Bobo doll experiment.
- Imitation is a subtype of observational learning.
- Mirror neurons are the putative biological basis of observational learning.

End of Chapter Practice

The best MCAT practice is **realistic**, with a focus on identifying steps for further improvement. For those reasons, we recommend completing practice questions in an online setting that simulates the real MCAT interface, and taking advantage of advanced analytic features to help you determine how best to move forward in your MCAT study journey.

With that in mind, **online end-of-chapter questions** are accessible through your Next Step account.

As a further supplement, given the importance of active learning for effective studying, we also suggest that you consult the Must-Knows as a basis for creating a study sheet, in which you list out key terms and test your ability to briefly summarize them.

This page left intentionally blank

This page left intentionally blank.

Motivation, Attitude, and Personality

CHAPTER 7

0. Introduction

While emotions and moods tend to be relatively short-lasting, the human psychological makeup includes more stable and longer-lasting features such as motivation, attitude, and personality. These concepts are often used similarly in everyday speech, but they're distinct from the point of view of psychology, as we'll explore in this chapter.

1. Motivation

We can define motivation as the underlying purpose for our actions. As we explore this topic in greater depth, we'll see that numerous explanations have been proposed for motivation, but a useful distinction to make at the start of this discussion is between intrinsic motivation and extrinsic motivation. In a nutshell, **intrinsic motivation** comes from inside oneself, and **extrinsic motivation** comes from outside oneself. More specifically, intrinsic motivation occurs when we find a certain activity to be enjoyable and rewarding on its own terms, like how someone might just love running, or reading, for its own sake. Intrinsic motivation is often involved in people's hobbies, but also helps explain why children and even animals play. Extrinsic motivation, instead, comes from some other reward. A very direct example is how money can motivate you to do tasks you'd otherwise not do as part of a job. Less directly, intangibles like prestige, social recognition, and stability can also serve as external motivators. It would be somewhat of an oversimplification to say that one kind of motivation is inherently better than the other. At the same time, though, educators have invested a lot of effort into trying to figure out how to foster internal motivation, because internal motivation is more likely to be self-sustaining and resilient in the face of obstacles, whereas external motivation vanishes as soon as the incentive does.

> **MCAT STRATEGY > > >**
>
> Throughout this chapter (and others!), we'll be covering a terminology which can seem like a jumble of terms that all sound similar or that sound like normal conversational English words. They aren't! Learn the technical definitions!

I. Instincts

Instincts, which are hardwired, fixed behavioral patterns that are somewhat more complex than reflexes, are perhaps the simplest level of motivation. We see instincts all the time in the animal kingdom, affecting patterns of movement, like flight in birds, or courtship and mating rituals, just to take a few representative examples. The degree to which humans have instincts is much more debatable, because humans have the remarkable power to make things complicated. To qualify as a human instinct, we need to find a behavior—not an urge—that happens automatically, regardless of cultural context. Such examples are surprisingly difficult to find; for example, basic biological functions like urination and defecation might seem like obvious candidates, but upon closer examination, notice how we use the term toilet *training* to describe how children learn to manage these processes? Even something so basic is subject to cultural learning. In fact, the most solid examples of instinctive behavior in humans are in infants, like their bodily functions, or how they cry to express distress.

II. Drives

Since we defined an instinct as a behavior, something like hunger or thirst wouldn't count as an instinct. But these are obviously powerful motivators, which we describe using the term **drive**. To frame the concept more precisely, one of the early researchers into drive theory defined a drive as an "excitatory state produced by a homeostatic disturbance." To understand this definition, we might need to refresh our memory on the concept of homeostasis, which refers to how our bodies regulate themselves to maintain a stable internal environment. This concept comes up frequently in endocrinology, for instance, since hormones are involved in maintaining homeostasis of physiological parameters such as blood glucose levels, fluid and electrolyte concentrations, and so on. So, in other words, a drive is an urge that we have to return some parameter of our body to homeostasis, and the logically-named **drive reduction theory** posits that we are motivated by our drives to act in ways that resolve uncomfortable discrepancies between our current state and a state of homeostasis. Thirst would work as a very simple—albeit biologically driven—example. We experience thirst, and are then motivated to drink. Drinking then alleviates the drive of thirst, in an example of a negative feedback loop.

Within the framework of drive reduction theory, it's common to distinguish **primary drives** and **secondary drives**. Primary drives are things like hunger, thirst, and the need to avoid extreme heat or cold - that is, they're basic, biologically-grounded needs. Secondary drives are less basic; examples might include the desire for recognition, or a socially prestigious career, or even to a certain extent money, although money is sort of a gray area in that money can pay for non-essential goods and services, the typical fodder of secondary drives, or for things like food and drink that satisfy primary needs.

The problem with the concept of secondary drives, though, is that trying to apply the definition of a drive as a homeostatic disturbance becomes increasingly dubious as we extend the scope of secondary drives to include things like social prestige, love, and so on. With this in mind, some theorists have instead spoken of needs. The most famous need-based theory of motivation was proposed by **Abraham Maslow**, who arranged human needs in a pyramidal hierarchy. Maslow's **pyramid of needs** arranges more basic needs at the bottom and more psychologically complex needs at the top, and the idea is that we can't really focus on the higher-up needs until our more basic needs are satisfied. At the bottom of the pyramid are physiological needs, like homeostasis, breathing, food, and water. Next up is safety, so things like the security of one's own body and resources, a place to live, safety of one's family, and so on. Then comes love and belonging, corresponding to needs like friendship, familial support, and sexual intimacy. The next highest level is esteem, including both self-esteem and respect from others. At the very top of the pyramid, we find self-actualization, including phenomena like morality, creativity, and so on. Maslow's hierarchy has received some serious criticism from research psychologists, but it's also probably one of the best-known psychological theories among the general public, so it's safe to say that it resonates with many people's experiences.

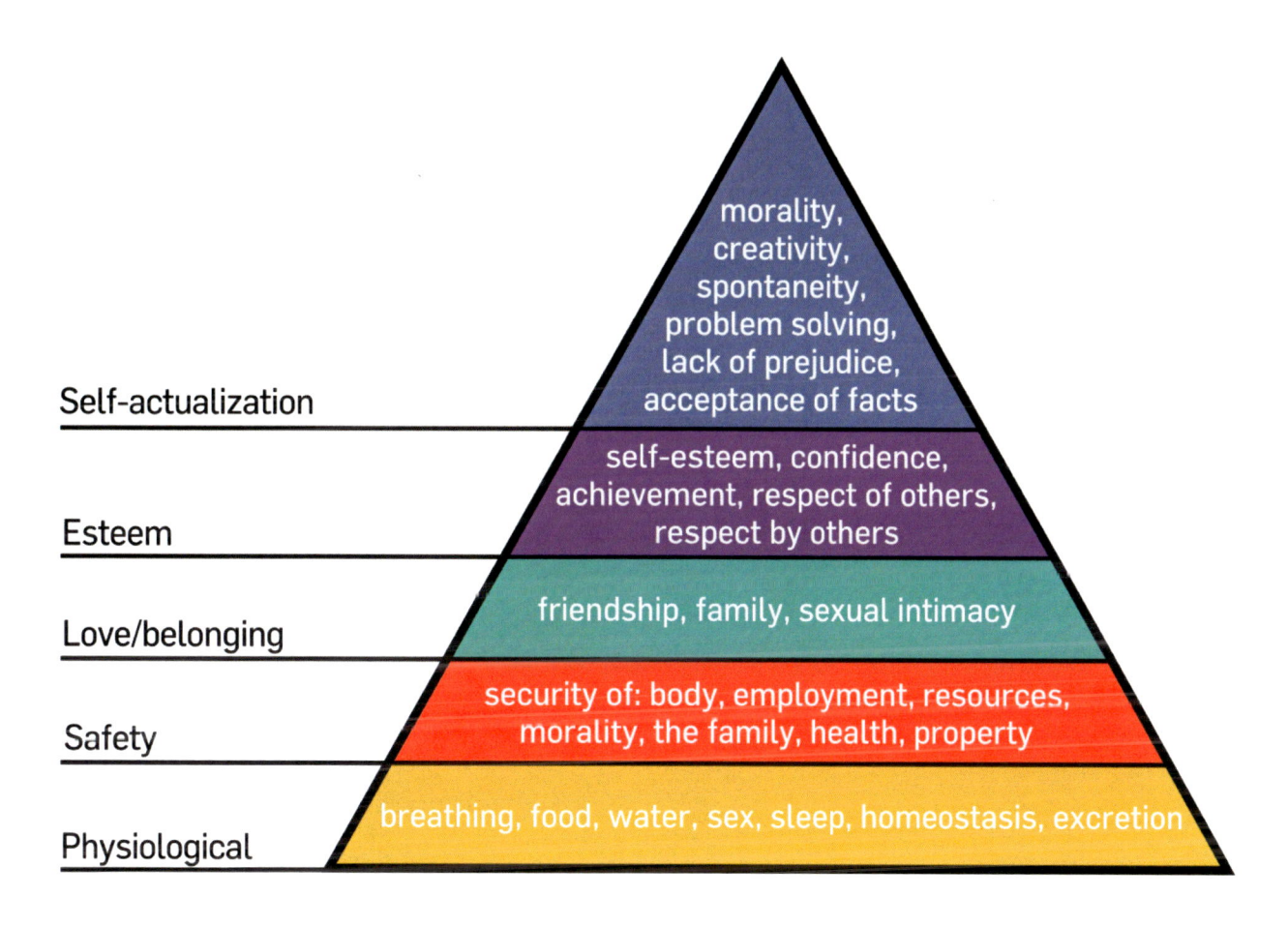

CHAPTER 7: MOTIVATION, ATTITUDE, AND PERSONALITY

Figure 1. Maslow's hierarchy of needs.

III. Other Approaches to Motivation

Motivation has also been linked to the phenomenon of **psychological arousal**, which can be summarized in simple terms as alertness and engagedness. The idea here is that people are motivated to engage in actions that optimize arousal. In other words, we don't like to be bored, and we don't like to be overwhelmed. This has an interesting echo in the **Yerkes-Dodson law**, according to which our performance at various tasks is optimized at medium levels of arousal.

In addition to the key concepts and theoretical proposals regarding motivation that we've covered, there are some other theories to be aware of. The **incentive theory of motivation**, as the name suggests, posits that humans respond rationally to external incentives. As such, this theory focuses largely on extrinsic motivation. Common to both the incentive theory of motivation and the drive reduction theory is the idea that reinforcers play an important role in shaping behavior, albeit in a less structured way than in a behaviorist framework. Much like the distinction between primary and secondary drives, **primary reinforcers** are rewards that correspond to basic physiological needs, like food, drink, and so on, while **secondary reinforcers** are more psychologically complex concepts, like recognition or appreciation.

Next, **expectancy-value theory** views motivation as reflecting a balance between expectancies and values. In this theory, the term "expectancy" refers to the degree to which someone anticipates being able to succeed at a task, and "value" refers to whether the task in question is seen as worthwhile. The idea is that people are maximally motivated

127

to engage in activities if they view themselves as likely to be successful and if they view the activity as being worthwhile, and that conversely, reducing either of those factors decreases motivation.

Self-determination theory is rooted in the distinction between intrinsic and extrinsic motivation, and its major goal is to understand the factors that contribute to intrinsic motivation. In particular, this theory focuses on the need for **competence**, **autonomy**, and **relatedness** as factors that promote intrinsic motivation. In other words, people feel inherently motivated to engage in tasks that they are competent at performing, that they are empowered to carry out relatively independently, and that they feel are relevant and important. Correspondingly, an organizational culture that diminishes those needs is likely to result in decreased intrinsic motivation. Since employers and educational institutions have a vested interest in encouraging intrinsic motivation, these factors have received quite a bit of attention. You may personally have seen how fostering these factors creates a good experience, as well as the destructive effects that take place when people's sense of their competence is eroded, restrictions are placed on their ability to make independent and meaningful decisions, and they are forced to funnel energy towards tasks they find meaningless. If you haven't yet seen those dynamics in practice, keep an eye out, as unfortunately these patterns contribute to burnout among medical students and even practicing physicians.

The final theory relating to motivation that we should mention is **opponent-process theory**. The idea here is that if a certain experience initially provokes an intense reaction of one form or another, as the experience continues over time, the opposite reaction tends to predominate. This is often exemplified by addiction, as the initial pleasurable experiences give way to the negative experiences of withdrawal, which induce an addict to keep using. Initially scary recreational activities like roller coaster riding or skydiving also furnish examples of this dynamic, as the initial experience of fear fades and is replaced by enjoyment.

Although several distinct theories have been proposed to explain motivation in humans, and it is necessary to keep track of which is which, it might be helpful to conclude this discussion by zooming out and looking at the big picture. In particular, both biological and sociocultural motivators shape people's actions. Straightforward examples of biological motivators include drives like hunger, thirst, and the sex drive, but researchers are paying increasingly more attention to the biological underpinning of phenomena such as addiction, obesity, and compulsive behaviors in general. Sociocultural motivators also play an important role in influencing people's behavior, and it's also important for future physicians to be aware of how some of the details regarding sociocultural motivations can vary from one culture to another, because understanding patients' motivations and behavioral patterns is a huge component of being an effective clinician.

2. Attitudes

Although many theories about motivation have been proposed, a common thread is the idea that people feel specific ways about a certain task or goal. That leads us to the topic of attitudes, which we can define as psychological orientations that we have towards a certain person, activity, or even topic in general. Attitudes are a very broad concept; essentially, if we can direct our attention towards something, we can have an attitude about it.

I. Components of Attitudes

Attitudes are understood to have three components, which we can remember by the handy mnemonic "ABC": **affective**, **behavioral**, and **cognitive**. Affective—with an "A", as we see elsewhere in psychology—means emotional, so this component of attitudes has to do with the feelings that we have towards something or someone. As the name implies, the behavioral component of attitudes refers to how we act, and the cognitive component refers to our underlying analytical perceptions of the object of the attitude. So, let's say somebody really likes chocolate—that would be affective. Maybe this person eats chocolate once every few days for desert—that would be behavioral. And if they were to recognize that chocolate-based desserts are tasty, but not the best for their health over the long-term, that would be cognitive. This is fairly straightforward. The one slight complication here is that not just any behavior can count as the behavioral component of an attitude; instead, we're looking for a behavior that is shaped by the affective and cognitive components of the attitude. For example, the choice to eat chocolate-based desserts a couple times a week might reflect a balance between an affective like of chocolate and a cognitive recognition that overdoing it isn't a good idea.

II. Behaviors and Attitudes

Karl Marx, the famed 19th-century political philosopher, once wrote that "philosophers have hitherto only interpreted the world in various ways; the point is to change it." In a similar spirit, theoretical analyses of attitudes are often ultimately aimed at figuring out ways to change them.

It's been well-established that behavior can affect attitudes. An accessible example is the **foot-in-the-door technique**, which is used to induce compliance with a large request by first getting someone to agree to a small request. The idea is that the behavior of carrying out that first small request will make someone more amenable to a subsequent request -- that is, it will shift their attitude. **Role-playing exercises** have a similar impact, in that simulating a certain behavior can shape one's attitudes. This applies both to role-playing exercises that are deliberately constructed and implemented for educational purposes, and—perhaps somewhat less obviously—to role-playing as an important developmental process through which children foster the ability to see others' viewpoints.

As we've already noted, attitudes can also influence behavior. In this context, it's worth mentioning the **Thomas theorem**, which articulates an important principle of social psychology: namely, that if people define situations as real, those situations have real consequences. In other words, attitudes—like whether something is defined as real—can have behavioral impacts.

III. Cognitive Dissonance Theory

Cognitive dissonance theory describes what happens when someone with a certain attitude or behavior is confronted with conflicting evidence. In particular, the idea is that people strive on some level for consistency, and therefore may modify either their behaviors or attitudes to minimize internal perceptions of inconsistency. **Cognitive dissonance** is traditionally exemplified by unhealthy behaviors that are addictive, or at least compulsive. For example, what happens if a smoker with a self-perception of being otherwise health-conscious is confronted with evidence about the terrible health impacts of smoking? Well, one option would be for the smoker to acknowledge that information and rededicate himself or herself to the goal of smoking cessation, thereby changing behavior. But let's face it, that outcome doesn't always happen. Another possibility is that the smoker might appeal to justifications of the habit, along the lines of how smoking can be relaxing, or that it's better than other addictive habits, like injection drug use or alcoholism. (In all seriousness, the latter point is often made in substance abuse programs, many of which don't view cigarette or caffeine use as a high priority for people wrestling with other addictions that pose a more immediate threat to their health or even to their lives) A third possibility is to acknowledge the risk, but introduce other hypothetical considerations or plans to mitigate it. This would mean saying something like "yes, smoking is bad, and I'd like to quit, but now is a really bad time, so I'll quit when things get less stressful in my life." A fourth option is to downplay the risk, through statements like "well, my grandfather smoked like a chimney and lived to be 90 years old, so I clearly have good genes and don't have to worry about it." Alternatively, someone might directly cast doubt on the risk by expressing skepticism about the medical establishment, and whether the evidence for the harms of smoking is that strong anyway.

It's worth familiarizing yourself with the mechanisms of cognitive dissonance, for a couple reasons. First, they might resonate with you in your own life. Second, the MCAT might require you to recognize which hypothetical cognitive and behavioral responses could be expected from someone experiencing cognitive dissonance. A final interesting point about cognitive dissonance is that although it's a pretty old framework in psychology, it also aligns well with recent research into the neurobiology of addiction and compulsive behavior. It's not random that such behavior is often used to illustrate cognitive dissonance; this really does seem to be a situation in which biological patterns and higher-level psychological phenomena go hand-in-hand. That said, cognitive dissonance theory is not limited to addictive or compulsive behavior. A highly relevant example for future physicians is furnished by the anti-vaccine movement in recent years. Physicians and other medical professionals have experienced tremendous frustration at how difficult it is to convince parents to vaccinate their children using scientific evidence, and the mechanisms outlined in cognitive dissonance theory capture many of the ways in which skeptical parents respond to attempts to confront them with evidence of the efficacy and importance of vaccination.

IV. Elaboration Likelihood Model

Given the gloomy picture we've just painted of cognitive dissonance theory, it almost seems like we're just stuck with our fixed opinions and behaviors. Luckily, people's attitudes do change, both spontaneously and in response to persuasion. The **elaboration likelihood model** was developed as a way to try to explain the different ways can be persuaded. It posits a distinction between the central route of processing and the peripheral route. The **central route** involves making a rational decision based on a thorough consideration of the advantages and disadvantages of possible choices. As such, it requires deep cognitive engagement, and it tends to lead to more stable outcomes, both cognitively and behaviorally. In contrast, the **peripheral route** is more superficial; it involves making decisions based on gut reactions, informed by surface-level characteristics, and often in response to cues regarding the credibility or desirability of the message, the attractiveness and charisma of the person delivering the message, and so on. Decisions made based on the peripheral route are less stable, and more vulnerable to competition from other messages trying to appeal to this route.

> **MCAT STRATEGY > > >**
>
> "Elaboration likelihood model" is a good example of a technical term whose name is misleading. If you haven't memorized it and you encounter it on a test, you may start to think about "elaboration" in the sense of something that's elaborate or complicated. Instead, it refers to how people are persuaded by various techniques.

As an example of this theoretical perspective, the central route would be used if someone bought a computer based on a careful consideration of the processing power, storage, graphics capacity, and RAM needed for their tasks, duly balanced with the cost tradeoffs. The peripheral route would be used if someone bought a brand-new shiny computer in response to slick marketing, because it's associated with a desirable lifestyle, or because it happened to be sold in a store with a very appealing atmosphere. In a nutshell, central-route processing is what the educational system tries to teach you to do—at least in an ideal world—and peripheral-route processing is the bread-and-butter of the advertising industry.

If we carefully examine our own experiences, most of us will find that we engage in both modes of processing. That is, we might think that central-route processing sounds smart, and resonates with the kind of deeply-informed and rational future physician we want to be. But let's be honest with ourselves here, it'd be hard to make every decision based on a careful analysis. So, what affects our likelihood of using one processing strategy or the other? Central-route processing requires a certain amount of **motivation** and **capacity**, where capacity refers both to the intellectual skills needed to engage in the reasoning of central-route processing and the attentional and time-related resources necessary to do so at a certain time. In other words, investing the cognitive effort needed to engage in central-route processing requires both that we have the ability to do so and that we care.

V. Social Context of Attitudes

Of course, attitudes don't exist in a vacuum. Our larger social context plays a major role in shaping our attitudes and the ways in which we are likely to change them. Both consciously and unconsciously, we often imitate the people who surround us, so modeling desired attitudes and behaviors can be a very powerful way of changing attitudes over the long term. Likewise, the establishment of social norms can be very powerful in this regard. We previously explored smoking as an example of cognitive dissonance, and it's also an effective illustration of this point. In the United States and many other developed countries, social norms regarding smoking have changed dramatically in the past decades, such that smoking is no longer allowed in many settings where it used to be routine, like in bars, restaurants, or even in hospitals—and what's more, that's not just a technical rule, but a full-on norm with social penalties for violating it. If you were to just light up in a restaurant these days, you would get nasty looks at best, and no one's likely to sympathize with you if you get kicked out. People's attitudes and behaviors can align with these norms without much conscious effort, so activists seeking to accomplish changes in social attitudes often seek to mold social norms as a powerful way to reach such goals.

Taken collectively, all these observations about human attitudes and behavior constitute a powerful toolkit for anyone interested in making a difference in the world, because doing so generally involves attitude and behavior modification. Effective strategies to do so include shifting behaviors and norms in ways that support certain attitudes, crafting the characteristics of a message to appeal to central-route or peripheral-route processing, targeting a message to the appropriate group, and accounting for relevant social factors. Of course, people can also resist persuasion, both due to principled rejections based on central-route reasoning and due to the patterns of denial and minimization that can result from cognitive dissonance. So although there may be no sure-fire rules here, this is an area of psychology with powerful implications for physicians, since patient care often involves attempts to modify attitudes and behaviors to be more healthful. Hopefully the topics we've covered in this discussion will be food for thought for you in this regard during your future career.

6. Personality

Personality refers to an aspect of our psychological constitution that is even more stable than motivation and attitudes. As such, psychologists have developed several schools of thought to account for how our personalities develop and for the phenomenal variety that exists in adult personalities.

I. Erikson's Stages of Development

It's obvious to even a casual observer that the human lifespan involves a certain trajectory. The physical and cognitive developments that accompany our journey from infancy to adulthood are perhaps the most immediate examples, but with some careful thought and observation, we can note that certain stages of life tend to recur. This is actually a pretty ancient idea, but one of the most important modern theorists of personal and psychological development across the lifespan is a researcher named **Erik Erikson**, who proposed that life is characterized by a series of stages. According to Erikson, at each stage of life, an individual is faced with a certain conflict to resolve, and doing so successfully is a prerequisite for healthy development. Correspondingly, failure to resolve a conflict is thought to lead to negative psychological outcomes.

The first of Erikson's life stages occurs in the first year of life, and is marked by the conflict of **trust vs. mistrust**. As the name of the conflict implies, this is the period where, based on interactions with caregivers, an infant learns to have either a trusting or a suspicious attitude towards the world. The next stage, **autonomy vs. shame/ doubt**, happens in toddlerhood, from 1 to 3 years of age. During this period, children begin actively exploring the world, and depending on whether they are appropriately supported in doing so, they can develop either a sense of autonomy—that is, a sense that they can explore the world and learn new tasks as an independent being—or a sense of self-doubt and shame about themselves, with consequences that can persist into later life. Expanding in scope a little bit, but still within the domain of early childhood, the next stage takes place between 3 and 6 years of age, and this time the conflict is **initiative vs. guilt**. Here, a child is starting to engage in more purposeful, goal-oriented tasks that may involve planning, self-control, and executive function. The idea is that if this goes well, a child will develop a healthy sense of initiative—that is, self-confidence and interest in engaging in self-directed activities—and if not, a child may develop a sense of guilt about his or her own interests and activities.

Between 6 to 12 years old, children are faced with the conflict of **industry vs. inferiority**. This is a time in life where children are often given tons of various tasks to complete, as well as opportunities to make and create things. Resolving this conflict successfully will promote diligence, discipline, and an an ability to defer immediate gratification to pursue a multi-staged task. Not resolving this conflict successfully will result in children having a sense of being inadequate, lacking self-confidence, and not viewing themselves as capable.

All four of Erikson's stages that we've seen are sort of building on a theme—as children get older, they start exploring and engaging in the world in greater depth, and they are either encouraged and supported in doing so, which leads to confidence and a further tendency to actively engage, or their attempts to do so are undermined, resulting in a lack of self-confidence and a certain level of distrust towards both oneself and the surrounding world. The details of these four stages vary based on the cognitive sophistication of children at various ages, but the underlying concepts remain similar.

This changes, though, starting with adolescence. During this period, which Erikson defines as lasting from 12 to 20 years of age, the main conflict that we undergo is termed **identity vs. role confusion**. Essentially, in this period, adolescents are coming to terms with who they really are on a deep level, and part of this process involves experimenting with different activities, perspectives, and even identities. Successfully resolving this conflict leads to having a stable, authentic sense of one's core self, while failure to resolve this conflict leads to a certain sense of indecisiveness and instability, or confusion about one's role in society, as manifested by the term "role confusion". It doesn't always work this way in psychology, but in this case—and for Erikson's stages in general—the terminology itself provides a fairly accurate summary of what's at stake.

The next stage occurs in early adulthood, from roughly 20 to 39 years of age. This stage involves the conflict of **intimacy vs. isolation**, and as the name implies, it essentially describes whether, and how, we make commitments to others—perhaps most traditionally in terms of stable romantic relationships or marriage, but also in terms of how we relate to groups of friends or even close colleagues. Successfully resolving this conflict means integrating ourselves into reciprocal and deep relationships that may require commitment and sacrifices, but are ultimately rewarding. Failure to successfully resolve this conflict leads to, as the name of the conflict itself implies, a sense of unwanted isolation from others.

Middle age—understood as 40 to 65 years of age—is characterized by the conflict of **generativity vs. stagnation**. The idea here is related to whether a person can make his or her life count. This means broadening one's focus beyond oneself, to focus on making contributions to society through work, other non-work roles like volunteering or community engagement in some other form, or raising a family. Successfully resolving this conflict means fully participating in society as a contributing member, and not doing so means continuing to live a life focused on one's own momentary pleasures, often accompanied by a deeper sense of dissatisfaction.

Finally, old age—that is, 65 years and older—involves the conflict of **integrity vs. despair**. This is the point of life where people look back and take stock. Integrity in this context refers not to whether one makes ethical decisions, or whether one's word can be trusted. Instead, it refers to whether a person feels like his or her life has made sense and been worthwhile. Sometimes, this question is posed as "Is it okay to have been me?", which is an interesting way of looking at things. Successfully resolving this conflict brings wisdom, and a readiness to wrap up one's affairs and move on, while failure to resolve this conflict might plunge an individual into a cycle of despair and regret.

There's no doubt that Erikson's stages provide ample food for thought, and we may be able to recognize our own experiences and those of our loved ones in some of these descriptions. On the other hand, though, some of these descriptions might really not resonate for you, and that's OK too. Erikson's stages involve a combination of dynamics that are probably fairly universal, since they're grounded in the biological fundamentals of how children develop, mixed in with some factors that are pretty culturally specific, like how adolescence works, when and how people embark upon careers, how romantic relationships are constructed and negotiated, and so on. What's more, you should learn the age ranges that we quoted for test-taking purposes, but it's worth understanding that especially in the older ranges, they're not set in stone. It's not like some switch is toggled in people's brains when they turn 40 that says "hey, OK, enough with intimacy vs. isolation, we've dealt with that, now it's time for generativity vs. stagnation." In reality, there can certainly be overlap between these stages, especially as we age. But as is often the case when studying psychology for the MCAT, the main goal is to be able to associate specific conflicts with the corresponding age ranges, accompanied by a general understanding of what's at stake with each conflict.

AGE	Stage of Development (Conflict)	Central Question	Positive resolution
Birth to 1	Trust vs. Mistrust	Can the world be trusted?	Hope
1 to 3	Autonomy vs. Shame/Doubt	Is it acceptable for me to be myself?	Will
3 to 6	Initiative vs. Guilt	Is it acceptable for me to take initiative?	Purpose
6 to 12	Industry vs. Inferiority	Do I have a shot at making it in the world?	Competence
12 to 20	Identity vs. Role Confusion	Who am I and what is my potential?	Fidelity
20 to 40	Intimacy vs. Isolation	Am I able to love another person and to commit myself to people and things?	Love
40 to 65	Generativity vs. Stagnation	Am I able to live and work in a way such that my life matters?	Care
65 to Death	Integrity vs. Despair	Did I live a good life?	Wisdom

Table 1. Erikson's stages

MCAT STRATEGY > > >

Make a study sheet out of the chart of Erikson's stages!

III. Kohlberg's Stages of Moral Development

We live in a society of laws and rules, but for society to function, it's also absolutely necessary for people to engage in moral and ethical reasoning. A 20th-century psychologist named **Lawrence Kohlberg** was especially interested in how moral reasoning develops as we move from childhood to adulthood, and saw this as a developmental trajectory parallel to, and informed by, other processes of cognitive and personal development.

The methodology of Kohlberg's research focused on how people react to moral dilemmas, typically in which the need to help someone is placed in opposition to some rule governing society. A common example of this kind of dilemma is the perennially debated question of whether it's morally justifiable to steal food if you or your family is starving. An alternative scenario that could be posed to children is whether it's OK to disobey a parent's rule against climbing trees if doing so is necessary to save a cat that's stuck on a branch. Kohlberg's insight was that the ways in which people reason about these choices could provide valuable information about how they see themselves in relation to others and the surrounding world as a whole.

Kohlberg distinguished three basic phases of morality: preconventional, conventional, and postconventional. As we'll see, each of these phases is subdivided into two stages, resulting in a total of six classifications.

Preconventional thinking is characteristic of childhood. The first stage, **obedience**, refers to a self-oriented perspective that is simply focused on the negative consequences of disobeying a rule for oneself. This is reflected in the classic childhood dynamic of needing to do what a parent or teacher says, because not doing so could result in a punishment like a time-out or loss of a privilege. Stage two, **self-interest**, is still a self-oriented perspective, but it's now focused on achieving benefits or rewards. On a very simple level, a child might behave well in expectation of being rewarded by a treat, or on a more complex level, the "self-interest" mindset is also exemplified by a student reasoning that he or she should diligently do homework and complete other obligations in school in order to get good grades, get into a good college, and so on.

According to Kohlberg, **conventional morality** tends to emerge around adolescence. Conventional morality is distinguished from preconventional morality because it begins to incorporate the perspectives of others. The first stage of conventional morality is **conformity**, and at this stage, an individual is essentially concerned with the approval of others based on social expectations. This can manifest either by direct concerns about whether peers or family members would approve, or more indirectly in the form of internalized expectations about what a good sibling, child, or student is expected to do. The next stage, **law and order**, incorporates the understanding that social expectations and rules play a major role in ensuring the stable functioning in society. To return to the example of a person in need stealing food, this perspective would point out that a system in which unfettered theft was permissible based on economic would descend into chaos.

The next phase is **postconventional morality**. Kohlberg actually didn't think that everyone progresses to this stage, but instead viewed it as a possible direction of development after completion of the law and order stage. The hallmark of postconventional morality is the ability to reason about laws from more general principles. In the **social contract** stage of postconventional morality, laws are seen as ways to reinforce the greater good through a complex network of interrelated rights and responsibilities. This perspective leaves open the possibility of adjusting laws in response to evolving social circumstances. In the final stage, **universal human ethics**, an individual can make abstract ethical judgments and engage in reasoning based on justice, to the point that laws can only be considered valid if they accord with principles

Kohlberg's stages are thought-provoking, but as you can imagine, they've been subjected to extensive criticism. For one, it's not clear that stage six, or "universal human ethics," exists in an empirically meaningful way outside of the context of university philosophy departments. For two, Kohlberg's stages are highly specific to a certain culture and time. They reflect a strong imprint from Western European and North American traditions of ethical philosophy, and may not generalize well to other places and times. In fact, a case can be made that Kohlberg's stages, along with many other developments in mid-20th-century, are best understood as part of a collective intellectual project to rationalize and learn from the atrocities of World War Two, which ended in 1945. Nonetheless, Kohlberg's research has inspired extensive inquiry into the topic of moral development, and his basic point that moral development should be seen as occurring in tandem with cognitive and personal development has stood up fairly well to time.

AGE	PHASE	STAGES
Preadolescence	Preconventional Morality	1. Obedience 2. Self-interest
Adolescence to Adulthood	Conventional Morality	3. Conformity 4. Law and order
Adulthood	Postconventional Morality	5. Social contract 6. Universal human ethics

Table 3. Kohlberg's three phases and six stages of moral development.

III. Psychoanalytic Perspectives on Personality

A man named **Sigmund Freud**, who lived from 1856 to 1939, is probably the most famous psychologist of all time. In the late 19th century and the first decades of the 20th century, Freud made some revolutionary proposals regarding the human personality and its development that completely overturned previous research in the field and set the agenda for discussions in psychology that continued for decades after his death, and to some extent to this day. It should be noted that Freud's views are no longer considered valid by most psychologists, but they're considered to be worth studying for historical reasons, given their extremely intense influence on 20th century psychology and literature.

Freud viewed the human psyche as consisting of three structural components: the id, ego, and superego. From Freud's point of view, the **id** is basically a bundle of basic, unconscious urges, including instincts to survive and reproduce, but also extending to the urge to receive immediate gratification in any relevant form. The latter tendency is known as the **pleasure principle**. Of course, it is not always possible to gratify the id's desires, and mental escapes into id-driven fantasies are known as **wish-fulfillment**. It's also worth noting that the id's desires, according to Freud, can be quite complex: it's not as simple as just wanting a range of fairly obvious things like food, drink, sex, and so on. Freud also makes a distinction between "Eros", or life-affirming desires, and "Thanatos," a term that literally means "death" in Greek and in Freudian thought refers to an unconscious drive for death and destruction that, according to Freud, also drives much human behavior.

In Freudian terminology, **ego** refers to something a bit distinct from how we usually use the term in everyday speech. In Latin, "ego" means "I", and Freud uses it in more or less this sense; the ego is the component of our personality that interacts with the world, makes decisions, and so on. In contrast to the pleasure principle that regulates the function of the id, the ego works according to the **reality principle**; that is, it navigates conflicts between the unruly demands of the id and the constraints of what is actually possible in the real world.

Finally, the **superego**—literally the "above I"—is, more or less, the "should" part of our personality. It focuses on what we are supposed to do, and is the emblem of our ideal version of ourselves, or our **ego-ideal**. The superego drives us to perfectionism; it can sort of be seen as an internalized authority figure that pushes us towards socially-internalized ideals. As such, it often conflicts with the id. For instance, according to Freud, the id might be pushing us to indulge in intense emotional displays, unrestrained food and drink, sexual pleasure and so on, while the superego is telling us to keep all of that in check so that we can get into med school, please our parents, and earn lots of money.

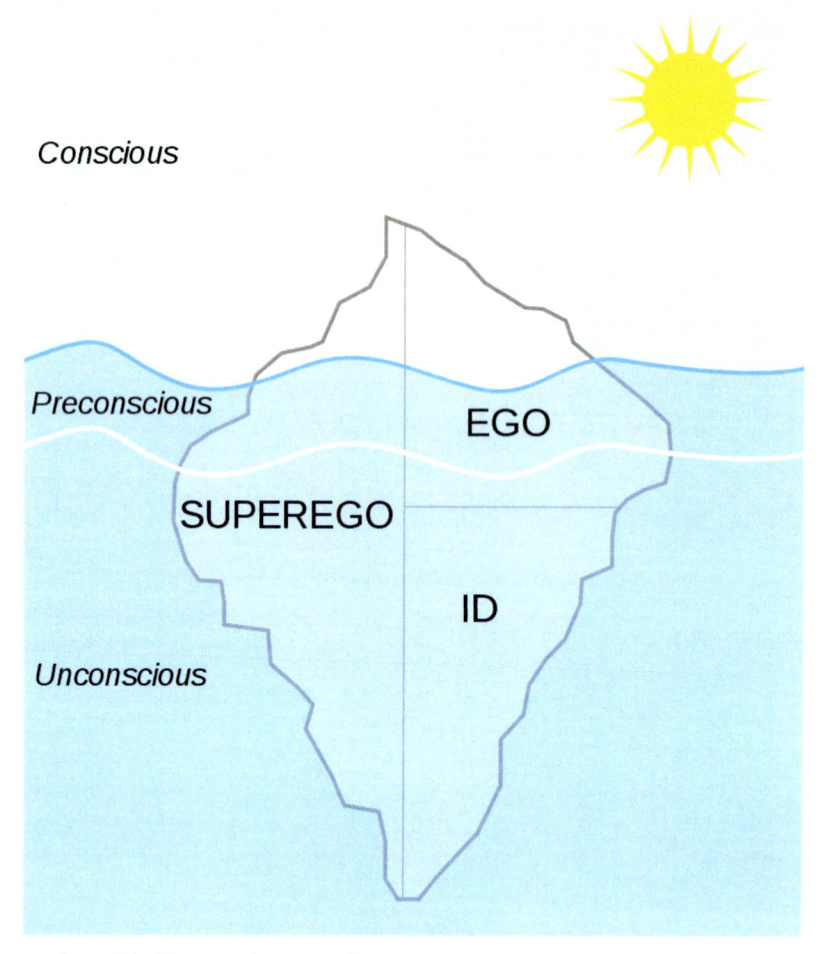

Figure 2. Freud's structural model, illustrated as an iceberg.

From Freud's point of view, conflicts between the id and superego are at the heart of human existence, and he argued that we have several defense mechanisms to help us cope with that stress. For instance, **regression** involves returning to an earlier developmental stage. The vaguely named phenomenon of **reaction formation** refers to an unconscious transmutation of unacceptable desires into their opposite. So, for instance, attraction to a forbidden figure might be converted into overt hatred or dislike of them. **Displacement** occurs when a desire has an unacceptable object, and involves transferring the desire to a more acceptable object. This dynamic is thought to explain the familiar phenomenon of how stress at work can cause a person to be irritable with his or her family. **Sublimation** refers to the redirection of desires that are felt to be unacceptable or inappropriate into another behavior. The classic example of this is that if adolescents are raised in an environment where their emerging sexual desires are felt to be "bad" for whatever reason, that energy might be channeled into something else, like schoolwork—but at the cost of deep dissatisfaction and lack of fulfillment. In projection, an individual attributes unwanted or uncomfortable feelings or behavior to someone else. For example, someone who is on some level concerned with their own substance abuse problem might nitpick other people's use of alcohol or other drugs. Another classic example is how someone who is deeply ashamed of their own sexuality might aggressively police the sexuality of others. **Rationalization** is the familiar process through which we come up with excuses for feelings or behaviors that we consider problematic. Finally, one way to handle a conflict is to try to make it go away. **Suppression** refers to conscious attempts to disregard uncomfortable feelings, and **repression** refers to the same basic tendency, but operating through an unconscious mechanism.

Freud pioneered an approach to treating psychological conditions known as **psychoanalysis**, which places a strong emphasis on intense and wide-ranging conversations between the patient and therapist, with the goal of uncovering unresolved conflicts, discussing them, and thereby resolving them through insight. Thus, the above ideas are known, broadly speaking, as the psychoanalytic perspective on personality.

Freud also had some influential ideas about personality development. Sometimes Freud's perspective on development is known as the **psychosexual perspective**, because he believed that the human libido—often used synonymously for "sex drive", but in the Freudian context more broadly incorporating the drive for constructive human behavior—persisted throughout life. Freud noticed that as children develop, their bodily behavior tends to center around different body parts. On this basis, Freud divided the lifespan into five stages: oral, anal, phallic, latency, and genital, and posited that frustration or excessive indulgence at any stage would lead to fixation at that stage, resulting in anxiety and psychological conflicts that can persist into adulthood with impacts on one's personality.

The **oral stage** lasts from birth to around 1 year, as infants derive pleasure from feeding and exploring the world through their mouths. As such, according to Freud, the mouth is the locus of oral gratification at this stage. Fixation at this stage can allegedly lead to the development of an immature, passive personality, as well as behavioral tics like gum chewing, smoking, and excessive eating and drinking.

Next, in the **anal stage**, which lasts from roughly 1 to 3 years, children focus on learning to control their bladder and bowels. Frustration or excessive gratification at this stage can lead to an **anal-retentive** personality, characterized by a preoccupation with order, or an **anal-expulsive** personality, which manifests as defiance, recklessness, and so on.

In the **phallic stage**, which lasts from about 3 to 6 years of age, children become aware of their own genitalia and those of the opposite gender, and experience increasingly strong effects of gender roles. At this stage, according to Freud, boys undergo a psychosexual struggle with their fathers to metaphorically possess their mothers. This conflict is known as the **Oedipus conflict,** named after the hero of a Greek play who—accidentally, it should be said—kills his father and marries his mother. Freud's disciple, Carl Jung , proposed that girls undergo an analogous struggle known as the **Electra complex**. According to Freud, successful resolution of this process takes place through **castration anxiety** in boys and **penis envy** in girls, resulting in identification with the same-sex parent.

Next, from about 6 years of age until puberty, the **latency phase** occurs, in which sexual urges enter a sort of dormancy. Fixation in this stage, according to Freud, can lead to a lack of sexual fulfillment. Then, at puberty, people enter the **genital stage** for the rest of their lives, in which libidinous pleasure is centered at the genitals. Problems in this stage can include a lack of sexual desire or difficulties engaging in the physical act of sex.

AGE	STAGE	DESCRIPTION
0-1	Oral Stage	Libido centered in mouth
1-3	Anal Stage	Libido centered in anus
3-5	Phallic Stage	Libido centered in genitals
5-Puberty	Latency Stage	Relatively stable, libido sublimated
Puberty-Adulthood	Genital Stage	Normal sexual relationships, given previous stages have been resolved

Table 2. Freud's five stages of psychosexual development.

As you can tell, therefore, Freud's theories provide a framework for explaining a very broad range of human behavior; perhaps too broad, since, after all, making falsifiable predictions is a characteristic of good science. In any case, though, Freud is mostly studied for historical reasons. A final interesting note about Freud before we move on, though, is that he ingested a lot of cocaine. A whole lot. In fact, he was one of the people most responsible for introducing cocaine to Western Europe and North America, and even published a work known as "On Coca" in 1884 in which he essentially argued that cocaine was a miracle drug. Whether that background information provides any additional insight into his theories is up to you.

To a great extent, the psychoanalytic perspective on personality is synonymous with Freud, but he launched a whole school of psychological research, and many of his students either expanded upon his ideas or disagreed with him. We briefly mentioned **Carl Jung**, who was probably Freud's best-known student, although Jung did sharply dissent from Freud's views in certain ways. A key distinction between Freud and Jung is that according to Jung, humans are able to access a **collective unconscious** that contains various archetypes, or universal patterns of thought and behavior, that structure our personalities and behavior. These archetypes for Jung included the **persona**, or how we present ourselves to the world; the **shadow**, or our hidden desires; and the **anima or animus**, a sort of internalized image of the opposite gender that shapes how we interact with the collective unconscious. Other archetypes might include figures like the father, wise old man, hero, trickster, and so on; these figures often appear in folk tales across cultures, which Jung viewed as evidence for their universality as part of human nature. Jung viewed the self as a sort of unifying process that helps integrate these disparate components into a coherent whole.

> **MCAT STRATEGY > > >**
>
> Freud's theories may not be seen as very scientific today, but the MCAT will expect you to be familiar with the structures of personality he laid out.

IV. Other Perspectives on Personality

Numerous other perspectives on personality have been articulated over the decades.

Behaviorism emerged in the 1930s under the intellectual leadership of a psychologist **B. F. Skinner**, and in some ways can be thought of as an extreme reaction to the tendency of psychoanalytic perspectives to posit extensive, but not directly verifiable, structures within the human mind. Instead, Skinner argued that objectively observable behavior and learning comprised the sole reliable sources of knowledge about humans, rejecting any theories about internal mental states or structures within the mind. From Skinner's point of view, everything in psychology boiled down to either reflexes or conditioned learning. Behaviorism was a surprisingly successful school in some regards, and has definitely generated some practical applications in contexts where the goal is to change or modify behavior, but very few psychologists would now agree with Skinner's complete rejection of phenomena like emotions and self-image as lenses into personality.

Humanistic psychology developed as, in a certain sense, as a reaction against both the psychoanalytic perspective and the behaviorist perspective, which respectively tended to view the human personality as either fundamentally sick and disordered or as virtually nonexistent as an entity distinct from a person's measurable behaviors. The humanistic school emphasized the importance of empathy as a therapeutic technique, with respect for creativity and free will. The pioneering psychologist **Carl Rogers** introduced the concept of **unconditional positive regard** into therapy, in which the therapist accepts the client completely and verbalizes that acceptance and care. Rogers' approach to therapy can be described as person-centered, and was non-directive in the sense that Rogers believed in people's freedom and right to shape the trajectories of their own lines. This stands in sharp contrast to perspectives like that of Freud, who essentially viewed life as a series of stages to navigate carefully, with perils lurking at every turn. Rogers and other humanistic psychologists were very interested in the concept of **self-actualization**, or the ability of people to fully live up to their personality; in fact, humanistic psychology research ultimately spurred Abraham Maslow to develop the well-known Maslow's hierarchy of needs, which is discussed above.

Trait theories of personality have attempted to atomize personalities into a more limited set of traits that combine in different ways in different people. Various theorists have approached this task in distinct ways, but the most widely used such theory is known as the "**Big Five**" theory, which classifies people according to their degree of **openness, conscientiousness, extraversion, agreeableness,** and **neuroticism**, forming the handy mnemonic OCEAN. Most of these terms can be understood reasonably well based on their use in everyday language, but it's worth mentioning that in the context of personality studies, "neuroticism" has a precisely defined meaning of the degree to which a person experiences intense emotions in stressful situations. The Big Five personality traits developed as an extension of a theory called the "**PEN model**" that was developed by **Hans and Sybil Eysenck** and used three factors: **psychoticism**, which for the Eysencks meant nonconformity, **extraversion**, and **neuroticism**.

Another approach to classifying personalities is to divide them into different types. Astrology is a commonly-encountered embodiment of this phenomena, as the claims made by astrological traditions include that people born at different times of the year will have distinct personalities. The distinction between "type A" personalities, who are highly organized and competitive, versus laid-back "type B" personalities, is another distinction that people make in everyday life. As our examples might suggest, **type theories of personality** are generally thought to be less scientifically valid than trait theories. The **Myers-Briggs Type Inventory**, or **MBTI**, straddles the border between type and trait theories; it uses Jungian theory to divide people into 16 types based on binaries between introversion and extroversion, intuition and sensing, thinking and feeling, and judging and perceiving; the latter category, by the way, refers more or less to how organized someone is, not to whether he or she is judgmental of others in the sense that we usually use the word. MBTI types are expressed as four-letter combinations, like INTP for introverted, intuition, thinking, and perceiving.

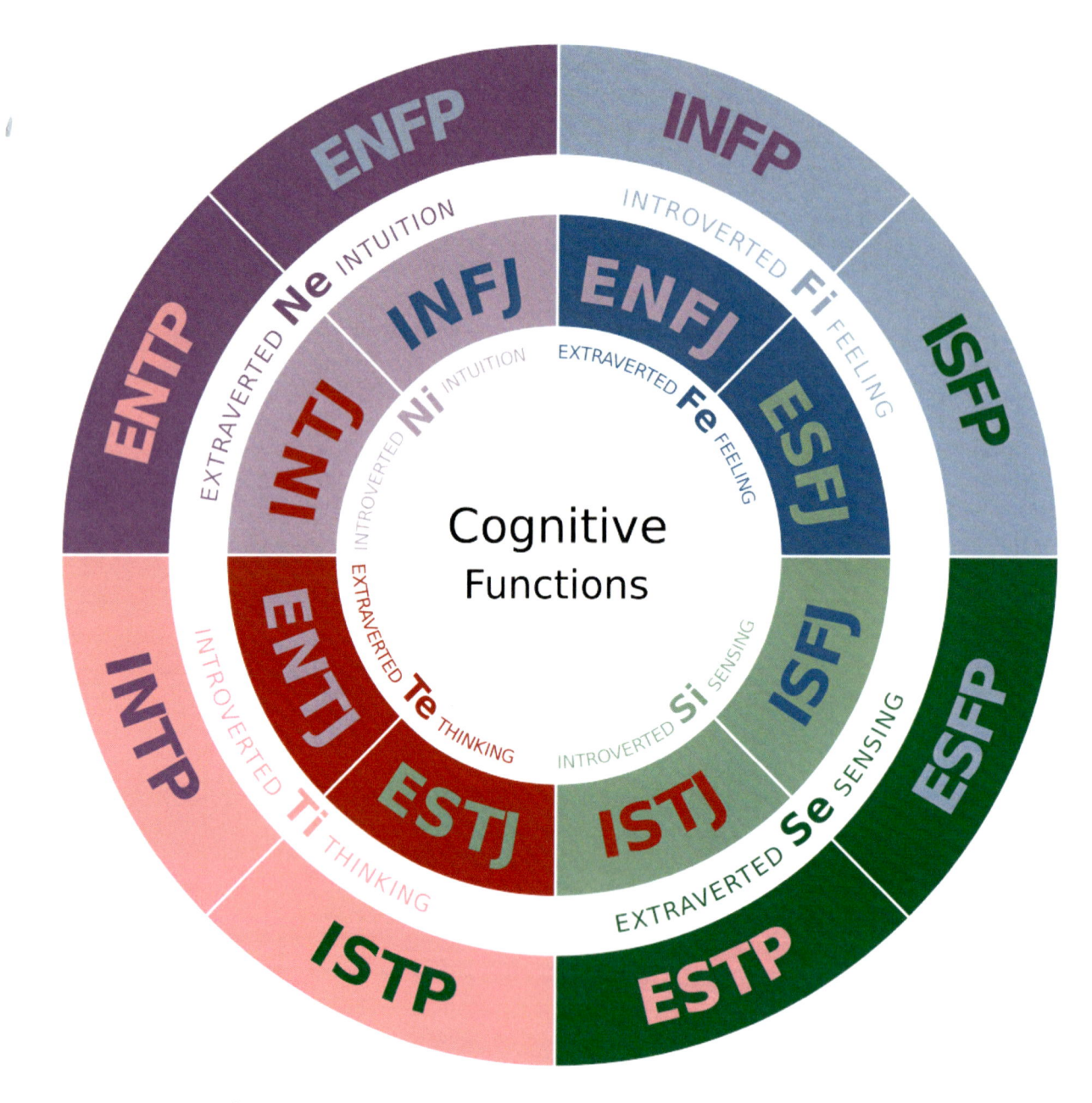

Figure 3. The cognitive functions of each MBTI type

One of the issues faced by both type and trait theories of personality is the need to account for how behavior, and even broader personality-level tendencies, can vary across situations based on contextual cues. Ideally, a personality test would yield the same results every time a person takes it, but that's not always the case. One of the reasons why the "Big Five" approach is considered valid, though, is that it uses a statistical technique called factor analysis to cluster together behaviors that tend to co-occur, minimizing the effects of somewhat random variation on personality classification.

Other theoretical perspectives within psychology also have implications for personality. For instance, the **social cognitive perspective** promoted by psychologists such as Bandura in the context of learning has ramifications for how people develop their personalities. Bandura in particular, who is most famous for the Bobo doll experiment in which children learned to beat up a doll by imitating an adult's behavior, developed the concept of **reciprocal determinism** to describe the interrelationships between our behaviors, choices, and personalities; for instance, our personalities might influence our choice of a career, and then shape our actions within that career. Finally our career—and the experiences we have in the workplace—in turn influence our personality. For Bandura, the fact that we learn from other people is always essential. A biological perspective on personality focuses on the impact of genetic factors on personality; this is certainly relevant, of course, although distinguishing between "nature" and "nurture" can be especially challenging in the setting of research into personality.

As a final note, it's worth mentioning a few researchers whose work bridged the domains of personality, learning, and identity. A researcher named **George Herbert Mead**, who was also a founder of the school of symbolic interaction in sociology, proposed that our psychological development involves an interplay between the "**I**", or our internal selves, and the "**me**", or the version of ourselves that the environment reflects back at us. This has some overlap with psychoanalytical approaches that emphasize the id and superego, as the "I" is like Freud's ego, with some influence from the id, and the "me" is somewhat like Freud's superego, but with a greater emphasis on input from others on one's identity as a whole and less of a strict emphasis on "should." The Russian psychologist **Lev Vygotsky** also emphasized the role of the other in personal development, focusing on how the "more knowledgeable other" could help a child develop new skills. In Vygotsky's thought, new skills that are in the process of development constitute a child's zone of proximal development. On one hand, Vygotsky's focus on cognition provides a closer parallel with Piaget than with the theorists who focused primarily on personality, but Vygotsky's approach also places an important emphasis on the role of others in how a child's sense of self is shaped, providing a useful bridge between these ways of looking at development.

7. Must-Knows

- Motivation: drives our actions. It can either be extrinsic and intrinsic; instincts = fixed behavioral patterns
- Drive reduction theory: we're motivated to return our body to homeostasis; disturbances of homeostasis produce signals called drives that we seek to reduce.
  - Primary drives are physiological, while secondary drives are psychological.
- Maslow's hierarchy of needs: physiological needs must be satisfied first, followed by safety, love and belonging, esteem & self-esteem, and self actualization.
- Expectancy-value theory: motivation will be highest if you expect to succeed and if goal is worth it.
- Self-determination theory: focuses on competence, autonomy and relatedness for intrinsic motivation.
- Opponent-process theory: after an initial intense reaction, the opposite reaction tends to dominate.
- Attitudes have ABC components: affective, behavioral, and cognitive
- Thomas Theorem: if people define situations as real, they have real consequences
- Cognitive dissonance theory: how we resolve conflicts when beliefs/knowledge don't align with our actions
- Elaboration likelihood model: central route persuasion (relies on reason) is effective for lasting change, but more difficult to achieve; peripheral route persuasion relies on emotional appeal but creates superficial change
- Erikson's life stages: trust vs. mistrust (0-1), autonomy vs. shame/doubt (1-3), initiative vs. guilt (3-6), industry vs. inferiority (6-12), identity vs. role confusion (12-20), intimacy vs. isolation (20-39), generativity vs. stagnation (40-65), integrity vs. despair (65+)
- Kohlberg's stages of moral development: preconventional morality (obedience, then self-interest), conventional morality (conformity, then law and order) and postconventional morality (social contract, then universal human ethics)
- Psychoanalytic perspective on personality: id (basest wants, operates on pleasure principle, fantasies called wish-fulfillment), ego (reality principle, navigates wants of id through real world), and superego (who we think we should be, our ego-ideal)
- Freudian defense mechanisms:
  - Regression: a return to an earlier developmental stage
  - Reaction formation: an unacceptable desire turned into its opposite
  - Displacement: taking stress out on someone else
  - Sublimation: redirection of strong unacceptable desires into a more appropriate behavior
  - Projection: placing one's own uncomfortable feelings onto other people
  - Rationalization: Coming up with excuses for feelings
  - Suppression: Consciously disregarding uncomfortable feelings
  - Repression: Unconsciously disregarding uncomfortable feelings
- Freud's psychosexual perspective on human development posits that humans go through five stages: oral, anal, phallic, latency and genital; failure to successfully navigate stages can cause lasting complexes
- Carl Jung: collective unconscious containing archetypes such as the persona, shadow and anima or animus
- Behaviorism: concerned with only observing overt behaviors, not speculating about internal states
- Humanistic psychology introduced the importance of empathy, the idea of unconditional positive regard and a focus on self-actualization
- Trait theories of personalities such as the Big Five personality traits and the PEN model divide personalities into a small set of traits
- Type theories such as astrology or the Myers-Briggs Type Inventory focus on discrete types; are generally considered to be not very reliable
- Social cognitive perspective spawned the idea of reciprocal determinism, the idea that our relationships shape our behavior and our behavior shapes our relationships
- Biological perspectives of personality focus on genetic factors

End of Chapter Practice

The best MCAT practice is **realistic**, with a focus on identifying steps for further improvement. For those reasons, we recommend completing practice questions in an online setting that simulates the real MCAT interface, and taking advantage of advanced analytic features to help you determine how best to move forward in your MCAT study journey.

With that in mind, **online end-of-chapter questions** are accessible through your Next Step account.

As a further supplement, given the importance of active learning for effective studying, we also suggest that you consult the Must-Knows as a basis for creating a study sheet, in which you list out key terms and test your ability to briefly summarize them.

This page left intentionally blank.

Psychological Disorders

CHAPTER 8

0. Introduction

Psychological disorders are a topic where the MCAT does not expect you to be an expert—that comes in your future, in medical school—but it does require you to have a general sense of major disorders, how they're diagnosed, and conceptual frameworks for understanding them.

Of note, psychological disorders are fairly common in the population, and their treatment is a mainstay of primary care medicine. In any given year, approximately one-fourth of the population is thought to be affected by a psychological disorder, with some especially common disorders including social anxiety disorder and major depressive disorder.

1. Classification

Two major approaches exist for conceptualizing and analyzing psychological disorders: the **biomedical approach** and the **biopsychosocial approach**. The biomedical approach understands psychological disorders as physically-based conditions, for which biologically-grounded treatments are appropriate. The biopsychosocial approach recognizes the importance of biological causative factors, but also emphasizes the role played by psychological factors, such as emotions and self-concept, and sociological factors like the presence or absence of social support and the social stigma associated with mental illness.

> **MCAT STRATEGY > > >**
>
> While the MCAT generally refrains from making value judgments, be aware that the biopsychosocial approach is generally seen as a superior, more comprehensive model.

With this in mind, we might ask how a psychological disorder is defined. A broad definition would be that a **psychological disorder** is a mental or behavioral pattern causing significant distress to a person or impairing their ability to function within society. A more pragmatic definition would follow the classification presented in the DSM-5, or the fifth edition of the Diagnostic and Statistical Manual of Mental Disorders. In clinical settings, the most up-to-date edition of the DSM is generally considered to be the definitive resource for information on the classification and definition of psychological disorders. Of note, psychological disorders are fairly common in the population, and their treatment is a mainstay of primary care medicine. In any given year, approximately one-fourth of the population is thought to be affected by a psychological disorder, with some especially common disorders including social anxiety disorder and major depressive disorder. The DSM-5 classifies various psychological disorders based on their symptoms, and does not make any claims regarding the biological underpinnings of mental illness. As suggested by this choice, research into the correlations between clinically defined conditions and neuropsychological phenomena is an ongoing area of interest, and may be an area of future breakthroughs. It's also worth noting in this context that the definitions of psychological disorders are culture-specific, both in the sense that they vary throughout the world and in the sense that the understanding of such disorders can change over time even within the same culture. For instance, the DSM-5 contains some important differences from the previous, fourth edition, and early editions of the DSM, from 1952 to 1974, classified homosexuality as a mental disorder instead of as a sexual orientation. In this discussion, we'll be presenting information on psychological disorders in accordance with the criteria presented in the DSM-5, but it's useful to keep in mind that our understanding of psychological disorders is constantly evolving.

In this discussion, we'll review depressive disorders, bipolar-related disorders, anxiety disorders, obsessive-compulsive disorder, trauma- and stress-related disorders, conversion disorders, schizophrenia, dissociative disorders, and personality disorders, and then briefly discuss the biological basis of certain of these disorders. Before we get started, it's worth emphasizing that our discussion will be concise, with a primary focus on presenting terms that you need to recognize and relevant clinical definitions. Be on a lookout for diagnostic criteria and cases in which disorders have similar-sounding names, or where a discrepancy exists between everyday linguistic usage and technical psychological terminology.

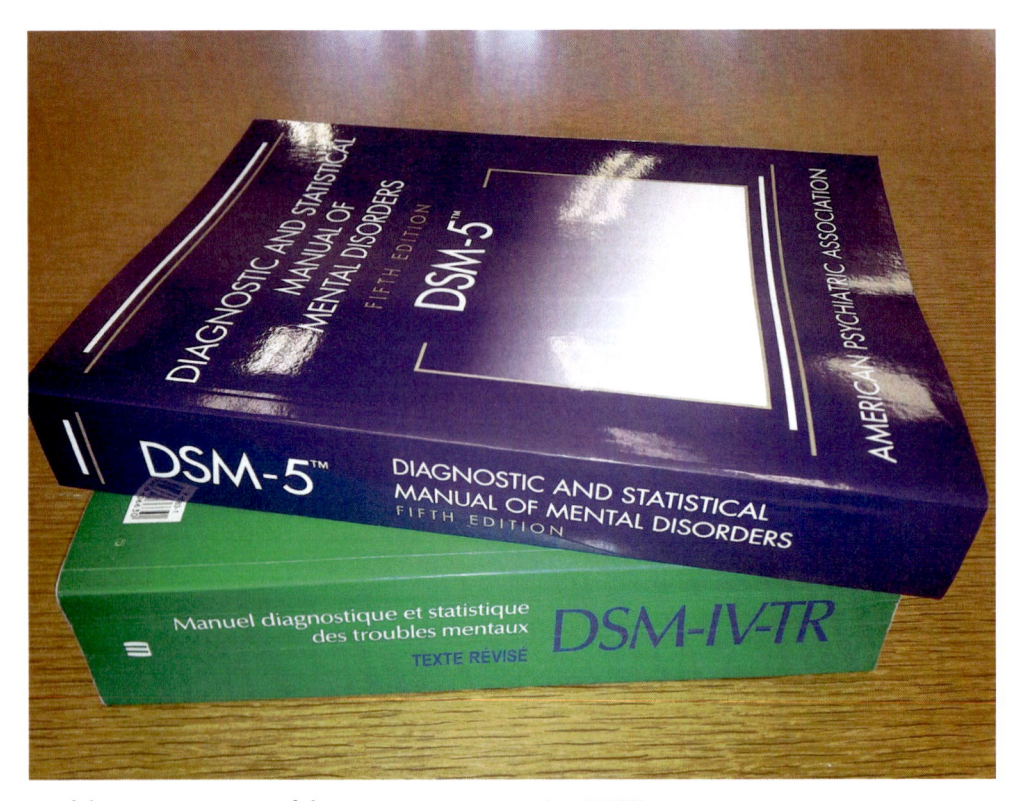

Figure 1. A copy of the DSM-5 on top of the previous version, DSM-IV-TR.

2. Depressive Disorders

There are a few depressive disorders to be aware of, which fall into the broader rubric of mood disorders. **Major depressive disorder** is defined by the presence of at least one **major depressive episode**, which is in turn defined as a two-week period including five or more of the following symptoms: intense sadness or a depressed mood; anhedonia, or lack of interest in activities previously felt to be enjoyable; weight changes; sleep disturbances; appetite disturbances; feelings of excessive guilt or worthlessness; reduced energy; psychomotor symptoms; difficulties in focusing one's attention on something; and thoughts of death or suicidal ideation or attempts. The two-week cutoff for these symptoms is essential, as is the fact that a depressed mood or anhedonia must be among the symptoms. **Dysthymia** is a less-intense form of depression that occurs for at least two years; together with long-lasting major depressive disorder, the category of persistent depressive disorder can be applied to people who experience significant depressive symptoms for two years or longer. **Seasonal affective disorder** can be thought of as major depressive disorder with a regular seasonal pattern of onset, usually occurring in the winter months.

3. Bipolar Disorders

Bipolar disorders involve both **depressive** and **manic episodes**. A manic episode is defined as a period lasting at least one week in which a person experiences an unusually elevated mood and at least three of the following symptoms: grandiosity or unrealistically inflated self-esteem, sometimes to the point of delusions; a reduced need for sleep; high levels of distractability; agitation; rapid speech or abnormal loquaciousness; flights of ideas or racing thoughts; and a tendency to engage in high-risk behavior. Manic episodes may also involve experiences of psychosis. **Bipolar I disorder** is primarily characterized by mania, with depressive episodes that may not reach the threshold required for major depressive disorder. In contrast, **bipolar II** is primarily characterized by depression, with the combination of at least one major depressive episode with hypomania, or a less intense experience of mania that may not dramatically interfere with life functioning. **Cyclothymic disorder** is similar to bipolar II in that it involves hypomania, but has a lower intensity of depression.

> **MCAT STRATEGY > > >**
>
> Psychological disorders, and mood disorders in particular, are especially good fodder for making study sheets to quiz yourself. They tend to sound similar, and the MCAT will expect us to know the exact definition.

4. Anxiety Disorders

Several anxiety disorders have been defined, the broadest of which is **generalized anxiety disorder**, which involves a disproportionate level of stress and worry regarding a diverse range of otherwise routine aspects of daily life. **Social anxiety disorder** entails intense feelings of stress linked to social situations, often linked to fears of embarrassment. **Illness anxiety disorder** manifests as excessive concern about medical conditions in the absence of physical symptoms. This condition was previously known as hypochondria. Specific phobias, or fears, also fall into the category of anxiety disorders. Common examples include arachnophobia, or the fear of spiders, and agoraphobia, or the fear of leaving one's residence and spending time in a public space. Now, a key point to make about these disorders is that not liking something is not equivalent to having a linked anxiety disorder. One can be an introvert without having social anxiety disorder, one can have dislike spiders without having arachnophobia, and so on. A key fact about anxiety disorders is that they can be functionally debilitating, and also involve sympathetic nervous system activation as a physical response, with manifestations including a fast heart rate, sweating, trembling, and so on. These symptoms are especially intense in **panic attacks**, in which affected individuals also may experience symptoms like hyperventilation and a sense of impending doom. Persistent panic attacks are characteristic of an anxiety disorder known as panic disorder.

5. Obsessive-Compulsive and Related Disorders

ISeveral disorders that were previously categorized as anxiety disorders are now considered to be separate entities in the DSM-5. **Obsessive-compulsive disorder**, or OCD, is a notable example. As the name implies, OCD consists of obsessions and compulsions. The basic distinction is that obsessions are thoughts—more specifically, intrusive, impulsive, persistent thoughts—and compulsions are ritualistic and repetitive behaviors that result from those obsessions, and generally function as temporary ways to gain relief from the anxiety induced by obsessions. For instance, the compulsive behavior of repeated hand-washing may serve as a way to reduce the anxiety induced by intrusive and persistent anxiety about germs. **Body dysmorphic disorder** was previously classified as a somatic disorder—more about those later—but is now considered to be related to obsessive-compulsive disorder. This condition is characterized by an obsessive focus on a perceived flaw in one's appearance that is more objectively minor or nonexistent.

6. Trauma and Stress-Related Disorders

Trauma and stress-related disorders form a distinct category. **Post-traumatic stress disorder**, or **PTSD,** is perhaps the best-known condition in this category. In people who are exposed to intense acute or chronic trauma, PTSD is characterized by a pattern of intrusive recollections, whether auditory, visual or otherwise, avoidance of stimuli related to the trauma, negative changes in mood and cognitions related to the traumatic event, and altered patterns of reactivity and arousal. These symptoms must persist for more than a month and cause significant impairment in daily life.

7. Somatic Disorders

Somatic disorders involve physical symptoms. Within this category, **somatic symptom disorder** refers to an excessive preoccupation or focus on a physical symptom, while **conversion disorder** describes physical symptoms involving the impairment of sensory of voluntary motor function that do not appear to have a biological cause. The onset of these symptoms usually occur shortly after a high-stress event.

8. Dissociative Disorders

Dissociative disorders are another category that were formerly grouped together under the rubric of anxiety disorders, but are now considered to be separate. The hallmark of dissociative disorders is disconnection from one's routine state of consciousness and/or personality. The best-known example of a disorder in this category is **dissociative identity disorder**, in which an individual has two or more distinct personalities that appear at different times. This condition was previously labeled "multiple personality disorder". It's been the subject of extensive debate, but one recurring thread is it tends to occur in people who were subjected to extreme trauma, including physical and sexual abuse, as children. **Dissociative amnesia** is a form of retrograde amnesia in which people lose episodic memories about their own lives. Finally, **depersonalization/derealization disorder** refers to a pattern in which people feel a sense of unreality about their own existence, as if they're observing themselves and their surroundings from a distance.

9. Schizophrenia

Schizophrenia has traditionally been considered the best-known example of a psychotic disorder, which are characterized by symptoms including hallucinations, delusions, disorganized thought and behavior, and abnormal movement patterns (also known as catatonia). These symptoms are known as **positive symptoms**, not because they're beneficial in any meaningful sense of the word, but because they reflect the addition of something extra onto one's baseline patterns of experiencing and interacting with the world. Schizophrenia can also be characterized by various **negative symptoms**, which reflect the lack or absence of aspects of one's baseline experience, such as diminished levels of emotional intensity or initiative. The peak age of schizophrenia development in both men and women is in the early 20s; however, especially in women, schizophrenia may develop later in life as well, although new-onset schizophrenia is rare beyond the age of about 50 or so in both sexes. The development of full-fledged schizophrenia may be preceded by a so-called **prodromal phrase**, in which a person displays a pattern of poor social adjustment and integration. Interestingly, in recent research, schizophrenia has been conceptualized as a spectrum, so the prodromal phase of schizophrenia can be difficult to distinguish from less severe manifestations of the disorder or other psychological difficulties. The treatment of schizophrenia primarily involves antipsychotic, or neuroleptic, medications, but therapy-based interventions have also been investigated and show promise.

We briefly listed some of the positive and negative symptoms in schizophrenia, but it's worth exploring them in more detail, both because schizophrenia is a disease with a major impact on public health and because the use of the terms positive and negative to refer to these systems sets a trap that the MCAT can use to target students who haven't actually studied this topic. We'll start with **positive symptoms**, which are again not "positive" in the sense of "good," but positive in the quasi-mathematical sense of involving the addition of something to one's baseline experiences.

The first positive symptom we mentioned was **hallucinations**, which involve the perception of an non-existent external sensory stimulus. Auditory hallucinations are the most common subtype in schizophrenia, including but not limited to the perception of external voices; however, hallucinations reflecting other sensory modalities, such as visual or even tactile hallucinations, can occur in schizophrenia and in other psychological conditions.

Delusions are defined as beliefs that conflict with reality and do not reflect a broader cultural consensus. Furthermore, in cases of schizophrenia, such delusions tend to persist regardless of evidence to the contrary. Several distinct subtypes of delusions are characteristic of schizophrenia. For example, delusions of persecution involve the conviction that powerful forces are acting against a person's best interests, or actively attempting to interfere with their lives. Delusions of grandeur refer to an outsized belief in one's exceptional nature, ranging from simply the conviction that one is unusually excellent to more specific delusions like being the incarnation of a religious or historical figure. Other delusions relate to perceptions about communication; for example, thought insertion describes the belief that thoughts can be transmitted into the affected individual's head, and its converse, thought broadcasting, refers to the belief that the affected individual's thoughts are, in some sense, visible to others. Delusions of reference refer to the belief that aspects of the publicly available external environment are specifically targeted towards the affected individual.

Disorganized behavior and thought are fairly self-explanatory concepts, although it's worth briefly noting that "disorganized" in both categories can refer to a level of disability that makes interactions with the outside world very difficult. For instance, disorganized behavior can include challenges with hygiene and erratic patterns of interactions with others, and disorganized thought can manifest itself as speech that is very difficult to understand. **Catatonia** is a very broad category of abnormal movement patterns, including energy-consuming but unusual movements that seem to occur without a specific external cause, the tendency to repeat others' actions and words (known as echolalia and echopraxia, respectively), and even the tendency to be very lethargic.

Several aspects of **negative symptoms** include disturbances of how emotion is expressed, known as **affect**. Remember that in psychologically, affect with an "A" is different from effect with an "E", in that affect describes emotions. Affect may be blunted or even flat in people with schizophrenia, meaning that they seem to show minimal to no emotional reaction in circumstances where such a reaction would be expected, or it can be socially inappropriate, reflecting a mismatch with social conventions.

Depending on when and if you've studied about schizophrenia in the past, you may have learned about various subtypes of schizophrenia, such as the paranoid, disorganized, and catatonic types. These types of schizophrenia were removed from the DSM-5 when it was published in 2013, and therefore are highly unlikely to appear on the MCAT. Instead, as mentioned earlier, the current consensus regarding schizophrenia is to consider it a syndrome with a diverse range of possible manifestations.

10. Personality Disorders

Personality disorders are also worth discussing in depth as a distinct category of psychiatric disorders. They describe maladaptive behavioral patterns that cause persistent problems in a person's life, but nonetheless may not be recognized as a problem by the affected person. Due to this property of personality disorders, known as **ego-syntonicity**, care is needed when diagnosing someone with a personality disorder to establish that the disorder really does cause significant problems in their lives. After all, personalities are diverse, and many fully-functional people may recognize aspects of personality disorders in themselves. When evaluating individuals, it is important not to over-diagnose these disorders, thereby medicalizing otherwise benign variations in human behavior. Also for this reason, personality disorders cannot be conclusively diagnosed in people under 18 years of age, because personality is thought to not fully crystallize until adulthood. Ten personality disorders are currently recognized, and are divided into three clusters, referred to as clusters A, B, and C.

The **cluster A disorders** are paranoid, schizoid, and schizotypal personality disorders. **Paranoid personality disorder** involves a high level of distrust towards others, jealousy, and a tendency to interpret innocent actions as involving malevolent intent. **Schizoid personality disorder** involves a marked preference for solitude, a tendency to form few relationships, and an overall tendency towards emotional aloofness, coldness, and a restricted range of emotions. **Schizotypal personality disorder** also involves intense discomfort in social contexts, but with the addition of unusual beliefs that may be reminiscent of delusions without actually rising to that level. Schizoid and schizotypal personality disorders are not the same as schizophrenia, although some of the patterns of cluster A personality disorders may also appear in the prodromal phase of schizophrenia.

Cluster B includes antisocial, narcissistic, histrionic, and borderline personality disorders. The most important thing about **antisocial personality disorder** is that it does not refer to being "antisocial" in the sense of preferring to stay in and watch TV or read a book instead of going to a party. Instead, it describes a pervasive pattern of disregard for the rights of others, often manifesting in violence and a lack of remorse. Antisocial personality disorder is relatively common among violent criminals, but perhaps unsurprisingly, it is also overrepresented among high-status individuals like CEOs and politicians. **Narcissistic personality disorder** includes a pervasive sense of one's unique talents, brilliance, and attractiveness, leading to fantasies about unlimited success and power, and is also associated with a pattern of shallow, conflict-driven relationships with others. Underlying narcissistic personality disorder may be low self-esteem and a need to seek validation in the form of status. **Histrionic personality disorder** describes a pattern of flashy, attention-seeking behavior, with exaggerated but perhaps not always fully sincere emotional expressions. **Borderline personality disorder** is characterized by a tendency for extremely intense, but unstable emotions and moods, as well as a cognitive pattern known as splitting, according to which people are seen as either totally good or completely bad, with no sense of shades of gray or ambiguity. Borderline personality disorder also often manifests through risky, impulsive behavior, which may be seen as attempts to cope with the often unbearable intensity of emotions associated with this condition.

Cluster C includes avoidant, dependent, and obsessive-compulsive personality disorders. The common thread uniting these conditions is that they are characterized by anxiety. **Avoidant personality disorder** involves a persistent sense of inadequacy and hypersensitivity to criticism that leads people to avoid social situations or challenges at school or in the workplace. **Dependent personality disorder** involves a profound need to be taken care of by others, even when it comes to otherwise routine life activities. It is very difficult for people with dependent personality disorder to be alone, and this condition places them at an elevated vulnerability to abusive relationships. Finally, **obsessive-compulsive personality disorder** sounds like, but is distinct from, obsessive-compulsive disorder. Instead, obsessive-compulsive personality disorder reflects an excessive concern with orderliness, rules, and regulations. This disorder is also characterized by perfectionism and a tendency to be controlling, inflexible, and stubborn.

Personality disorders are important to study for the MCAT both because of their inherent importance as psychological conditions and because they are structurally very testable due to their sub-clustering and the presence of multiple points of confusion with everyday language, as in antisocial and borderline personality disorders, or with other psychological terms, as is a danger when studying schizoid, schizotypal, and obsessive-compulsive personality disorders.

> **MCAT STRATEGY > > >**
>
> A good way to remember the clusters of personality disorders are the 3 W's: "weird" (cluster A, including more clearly non-narrative types of behavior), "wild" (cluster B, encompassing larger-than-life personalities), and "worried" (cluster C). Of course, these are purposeful stereotypes for the sake of memorization, and shouldn't be taken to heart, but are commonly used in medical training.

11. Biological Basis of Psychiatric Disorders

Finally, for the MCAT, you're expected to be familiar with the biological basis of certain conditions affecting the brain, including schizophrenia, depression, Alzheimer's disease, and Parkinson's disease. These are all hotbeds of ongoing research, so that the information we present here is not necessarily the last word on the topic; however, all the mechanisms presented below do reflect at least highly influential hypotheses.

As we've discussed elsewhere, **schizophrenia** has a strong genetic component and is highly heritable. It is also associated with excess levels of the neurotransmitter dopamine in the brain. Conversely, **Parkinson's disease**, which manifests by symptoms and signs including tremors, slow and shuffling movements, loss of facial expression, and a bent posture, is caused by cell death in a brain area known as the substantia nigra, leading to reduced dopamine expression. Therefore, care needs to be taken with medications affecting dopamine levels such as methamphetamines, as promoting excess dopamine levels can lead to symptoms reminiscent of schizophrenia in vulnerable individuals, and drug-induced parkinsonism can occur in response to a surprisingly broad class of medications, including but not limited to antipsychotics used to treat schizophrenia.

An influential proposal regarding the cause of **depression** is that it may be caused by deficiencies in the neurotransmitters serotonin and dopamine. Research is currently suggesting that the overall picture may be more complex, but it's worth being aware of this proposal—especially as involves serotonin—since **selective serotonin reuptake inhibitors**, or **SSRIs**, work to boost serotonin levels in the brain and are a major class of first-line antidepressants. Finally, **Alzheimer's disease** is a form of dementia that is not generally classified as a psychological condition but is worth mentioning since it does produce psychological symptoms, such as memory loss and emotional disturbances. The causes of Alzheimer's disease are complex and not fully understood, but key physical findings include masses of plaques of **beta-amyloid proteins** and fibrillary tangles of **tau proteins** in the brain. Reduced levels of the neurotransmitter acetylcholine are also observed in patients with Alzheimer's disease.

12. Must-Knows

- Biomedical approaches describe disease as purely biological, while biopsychosocial approaches see it as a multi-factorial phenomenon; the DSM-5 is the current standard for classification of mental disorders.
- Depressive disorders
  - Persistent depressive disorders are any depressive disorders lasting more than two years.
  - Major depressive disorder (MDD) is defined by at least one two week episode of major depression.
  - Dysthymia is less severe than MDD but lasts at least 2 years.
  - Seasonal affective disorder is depression with a regular seasonal onset.
- Bipolar disorders
  - Bipolar I is characterized by manic episodes and does not require depressive episodes to be diagnosed.
  - Bipolar II is characterized by at least one major depressive episode and one or more episodes of hypomania.
  - Cyclothymic disorder also involves hypomania, but usually less intense depression.
- Anxiety disorders
  - Generalized anxiety disorder involves extremely high levels of stress for everyday, routine aspects of life.
  - Social anxiety disorder is the onset of intense feelings of stress in social situations.
  - Illness anxiety disorder is excessive concern about medical conditions in the absence of physical symptoms.
- Obsessive-compulsive disorder is the presence of obsessions (intrusive thoughts) that can only be quieted temporarily by compulsions (ritualistic behaviors).
  - Body dysmorphic disorder: obsessive focus on a perceived flaw in appearance (negligible or not present).
- Post-traumatic stress disorder (PTSD): caused by intense acute and/or chronic trauma; intrusive recollections (not necessarily visual), avoidance of stimuli related to trauma, negative changes in mood and cognitions related to the traumatic event and altered patterns of reactivity and arousal (symptoms ≥1 month).
- Somatic disorders
  - Somatic symptom disorder is excessive preoccupation with a physical symptom.
  - Conversion disorder: impaired voluntary motor/sensory function with no apparent biological cause
- Dissociative disorders
  - Dissociative identity disorder: different personalities at different times within the same individual
  - Dissociative amnesia: retrograde amnesia in which people lose episodic memories of their own lives
- Depersonalization/derealization disorder: disconnection from own existence, as if observing onself
- Schizophrenia
  - Prodromal phase: period of poor adjustment before acute illness
  - Positive symptoms (added: hallucinations and delusions) vs. negative symptoms (subtracted: flattening affect, lethargy etc.). Catatonia is also common.
  - Biological cause of schizophrenia is thought to be primarily excess dopamine production. Schizophrenia is also highly heritable, with a major genetic component and a high concordance rate.
  - Treatment of schizophrenia usually involves antipsychotics, neuroleptics and therapy-based approaches
- Personality disorders: pervasive maladaptive behavior; ego-syntonic (patients don't perceive the problem)
  - Cluster A: paranoid, schizoid, and schizotypal personality disorders;
  - Cluster B: antisocial, narcissistic, histrionic, and borderline personality disorders
  - Cluster C: avoidant, dependent, and obsessive-compulsive personality disorders
- Biological causes:
  - Parksinon's disease: motor tremors, etc. Caused by cell death in the substantia nigra and reduced dopamine expression; can be induced by dopamine antagonists.
  - Alzheimer's disease: form of dementia with emotional disturbances; correlated with beta-amyloid plaques and tau protein fibrillary tangles.
  - Biological causes of depression: serotonin and dopamine deficiencies are currently thought to be the main cause of depression; selective serotonin reuptake inhibitors (SSRIs) increase serotonin levels in the brain and are currently the first line of treatment.

End of Chapter Practice

The best MCAT practice is **realistic**, with a focus on identifying steps for further improvement. For those reasons, we recommend completing practice questions in an online setting that simulates the real MCAT interface, and taking advantage of advanced analytic features to help you determine how best to move forward in your MCAT study journey.

With that in mind, **online end-of-chapter questions** are accessible through your Next Step account.

As a further supplement, given the importance of active learning for effective studying, we also suggest that you consult the Must-Knows as a basis for creating a study sheet, in which you list out key terms and test your ability to briefly summarize them.

This page left intentionally blank.

Social Psychology

CHAPTER 9

0. Introduction

So far, our discussion of human psychology has primarily focused on humans in isolation; that is, we've explored how individual minds work, but have yet to focus more explicitly on how people function in groups. However, humans are social animals, and as such, any exploration of human psychology would be incomplete if it did not consider this aspect of existence.

1. Group Effects on Individual Behavior

I. Social Facilitation

Let's ease our way into this topic by considering two comparison of solo behavior to behavior in group settings. These are bike riding and music playing. For bike riding, imagine that you're going for a bike ride around your town on a nice, warm spring day. It's an enjoyable experience, and your ride will probably be pleasant, but not necessarily the fastest or most efficient. Now let's imagine that some friends join you. You might pick up the pace, focus a little bit more on where you're going, and all in all ride more quickly and efficiently. Now imagine being in a race. You'll be more alert, on edge, and race with all your focus and strength -- so, you'll ride the fastest in these circumstances.

Switching gears, imagine that you're an intermediate-level guitar player with enough skills to have fun, but not really enough to impress anyone who has serious chops. Say you've just learned a piece that stretches your technical skills. If you're hanging out by yourself and try to play the piece casually, you may forget certain parts of it or make some technical mistakes because you're not paying complete attention. But if you want to show some friends the cool new piece you've learned, you'll probably focus more and play the piece to the best of your abilities. On the other hand, if you were put in front of a large and judgmental audience, your stress would probably get the best of you, causing your performance to suffer.

> **MCAT STRATEGY > > >**
>
> Although we tend to focus on the negative impact that the presence of other people has on human behavior, it can be positive as well. Remember that social facilitation makes people perform *better* at some tasks.

So, there are a couple things going on with these examples. In both of them, we started with a relaxed activity performed in a solo setting, and then gradually added more people and increased the level of **psychological arousal**, which is a term that refers to alertness and readiness to respond. For the bike-riding example, as we increased psychological arousal in a group setting, performance increased. Generalizing this example, the idea that we perform tasks better in group settings where psychological arousal is higher is known as **social facilitation**. But what about the guitar-playing task? In this context, social facilitation only worked to a certain extent. When the situation got *too* stressful, performance broke down. So what's the difference between bike riding and guitar playing? Well...remember that we specified that the guitar piece was one that stretched the player's technical ability. In contrast, bike riding is pretty simple. Once you've learned how to do it, you know how to do it. In contrast, playing a technical piece of music that you've just learned is more demanding and complex.

So, to summarize this information visually, consider a graph with increasing psychological arousal on the x-axis and performance on the y-axis. For simple or familiar tasks, like bike-riding, we'd just get a linear increase. This is social facilitation in action. For a complex task, like playing a difficult piece of music, we'd get an upside-down U-shaped graph, with the best performance being somewhere in the middle under conditions of moderate arousal. This U-shaped relationship is known as the **Yerkes-Dodson law**.

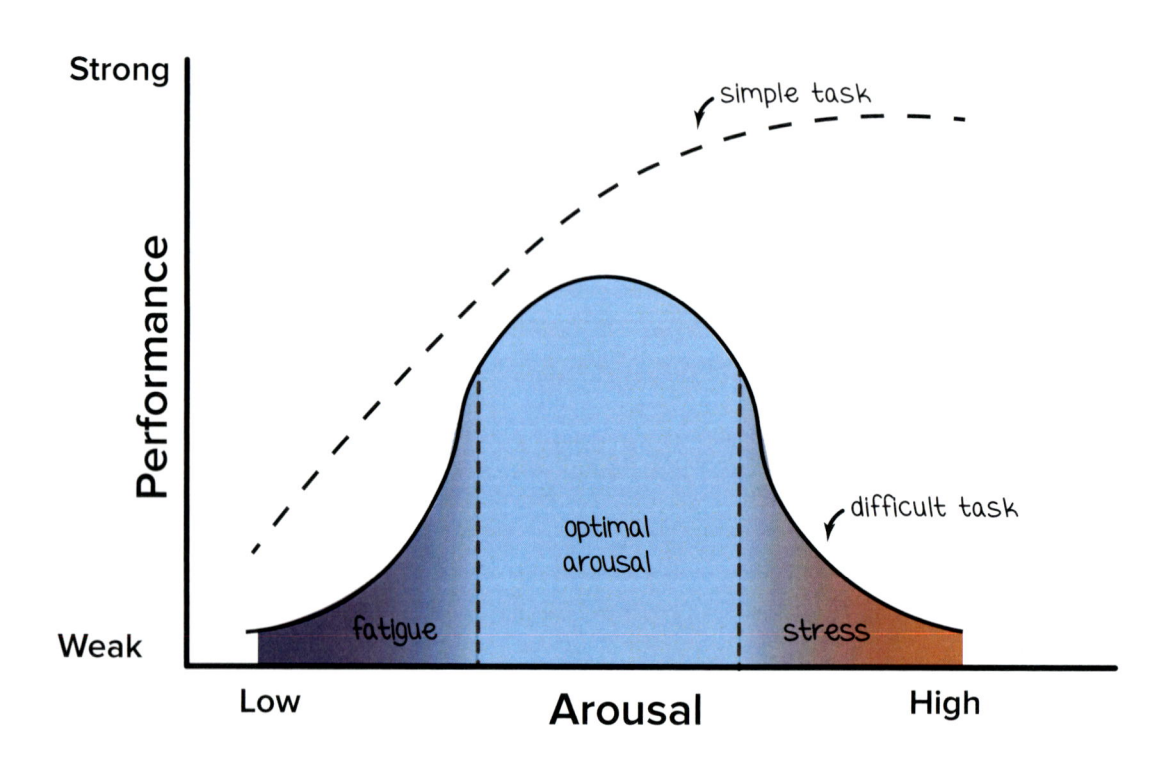

Figure 2. Yerkes-Dodson law.

II. Social Loafing

However, being in a group setting isn't always a *good* thing for our behavior. Another phenomenon, **social loafing**, is probably very familiar to anyone who is, or has ever been, in school. The idea is that you can work less hard, or be less productive, in a group setting because other people will pick up the slack. Group lab reports might immediately come to mind. That said, social loafing doesn't have to be a deliberate choice. For example, you might clap less loudly after a performance if you're part of an audience of 100 people than if you're part of an audience of only 5 or 10 people, but it's unlikely that you'd be making a deliberate choice to clap less intensely. The clapping example is worth noting both because it's subconscious and because it's not necessarily an example that would jump to mind when you think of "working hard". The example of slacking off in group projects is almost always used to illustrate this concept because we've all been there, but it's important to keep in mind that social loafing can be applied in any situation where there's some measurable output.

II. Bystander Effect and Deindividuation

On a gloomier note, the **bystander effect** is an especially famous example of the dark side of human behavior in groups. It refers to people's tendency not to offer help to someone in distress if other people, or bystanders, are present. One reason for this is the diffusion of responsibility within a crowd. That is, if many other people are present, especially strangers, it's easy to assume that you're not personally responsible for dealing with the situation and that other members of the crowd will step in to assist. A second reason is that we model our behavior on that of other people around us, so if something unusual happens on a busy street, but everyone else walks by as if nothing out of the ordinary is happening, it's likely that we'll do the same. Social etiquette also plays a role, since it may be considered impolite to pay too much attention to strangers in a public space. However, some factors have been found to increase the likelihood that we'll respond to a stranger in distress: namely, being in a group made up of acquaintances and recognizing that a situation is especially dangerous.

Research into the bystander effect was spurred by the murder of Kitty Genovese in 1964 in New York City. Genovese was stabbed to death at 3:15 AM in a public space, and the New York Times published a sensational story a few weeks later stating that many neighbors heard her screams but did not call the police because they assumed that someone else had already done so. More recently, it's been called into question whether that event actually went down the way the news story said it did, but regardless, it was an extremely influential news item that launched this whole area of research in psychology.

As a more general phenomenon, **deindividuation** describes how people tend to lose their sense of self-awareness in a large group setting, due to a high degree of psychological arousal and a low degree of perceived responsibility. These effects take place on a spectrum. Moderate deindividuation can take place in positive crowd experiences, like those you might have at a dance club, music festival, or rave. More intense deindividuation, with negative consequences, helps to explain the behavior of violent mobs. Three main factors contribute to deindividuation. First, there's **anonymity**, and in particular the sense that no one will know what you do in a crowd. Second, there's **diffused responsibility**, or the sense that you're not really responsible for what happens. Third, there's **group size**, which increases the effects of both anonymity and diffused responsibility.

To summarize, the conceptual thread that ties all of these examples together is the idea that an individual person may behave differently in an individual setting versus in a group setting, and the details depend on the situation, the type of group, and so on. Some of these findings, like those related to the bystander effect and deindividuation, might not be especially comforting, in that they suggest that the ways we behave in certain settings might not line up very well with how we like to think of ourselves. But in any case, it's food for thought, especially for future physicians and other health professionals, since group settings are such an integral part of the medical education process and how healthcare is delivered.

2. Group Polarization and Groupthink

In addition to how groups influence individual behavior, social psychologists have also explored how groups function in their own right. Two particularly important phenomena are group polarization and groupthink. For the MCAT, the biggest danger with these concepts is getting them confused, so we're going to define them, work through a few examples, and then discuss how to make sure that you can tell them apart in a testing situation.

Group polarization refers to the tendency of a group to make decisions or arrive at final opinions that are more extreme than the initial positions of the individual members of the group. This reflects a dynamic in which initial opinions get amplified over the course of a discussion. Imagine that you put five chocolate-lovers in a room and have them talk about chocolate, and maybe even prepare a little presentation about chocolate. Group polarization would predict that the participants would get each other all amped up about how great chocolate is, and then deliver a presentation that would be *extremely* positive about all the virtues of chocolate, even beyond their starting point.

On a more serious note, group polarization famously occurs when people talk about politics. In recent years, concerns have been raised about the so-called "echo chamber" effect of social media, in which people interact primarily with other people who they already agree with, and how this might create spaces where group polarization yields harmful effects for society as a whole. Two major factors contribute to group polarization: **informational influence** and **normative influence**. Informational influence refers to the idea that in a group discussion, people are more likely to express points of view in line with the dominant viewpoint, and the disproportionate attention paid to such information reinforces individuals' pre-existing viewpoints. Normative influence, in contrast, refers to our desire to be socially accepted, affirmed, or admired within a group. This is more easily accomplished by agreeing with people than by disagreeing with people, and this tendency towards agreement contributes to group polarization.

Groupthink is a similar-sounding but distinct phenomenon, in which irrational decisions are made within a group due to pressures towards harmony and individual conformity. An American psychologist named Irving Janis was the first scholar to research this phenomenon. Janis argued that groupthink played a crucial role in several disastrous decisions in 20th-century history, such as the decision of Nazi Germany to invade the Soviet Union, and the decisions made as part of American involvement in the Vietnam War. He proposed eight specific factors that are characteristic of groupthink.

The first of these, **illusion of invulnerability**, refers to the belief that no serious harm will happen to the group. This unjustified optimism can result in excessive risk-taking. Next, **illusion of morality** refers to a rigid, unbending belief in the moral righteousness of the group's cause, which helps blind group members to objections and leads them to overlook possible consequences of their action. A third illusion, **illusion of unanimity,** refers to the assumption that the majority opinions in the group are unanimous (i.e., that everyone in the group agrees). This factor is buffered by **self-censorship**, which means that members who *do* disagree don't share their opinion. This is in turn supported by **pressure on dissenters**, which means that members feel pressure not to express opinions contrary to the majority group. **Collective rationalization** refers to the tendency for group members to find reasons to ignore warnings and to avoid reconsidering their actions our assumptions. This is linked to **excessive stereotyping**, which means that negative views about outside opinions or viewpoints lead group members not to take other perspectives seriously. What's more, those opinions might not even make it to the group in the first place, thanks to our eighth and final factor: **mindguards**. This strikingly-named factor refers to a phenomenon where certain members of the group filter out information that could destabilize the group's consensus.

Janis' Eight Factors of Groupthink	Practical Definition
Collective rationalization	Group members ignore warnings and do not reconsider their actions, assumptions, or beliefs.
Excessive stereotyping	Negative views of outside or dissenting opinions render effective responses to conflict unnecessary.
Illusion of invulnerability	An unjustified and excessive sense of optimism encourages risk-taking.
Illusion of morality	Member of the group believe in the moral rightness of their cause and therefore ignore the consequences of their actions.
Illusion of unanimity	The majority views of the group are assumed to be unanimous.
Mindguards	Members of the group protect the group's cohesiveness by filtering out information that would be problematic.
Pressure on dissenters	Members are constantly under pressure to not express views or beliefs that are against those of the group.
Self-censorship	Members who do hold dissenting opinions do not share them.

Table 1. Irving Janis' eight factors of groupthink.

The concept of groupthink originally emerged from researchers trying to figure out why military and governmental policymakers, in particular, made bad decisions about war. But groupthink isn't limited to war, or even politics. For instance, groupthink can apply in corporate contexts, like when a company goes ahead with the release of a new product despite failing to research the market or think about trends in the industry, only for the new product to totally flop. It could also apply to situations in which an organization protects incompetent or abusive members of its inner circle, while dismissing calls for reform as coming from vindictive outsiders.

> **MCAT STRATEGY > > >**
>
> A scenario in a question or passage must satisfy the specific criteria of groupthink in order for it to be the correct answer.

What unifies these examples of groupthink is that they all involve irrational decisions made by a group due to the eight factors described in the model articulated by Janis, including delusions about being invincible and righteous, plus strong pressures towards harmony and conformity. It does *not* refer to all bad decisions made by a group, and it definitely doesn't refer to all situations in which a group kind of goes off track in terms of its thought process. But groupthink always must involve a decision.

In contrast, group polarization may be irrational—although the definition doesn't actually specify that, it just says that opinions get more extreme—and it may be the result of group-specific cognitive factors, but it doesn't require making a decision, and the specific group-internal factors don't have to line up with those described by Janis. Think about our example of chocolate-lovers: their eventual presentation on the extreme benefits of chocolate doesn't have to be motivated by anything more sinister than contagious enthusiasm.

3. Conformity, Compliance, and Obedience

In our next discussion, we'll be dealing with three concepts that describe how certain members of a group influence others: conformity, compliance, and obedience. In everyday life, we often use these words more or less interchangeably, so as always, we'll need to be more precise for the MCAT. This is especially true for this subject matter, because unfortunately, even psychologists researching these concepts haven't exactly always followed the guideline of using a single, clearly-defined, and distinct term for each concept.

I. Conformity

Conformity describes situations where someone's behavior, beliefs, or thinking changes to line up with the perspectives of others or with social norms in the community. Note the word "changes." This implies that we can't just observe someone behaving in the same way as the rest of a group, or the rest of the community, and conclude that it's an example of conformity in the technical sense. The term for such a situation, where someone's beliefs or behaviors just happen to line up with those of the group, is **convergence**—although you may also encounter **congruence**, which emphasizes that this concept refers to pre-existing overlap.

An interesting aspect of conformity is that sometimes it corresponds to a genuine change in someone's beliefs, which is referred to as **internalization** or **conversion**, but sometimes it doesn't. That latter situation, where someone just goes along with the group but internally dissents, is known as **compliance**. Now, let's take a second here to address a terminological point: This sense of the word compliance, as a subtype of conformity, is not the same as the kind of compliance that you will read about later in a separate subsection.

> **MCAT STRATEGY > > >**
>
> The two meanings of "compliance" can be a source of confusion, but try to rely on context. This is simply a case where a word is used in two different ways, like how "nucleus" has multiple meanings in biology.

There can also be a middle ground between internalization and compliance, where someone's behavior and beliefs change, but only kind of, and only in the presence of the group. This is known as **identification**. It's kind of a slippery concept, and can be counterintuitive because we often like to think of our beliefs as these core, never-changing parts of our identity, but in reality, things can be a bit fuzzier.

Conformity is not necessarily a bad thing, even though we often use the term with a pejorative implication. Most of us conform with norms about politeness, and society works better as a result. Along those lines, it's also worth noting that conformity doesn't have to literally involve a group of people right there in the room with you. In particular, you can conform to internalized norms even when no one else is present. For example, some people have internalized the norm of making their bed after getting up in the morning, and do so even when living alone. It's entirely up to you to judge whether this is a good or a bad thing, but in any case, conformity doesn't have to be dangerous, but it can be if it leads us to engage in risky behavior or act unethically.

The **Solomon Asch experiment** is a thought-provoking example of the power of conformity. In this experiment, each subject was shown a card with a line on it, then shown another card with three lines ("A," "B," and "C") and asked which of those three lines matched the length of the original line. Subjects were asked to perform this task in a group setting. However, all but one of the group members were confederates who knew the true purpose of the experiment. The subjects were asked to state their answer out loud in front of other group members. The confederates would report an incorrect answer for the matching line, and the subjects showed a strong tendency to repeat that incorrect answer.

II. Compliance

Compliance is a little bit more direct than conformity, in that it refers to responses to requests from someone who has no power to directly enforce that request. Note, again, that this concept is different from compliance as a subtype of conformity. There really should be two different words for these concepts (come on, get it together, psychologists!) but the good news is that the MCAT will always make it clear which one we're talking about. Marketing and sales pitches are common examples of the request-related form of compliance, although it's curious that we're exposed to so much advertising that we might not even consciously register how commercials, for example, essentially contain a request to buy a certain product.

Several tactics can be used to increase the likelihood of compliance to a request. The **foot-in-the-door technique** involves first making a small request of someone and then making a larger request. The idea is that positively responding to a small request makes it more likely that the person will then agree to a larger request. An example might be first asking your professor if you can turn in an assignment a little bit late, like at 9 am the next day if it's a midnight deadline, and then upping the request to get a longer extension. A more modern example could be asking people to follow you on social media before hitting them up for crowdfunding.

In contrast, the **door-in-the-face technique** involves making a large request at first that you know will be rejected, only to follow it up with a smaller, more reasonable-seeming request. So, imagine you're doing some fundraising for charity. You first ask people to make a $100 donation, knowing that that's a lot of money, and they'll say no—at which point your request for a $20 donation instead, which was your goal all along, will seem reasonable. Finally, the **low-ball technique** involves offering something at a low price, only to raise it at the last minute, once the customer is invested in the purchase. A common example of this technique is buying a car, in which the customer is often presented with a relatively low price at first, only to be presented with various last-minute expensive options after demonstrating interest in the deal.

III. Obedience

Obedience refers to a change in behavior in response to a direct request from someone who has power to enforce that request. Common examples include orders from law enforcement officials or one's boss. In a famous experiment conducted in 1961, a psychologist at Yale named **Stanley Milgram** decided to see how far people would go in terms of inflicting pain on someone in response to direct instructions. This line of research originated in attempts to understand the atrocities that had occurred in World War II.

The **Milgram experiment** involved a setup with three roles: experimenter, teacher, and learner. The experimenter and learner were always part of the research team, so each participant was always allocated the role of "teacher". The participant was told that he or she would be taking part in a study of memory and learning, and that the study was going to investigate the impact of punishment on a learner's ability to retain content. The learner was situated in a different room from the experimenter and teacher, and the teacher's job was to give electric shocks to the learner for failing to memorize a list of word pairs. The teacher would even get a sample shock to help convince them that the pain was real. The twist, of course, was that the learner wasn't receiving real shocks, but rather was just acting to convince the teacher that his or her actions were causing pain. Anyway, the "shocks" would get stronger and stronger, and they'd even simulate the learner screaming in pain, banging on the wall, and eventually going silent. Reluctant participants were told that it was essential to continue, or that they must go on. On the bright side, the participants were reluctant, did question the experiment, and showed physiological signs of stress. However, most subjects went through with it anyway, administering shocks all the way to the strongest level.

Spurred by similar questions, in 1971, a researcher named **Philip Zimbardo** ran an experiment at Stanford that simulated a prison environment. In the **Stanford Prison Experiment**, student volunteers were assigned to be either guards or prisoners. Prisoners went through a realistic intake process, including a simulated arrest by real members of the Palo Alto police department and the guards were instructed to treat the prisoners arbitrarily and harshly, but without actual physical violence. The principal investigator, Zimbardo, played the role of the prison superintendent. Things turned grim, fast. Within a week, some of the prisoners started showing signs of real suffering, and about a third of the guards demonstrated what Zimbardo felt to be genuinely sadistic tendencies. The experiment was planned to continue for two weeks, but was ended early, after just six days.

Some of you who've done research might have noticed how institutional review boards, or IRBs, have all sorts of requirements about scientific ethics, and it can be time-consuming and frankly even a little frustrating for researchers to document that they're complying with these rules. But the Stanford Prison Experiment is an important example of why such guidelines exist. In addition to the basic ethical issues involved in this experiment, its scientific validity has been questioned too, since Zimbardo was actively involved in the experiment, and guards were encouraged to behave in certain ways. But regardless of its ethical and even scientific issues, it's probably one of the most famous psychological experiments out there, and it's definitely thought-provoking about how the factors of conformity, compliance, and obedience can shape our behavior in frankly disturbing ways.

4. Social Norms, Deviance, and Socialization

I. Norms

Society is governed by norms, which are the rules (spoken or unspoken) that regulate the behavior, beliefs, attitudes, and values of members of society. The concept of **social control** refers to the myriad of ways in which those norms are taught, enforced, and perpetuated. **Deviance**, in turn, occurs when someone doesn't follow a norm. Norms are a very general concept, but we can make them more specific by breaking them down into subcategories. The first distinction to make is between **formal norms** and **informal norms**. A formal norm must be encoded somewhere, usually in a law or a regulation, and formal norms have specific penalties for violating them. Laws are an excellent example, but formal norms can also be found in places like employee handbooks or the charter of an organization or club. Informal norms, in contrast, aren't written down anywhere. They're just expectations, and they don't have fixed penalties for violating them.

Some informal norms are more important than others. The term **folkways** refers to relatively insignificant informal norms that typically involve small details of everyday behavior. For instance, fashion trends can be considered folkways. Violating folkways doesn't usually cause too much of a problem. So, for instance, if your footwear of choice is a combination of bright blue sandals with mismatching socks, you may not impress anyone with your fashion sense, but the direct consequences should be minimal.

In contrast, important informal norms are known as **mores** (pronounced like "morays"). There's not exactly a fixed definition of mores—remember that the defining feature of informal norms is that they're not codified—but a good rule of thumb is that mores are norms that you'll get some serious disapproval for violating. One example might be cheating on a romantic partner. Or being a jerk to people who work retail. None of these things are illegal, and it's not like you'll be cast out of society for doing those things, but the disapproval may be very real. Finally, **taboos** refer to the most restrictive norms, or things that you just don't do. Examples that apply in modern American culture include incest—even between consenting adults—and cannibalism. Taboos can be culture-specific, and examples from other cultures include restrictions on which foods can be combined with each other or what kind of sexual orientations are acceptable. A final note about taboos is that because violating them is perceived to be such a severe offense, they do kind of blur the line between formal and informal norms. That is, some taboos are forbidden by law, while others aren't.

We've touched on the idea that violating social norms has consequences, but let's articulate that idea a little bit more. In sociology, the term **sanctions** refers both to any punishment or negative consequence for violating a social norm *and* to any reward for following those norms. On a conceptual level, sanctions are closely linked with the idea of **social control**, and we can think of social control as being the more general phenomenon, while sanctions are the specific ways that social control manifests. **Peer pressure**, which we've all encountered (for better or worse) is another mechanism through which social control is exerted and refers to how the desire of approval from our peers—or the fear of disapproval from them—can be a particularly powerful motivator.

We may not always agree about norms in society, both for individual reasons (because some norms might rub us the wrong way) and because society changes pretty rapidly. At the end of the 1800s, a pioneering French sociologist named **Emile Durkheim** analyzed this latter issue, particularly in light of the rapid social changes that he had seen occur in his lifetime due to industrialization. He coined the term **anomie**, which refers to a situation in which there's no longer a good match between society's stated norms and the norms that an individual responds to. This is often framed as a weakening or withering of social norms, but in any case, such a mismatch results in a breakdown of traditional systems of moral regulation, sometimes accompanied by negative feelings of apathy or despair.

> **MCAT STRATEGY > > >**
>
> In sociology, "deviance" isn't a general term that just means weird behavior; instead, it must be defined relative to a specific social norm that is violated. Although deviance isn't necessarily negative, it is the case that theoretical approaches to deviance have focused on negative, criminal behavior.

II. Deviance

As we mentioned earlier, **deviance** refers to someone not following, or violating, a norm. Just like there are different levels of seriousness for norms, deviance can be relatively trivial or relatively serious. For a trivial example, consider how we have certain norms about which foods we eat at which meals. If you eat salad for breakfast and pancakes for dinner, that's deviating from those norms, but nobody is likely to raise a fuss. However, very serious crimes like murder are also forms of deviance. Deviance can even be positive, such as eschewing counter-productive social norms. Sociologists have tended to pay more attention to relatively serious types of negative deviance, but the MCAT expects you to understand deviance as a general concept.

Various theoretical frameworks have emerged to try to make sense of deviance, and the MCAT expects you to be familiar with a few of the highlights. First off, **differential association theory** focuses on deviance as behavior that's learned socially. To put it very bluntly, criminals become criminals by hanging out with other criminals and learning to commit crime from them. That might sound obvious, but it was actually somewhat revolutionary at its time, because previous perspectives on deviance explained deviant behavior as resulting from inherent deficiencies or flaws in a person—that is, instead of saying "people do bad things because they're awful human beings," differential association theory said "hey, maybe people do bad things because they learned to do so in some social setting." This theory draws from the **symbolic interactionist** school of sociology in terms of how it sees behaviors as learned phenomena with culturally-determined significance.

Another perspective derived from symbolic interactionism is the **labeling approach** to deviance, which focuses on how people's behavior is affected by being labeled as deviant. The idea is that being labeled as a deviant shapes people's identity in a way that increases the frequency of deviant behavior. In other words, it's kind of a compulsively defiant approach to deviance.

Within the labeling approach framework, a distinction exists between **primary deviance** and **secondary deviance**. Primary deviance refers to deviant acts committed before someone receives a label, while secondary deviance refers to such acts that are committed after someone has been labeled, partially in reaction to that label. As such, acts of secondary deviance are likely to be treated more harshly by society, and this concept has been found useful in trying to explain the process through which someone becomes a hardened criminal.

From more of a functionalist point of view, **strain theory** looks at why people engage in deviant behavior, and in particular focuses on the role of social and economic pressures in pushing people towards criminal behavior. Strain theory doesn't just say that people steal because they're poor, but instead would say that deviant behavior occurs in some people when there's a mismatch between socially acceptable goals and socially accepted ways to get there. So for instance, if we glorify wealth, no matter how it was attained, while making certain ways of getting wealthy illegal, we're going to see some people committing crime as a way to achieve that goal. To anticipate a possible objection here, strain theory doesn't say that everyone would commit crime under those circumstances, just that some would. More recently, this theory was expanded upon to create **general strain theory**, which hypothesizes that people who experience social, economic, or even personal stressors may have negative emotional experiences that push them towards deviance or crime.

CHAPTER 9: SOCIAL PSYCHOLOGY

As is often the case in sociology, these theories are not mutually exclusive. All of these theories can provide us with some potentially useful insights, but none of them really captures a whole picture or has fantastic predictive value. As always, the goal for the MCAT is to be able to recognize how these theories can be applied to explain a certain phenomenon, in this case deviance.

III. Socialization

Finally, there's one piece of the picture that we haven't really dealt with yet. How do we learn all these norms, anyway? The answer is the process of **socialization**, which refers to how we learn the whole dizzying range of informal and formal norms that govern society by interacting with other people and institutions. The first agent of socialization we encounter is the family, in which parents of young children will tell you that a huge amount of energy goes into setting expectations, defining behaviors, and so on. The educational system is another important agent of socialization that starts as soon as preschool or kindergarten. We also internalize a lot of information about social expectations from mass media, and we can't forget peers and the workplace as well. Any major social institution can serve as an agent of socialization. That is definitely food for thought as you go about your daily business.

5. Aspects of Collective Behavior

We've talked about deviance on an individual level, but deviant behavior can occur in a collective setting too. Collectives are short-term collections of people without close ties or exclusive membership, unlike groups, which are characterized by longer-term bonds and exclusivity. Examples of collective deviant behavior involve situations where very loosely-defined groups of people engage in behavior that doesn't match social norms for a limited amount of time, often reflecting what feels like a temporary surge of enthusiasm, panic, or anger.

Fads occur when a new behavior suddenly becomes extremely popular, and then its popularity fades. It's a lot like something going viral, but not as a phenomenon exclusive to the internet or videos and images—that is, the focus is more on the behavior or product itself, and less on the specific videos or images used to spread awareness and interest of it. One of the first well-documented fads was something called pole-sitting in the 1920s, in which the hip thing to do was to climb up on a pole and just stay there for as long as possible. (Guess you had to be there!) A good example of a product-oriented fad is how something called the Pet Rock became wildly popular in the 1970s. As the name implies, some marketing genius hit on the idea of taking literal rocks and selling them to people as pets. Again, the details of fads don't really age well. This tendency not to stand up that well to time is actually a characteristic of fads. In the modern media environment, fads are very common. A few examples include planking, dabbing, and various "challenges" that spread through social media.

Next, **mass hysteria** is sort of like a dark version of fads, where instead of a harmless dance move, or pole-sitting, or whatever, the behavior that spreads like wildfire is freaking out about some perceived threat, be it witches in the 1600s or the situation in 2016 where people throughout America were calling in sightings of evil clowns. Opposition to vaccination may fit into this category as well. The key point about mass hysteria is that it must be irrational, even verging on the point of a collective delusion. The real-life line between classic examples of mass hysteria and circumstances where the public's emotions are just whipped up about the controversy of the day isn't always crystal clear, but any example you get on the MCAT should be unambiguous.

Riots are even more temporary than mass hysteria or fads. Riots can be thought of as spontaneous episodes of civil disorder where people violently lash out against authority in some form or another, although in some cases the actual target of the riot is not clear. Vandalism and property destruction are common features of rioting. People often engage in riots somewhat spontaneously, and riots form a classic example of deindividuation—that is, of how anonymity and a feeling of reduced responsibility in a crowd can lead people to engage in atypical behaviors.

Even though fads, mass hysteria, and riots are collective phenomena, not individual behaviors, we can still see the same pattern that we identified for individual deviance, in which there's a spectrum between relatively harmless deviance, like fads, and more serious forms of deviance, like riots. The seriousness of deviance depends on the specific norms that are violated, so we can see that norms and deviance are two sides of the same coin, because without norms, the concept of deviance wouldn't make any sense.

6. Attributions

In most, if not all, social interactions, we form impressions of people or have those impressions confirmed or challenged. Another way to think about this is that we try to figure out why people act the way they do, and in part, we judge them based on those explanations. In social psychology, these kinds of down-to-earth explanations of people's behavior are known as **attributions**. An attribution is something like: "Brandon acted that way because he's a stellar human being" or "That customer who was rude must have been having an awful day"—everyday, familiar things, not explanations in the sense of diving into the whole constellation of biological, psychological, and social factors that shape our behavior.

The examples above, of someone named Brandon and a rude customer, illustrate a tremendously important distinction. When we said that Brandon acted a certain way because he's a stellar human being, that explains his behavior in terms of something internal, or inherent to his disposition or character. This is known as a **dispositional attribution**. Dispositional attribution can also be negative—we might attribute Brandon's behavior to being lazy or pretentious or something else. On the other hand, when we said that the customer was rude because he or she was having an awful day, that's an externally-focused explanation, which is known as a **situational attribution**. Whether we make dispositional or situational attributions has major implications for our relationships with people, because dispositional attributions draw on stable, inherent traits, for better or for worse, so we might judge people more intensely as a result, whereas situational attributions are fleeting and external, and don't really reflect core aspects of who someone is as a human being. This might predispose us to forgive bad behavior more easily, but also might lead us not to be as impressed by good behavior. Regardless, a considerable amount of research has gone into figuring out when we tend to make which kind of attributions.

If you've known someone for some length of time, you've probably had the chance to see how he or she acts in various situations. This means that in any given *new* situation, there will be various cues that guide whether you interpret that person's behavior through a dispositional or situational lens. For one, you might notice whether a given instance of behavior is consistent with how that person has behaved previously, over a longer stretch of time. These cues are known, reasonably enough, as **consistency cues**. The idea here is that the more consistent the behavior over time, the more likely we are to make a dispositional attribution. For example, imagine you have a friend named Susan. If she's always quiet and subdued, then that's probably just how she is. But if she's normally vivacious and talkative, but today is quiet and subdued, then you might infer that something's happened—that is, you might make a situational attribution. **Distinctiveness cues** are similar, but focus more on how someone behaves differently—or "distinctively"—in comparable situations. The idea here is similar—namely, that if someone shows uneven patterns of behavior in otherwise comparable situations, we're likely to make a situational attribution. The concept of consensus cues brings in the broader social context of norms and expectations, and here the idea is that if someone's behavior doesn't line up with what's socially expected, we're likely to make a dispositional attribution.

Several other interesting quirks in how we assign situational versus dispositional attributions have been observed by psychiatrists. Pay close attention here, though, because the terms that we're about to introduce are very commonly mixed up or confused. These are the actor-observer bias, the fundamental attribution error, and the self-serving bias. First, the **actor-observer bias** refers to the idea that we're more likely to make a dispositional attribution of someone else, but a situational attribution for ourselves, especially when explaining negative behaviors. In other words, if somebody else cuts you off in traffic, it's because he or she is a terrible driver and/or a generally inconsiderate person, but if you cut someone else off in traffic, there's probably some external reason for it—maybe you were in a hurry just this once, or maybe it was hard to see the other person's car there for some reason, or who knows. One explanation for this is that we're more aware of the situational circumstances that affect ourselves than of those affecting others. Another is that we might be more ready to apply negative labels to other people than to ourselves. Something called the **fundamental attribution error** reflects a similar basic insight, but applied only to other people—that is, we're more likely to apply dispositional attributions than situational attributions to other people. So these two concepts, the actor-observer bias and the fundamental attribution error, get at the same issue but from a slightly different perspective: the fundamental attribution error focuses on others, while the actor-observer bias additionally points out that there's also an asymmetry in how we explain our own behavior. Finally, the **self-serving bias** focuses just on ourselves, and the idea here is that we're more likely to make dispositional attributions of our own behavior if the outcomes are good, and situational attributions if the outcomes are bad. So, for instance, if you get a very high score on the MCAT, you tell yourself it must be because you're just that good, but if you were to get a much lower score than you had hoped, there probably was some external reason, you may have been tired, gotten unfortunate passages, and so on. More broadly, the self-serving bias can be extended to describe a general tendency for people to perceive themselves in a positive way that minimizes their flaws and failures.

The balance between dispositional and situational attributions of our own actions is affected by a concept called **locus of control**. People differ somewhat systematically in terms of whether they view themselves as having personal control over their circumstances. People with an internal locus of control do see themselves as being able to affect their personal situations, while people with an external locus of control tend to focus more on the impacts of factors outside of themselves, like luck, external circumstances, or even fate. The concept of locus of control is of interest in its own right as a predictor of people's behavior in various contexts, but it's also linked to self-serving bias, in that people with an external locus of control are even more likely than people in general to use situational attributions to explain poor outcomes.

Returning to the topic of how we see others, there are a few other important concepts to be aware of that are less specifically linked to the distinction between situational and dispositional attributions. The **halo effect** is one to watch out for in our everyday lives. It describes how positive—or negative—impressions of someone in one domain can expand out to affect judgments of them in other domains. A classic example of the halo effect has to do with the good impressions created by attractive people who dress well and behave charmingly. Those positive impressions can spill over into other judgments that people make, like about whether someone would be a good coworker, employee, business partner or friend. In other words, the halo effect is part of why people dress up for interviews. But, of course, the danger with the halo effect is that you can't always extrapolate one aspect of someone's life to make assumptions about other aspects.

The **just-world hypothesis** is another important phenomenon that impacts how we assess people. The idea here is that good things happen to good people, and bad things to bad people, so if you're in a good situation, you must be a good person, or have done something good to deserve it, and if you're in a bad situation, you must be a bad person, or must have done something bad to deserve it. Now, the name here is a little bit misleading, to the point that you would be best served to think of the name as a sarcastic joke. The logic here is clearly not airtight, and people may not necessarily believe exactly that, although some people do. Instead, the point behind the just-world hypothesis is that it's a bias that can affect how we see people, even if we wouldn't explicitly endorse it as a law of the universe. All things being equal, we tend to assume good things about people who are doing well in life, and the converse can hold about people who aren't doing well, or have had bad things happen to them. To some extent, this bias may stem from a tendency that many of us have to want the world to be just, which is challenged by situations where awful people do well in life and die a peaceful death at an old age, or where good people experience horrible things, so we try to minimize that discomfort by finding excuses for outcomes that challenge our assumptions and make us uncomfortable. It might also, to a certain extent, be an extension of the halo effect. In any case, it's something to watch out for, both in life in general and on the MCAT.

Culture can also play a role in shaping attributions. In particular, it's been suggested that people from collectivistic cultures—most commonly exemplified by traditional East Asian societies—are relatively more likely to make situational attributions than people from individualistic cultures, such as America and Western Europe, who are more likely to make dispositional attributions. In other words, people from an individualistic culture are more likely to interpret someone's actions in light of his or her inherent traits as an individual, whereas people from a collectivistic background are more likely to focus on the external factors that shape someone's actions. That said, there's also obviously more to culture than just this two-way distinction, and specific aspects of attributions can be affected by specific cultural assumptions and references. To take a small but telling example, attributions related to the behavior of tipping vary widely throughout the world, and are shaped both by general cultural attitudes and, perhaps more importantly, differences in how waiters and waitresses are compensated.

What's more, our perceptions of ourselves also shape how we perceive others. In a nutshell, as a rough-and-ready way of explaining why other people act the way they do is to try to imagine under what circumstances we would act that way. Now, there are obviously some limitations with this strategy, as many of us might have experienced in familial relationships, friendships, or romantic relationships, but it's a common knee-jerk reaction. Furthermore, our perceptions of the environment surrounding us can also shape how we perceive others' actions. For example, in a situation where the vibe just feels weird, like something's off, you might be more likely to read people's actions as threatening than in a comfortable, cozy, safe-feeling space. All in all, what it boils down to is that a lot of factors go into how we perceive people. For the MCAT, you should be very sure to understand the distinction between dispositional and situational attributions of behavior, as well as how the concepts of actor-observer bias, fundamental attribution error, and self-serving bias utilize that distinction to explain asymmetries in how we perceive ourselves and others.

7. Prejudice, Stereotypes, and Discrimination

The concept of attribution refers to how we explain individuals' behavior, or, in simple terms, how we judge people as individuals, but we also make judgments about groups, or about individuals based on the groups they belong to. This is where the concepts of prejudice, stereotypes, and discrimination come in. These phenomena exert a tremendous real-world impact on people's life experience, plus these terms have technical definitions in sociology that are more precise than how we use them in everyday life.

Before we really jump into things, as a background note, we should be aware that even though prejudice, stereotypes, and discrimination are most often talked about in the context of demographic features like race, gender, sexual orientation, religion, and age, they can actually apply to any group, including those defined by more or less voluntary characteristics, like wearing a mullet, or liking boy bands. Part of why we tend to focus on parameters like gender, sexual orientation, race, religion, and age is that prejudice, stereotypes, and discrimination based on these categories are pervasive and high-impact. But the flip side of that is that these can be sensitive topics, and we want to really have a laser-like focus on understanding the conceptual relationships going on here.

Therefore, we'll use a lower-stakes example as something to return to throughout this discussion: how people dress for job interviews. In many industries, the expectation is that interviewees should show up wearing fancy clothes, and not doing so can be an immediate problem. However, in some other industries—perhaps most notably tech companies on the West Coast—getting very dressed up for an interview isn't expected, and can actually work against you. As a shorthand, we'll refer to these two behaviors as suit-wearing and hoodie-wearing.

The term **prejudice** refers to irrational attitudes—positive or negative—towards various groups, or even objects. The key point is that prejudice is an affective, or emotional, response. Think of it as an immediate thumbs up or thumbs down response, the kind of thing that can hit you at a gut level before you even really have time to process why. Imagine that you're an interviewer, you open the door to go into a room to interview a candidate you haven't met before, and you see that he or she is wearing sandals and a hoodie. Is your immediate reaction positive or negative? Either way, that's prejudice in action.

Next, let's probe a little bit deeper into your reaction in the scenario that we just described. If you're on team hoodie-wearing, you might consider relatively informal attire at a job interview to be a positive sign that someone's not stuck up, and is likely to focus on the substance of the job, rather than spending a lot of time and energy looking nice. Overall, you just might get an authentic vibe from such a person. On the other hand, wearing a suit might suggest pomposity, a focus on looking good rather than building a good product, and overall insincerity. On the other hand, if you're on team suit-wearing, you might consider informal attire to be an indicator of carelessness or disrespect, and maybe a sign that someone won't put in the effort to get things right on the job, where on the other hand, formal attire might be a positive sign of someone being attentive to details, ambitious, and respectful. It doesn't really matter where you come down on this question—the point is that we all have certain opinions about what these choices signal about someone. Those, in a nutshell, are **stereotypes**. The key point about stereotypes is that they're contentful—that is, they contain specific content about what we assume about people. For that reason, stereotypes are often considered to be cognitive, in contrast to prejudices, which are affective, or emotion-related. Here, the stereotype would be, "Oh, the interviewee must have such-and-such characteristic because he's wearing a tie," whereas prejudice would be the visceral, emotional reaction to the interviewee walking into the room wearing a hoodie and flip-flops.

The concepts of prejudice and stereotypes can be difficult to disentangle because they generally co-occur in real-world situations, but let's try to imagine some situations where you might have one without the other. Stereotypes without prejudice could conceivably occur if you had a stereotype that was specific, but emotionally neutral. An example would be the stereotype that people from California like to surf, assuming that you really don't feel one way or the other about surfing as a hobby. For prejudices without stereotypes, you'd have to find a situation where someone likes or dislikes something, or a group of people, to an irrational extent, without having a clear reason for it whatsoever. However, it can be hard to find good examples of this, because it might always be the case that someone does have a stereotype that underlies a prejudice, but just can't articulate it.

Hopefully, we've been able to make this clear through the examples we've chosen, but it doesn't hurt to say it directly: Stereotypes often are negative, but they can be positive too. More specifically, the **stereotype content model** proposes that stereotypes of social groups can be arranged on two axes: **warmth and competence**, where warmth refers more or less to our fondness for the group in question, and competence refers to how capable we perceive that group as being. The combination of high warmth and low competence results in a **paternalistic stereotype**, which is applied to people who are low-status in society but not felt to pose a competitive threat. As the name implies, children can be an example of this, but also, interestingly, paternalistic stereotypes can be directed towards elderly people who require care. The combination of high warmth and high competence yields **admiration**, which is directed towards people who are felt to be high-status and not to pose a competitive threat—in other words, one's own in-group, or close allies thereof. The combination of low warmth and low competence is applied to people who are felt to be low-status and to pose a competitive threat of some sort. This corresponds to a **contemptuous stereotype**. Finally, the combination of low warmth and high competence is applied to high-status people who pose a competitive threat. This results in an **envious stereotype**. Both contemptuous and envious stereotypes are common features of angry political diatribes, but contemptuous stereotypes tend to be directed against more marginalized social groups, while envious stereotypes tend to be directed against groups perceived as elites.

Discrimination, in contrast, requires action: it occurs when someone is treated differently based on prejudices regarding their membership in a group. So, returning to the example from before, if you are interviewing someone who dresses in the wrong way, and choose not to hire him or her based on a gut-level reaction, that's discrimination. So, pulling the pieces together, prejudice refers to an initial reaction, stereotypes refer to the details of what I think the choice of a hoodie or suit says about someone, and discrimination refers to viewing clothing choice as a disqualification and not hiring people who make the wrong choice. Simple, right? Sure, but at the same time, mistakes on questions about these concepts are surprisingly common, so let's tackle a few misconceptions.

First off, in the interview example we just walked through, you might object that the choice not to hire someone because of inappropriate clothing isn't discrimination, because it's reasonable. Maybe wearing a hoodie to an interview at an investment bank or something would reflect a catastrophic lack of judgment for which it would be justifiable not to hire someone. This is a gray area, because discrimination is rooted in prejudices, which we do define as irrational attitudes—but people can disagree about which attitudes are rational and which are irrational, and social changes often shape those perceptions.

> **MCAT STRATEGY > > >**
>
> For the MCAT, don't worry too much about whether an attitude underlying potential discrimination is rational or irrational. Any examples you encounter should be unambiguous, with clues given in the passage or question stem.

A further important consideration is that there aren't really any fixed limits on what actions can constitute discrimination. Employment-related decisions are common examples, because discrimination in employment can have devastating outcomes, but really anything could be in scope, ranging from aspects of communication to making various opportunities available to people. So keep a close eye out. Just because an example given to you in a passage or question might not sound like familiar examples of discrimination doesn't exclude the possibility of discrimination taking place.

Yet another key factor is that for our purposes, discrimination has to involve actions or outcomes. If a scenario doesn't give you a description of actions or outcomes, you can't infer them. Period. Therefore, a scenario on the MCAT could present someone in a position of power with ludicrously strong prejudices and/or stereotypes, and then just say that that person doesn't make decisions or change his or her behavior based on those prejudices and stereotypes, and you just have to roll with it. In other words, discrimination is off the table as an answer choice, no matter how unrealistic you think it is that someone in that position could make unbiased decisions.

A final important distinction is between **individual discrimination** and **institutional discrimination**. As the name suggests, individual discrimination reflects behavior on the individual level - that is, ways in which a single person can treat other people differently based on their group membership. However, institutional discrimination refers to larger patterns of unequal behavior or outcomes, as mediated by entire institutions. Institutional discrimination can be overt, as was the case when racial segregation was legal in the United States, but it can also be more covert. For example, experiments have shown that job applications sent out with equal qualifications tend to get fewer responses when they're submitted under names that are associated with marginalized racial or ethnic groups. Education gaps and inequalities in health care have also been analyzed through the lens of institutional discrimination. Institutional discrimination is particularly tricky to target because it can be impossible to prove ill will from specific individuals, in the absence of specific policies openly targeting certain categories.

At this point, a logical question would be why prejudices, stereotypes, and discrimination exist in the first place. As we've discussed, prejudices have a major emotional component—and to a certain extent, are even defined as an emotional, or affective reaction—but they're rooted in the cognitive content of stereotypes. An influential argument was made in the mid-20th century that the cognitive background of prejudices—that is, the phenomenon of stereotyping—may be rooted in our subconscious attempts to organize our perceptions of the world around us. In other words, stereotyping may be a cognitive shortcut, or heuristic, that we use to streamline our processing of the world, given how overwhelming it would be to consider every social category we ever encounter from scratch and in depth. From this perspective, stereotypes and prejudice are unavoidable parts of the human experience, and our task is to minimize their harmfulness and impacts.

Circling back to the point we made at the beginning of this discussion, prejudice, stereotypes, and discrimination often involve demographic categories like race, sex, religion, sexual orientation, and age. These categories are deeply embedded in the socioeconomic hierarchy, and as such, prestige, power, and class often shape both which prejudices and stereotypes are formed and the ways that the resultant prejudices and stereotypes can shape outcomes by means of discrimination. In fact, even seemingly innocuous prejudices and stereotypes, like what we saw in the example of hoodie-wearing versus suit wearing at job interviews, can be seen through the lens of how we regulate access to opportunities and power, and what signals we consider to be appropriate for those who aim to rise through the social hierarchy. The point really is just that these phenomena don't take place in a neutral background.

As a final note, though, although it's important to appreciate some of the subtleties associated with these topics, we should never lose sight of the core definitions for the MCAT: Prejudice is an affective, or emotional response, stereotypes are a cognitive phenomenon, involving contentful but oversimplified ideas about various groups of people, and discrimination refers to actions or outcomes based on prejudices. Carefully applying those definitions will give you a huge edge on any questions that you encounter based on these topics.

8. Real-World Impacts of Stereotypes

As we've mentioned, the major reason why prejudice, stereotypes, and discrimination are emphasized for the MCAT is that they have very real impacts on people's lives, including in ways that are relevant for healthcare professionals. Moving beyond the general sense that discrimination is bad, there are a few specific phenomena related to how stereotypes play out in the real world that you should be aware of.

A **self-fulfilling prophecy** occurs when our perceptions of ourselves, usually but not always derived from other people's statements about ourselves, wind up shaping our behavior. A common example is that if children are told that they're bound to fail at something, that expectation causes them to behave in a way that makes failure likely, and conversely, expectations of success breed behavior that leads to success. This phenomenon is linked to stereotypes is that those expectations don't generally occur in a vacuum, especially when the self-fulfilling prophecy occurs in response to messages that people receive from authority figures like teachers or the mass media. In other words, with or without explicit encouragement from a parent or teacher, people can still pick up on stereotypes that apply to them and act accordingly. Of course, this isn't an ironclad law—obviously not everyone, and maybe not even most people in most circumstances, acts in accordance with stereotypical expectations, but the idea is that self-fulfilling prophecies can affect enough people, in enough circumstances, to be noteworthy as a sociological phenomenon.

Stereotype threat describes how this can occur even on a subconscious level. The idea with stereotype threat is that even just being reminded indirectly of relevant stereotypes can affect someone's performance. In the study that launched the concept of stereotype threat, a difficult verbal examination was administered to African-American and white test-takers, and it was framed in different ways: as a test that was diagnostic of intellectual ability, or as a test that was an intellectual challenge that was nondiagnostic of intellectual ability. The idea was that framing the test as diagnostic of intellectual ability would prime African-American test-takers to be aware of the stereotype of African-Americans having lower intellectual ability. In the results, all test-takers performed worse when the test was presented as diagnostic of intellectual ability, but this effect was stronger for African-Americans. This study, which was carried out in 1995, launched a tremendous wave of research—over 8,000 other articles have cited that original study—and broadly speaking, subsequent research has confirmed this phenomenon. **Stereotype boost**, on the other hand, occurs to how people can perform better if they're reminded of positive stereotypes that apply to them. Nonetheless, despite the huge amount of research that has investigated stereotype threat, the degree to which it contributes to longer-term, lasting inequalities is still a topic of investigation.

Stigma is a concept related to negative stereotypes. Stigma refers to intense disapproval that society directs towards certain identities and behaviors, and that disapproval also goes hand in hand with negative stereotypes about the people in question. Specific patterns of stigmatization can be affected by rapid social change —for instance, homosexuality, premarital sex, divorce, and marijuana use were intensely stigmatized in the mid to late 20th century, but the stigmas attached to these identities and behaviors have been greatly reduced since then. Other common examples of stigma include injection drug use and sex work. Broadly speaking, stigmatized people are likely to bear the brunt of discrimination and various negative outcomes. Even though we led off with examples where you may sympathize with the stigmatized groups, stigma also applies to groups that you're not likely to sympathize with, and you might even feel like that stigma is reasonable. For instance—even with full recognition of the overwhelming evidence supporting vaccination—it is nonetheless the case that anti-vaccine beliefs are stigmatized by health professionals. What's more, criminal behaviors like theft, murder, and domestic violence are stigmatized. But sociologists would point out that, if taken too far, even justified stigma can interfere with our ability to understand, and perhaps to prevent, the behaviors in question. As such, healthcare providers, social workers, and other professionals in relevant fields should be aware of how stigma might affect the services that they provide.

Ethnocentrism is another phenomenon that's intricately linked with stereotypes. Ethnocentrism refers to applying the norms and beliefs of one's own culture directly to another culture, or, in other words, judging other cultures by the standards of one's own. This often goes hand-in-hand with applying stereotypes of other cultures without deeper reflection. For our purposes, in any case, whenever you hear ethnocentrism, you should immediately contrast it with its opposite, **cultural relativism**. Although cultural relativism is often oversimplified as the idea that everything is acceptable in its own cultural context, or that you can't criticize anything in another culture, that's not quite what this concept refers to. Instead, the idea is that if we encounter a tradition or behavior in another culture that seems strange or uncomfortable, instead of immediately judging that behavior in the same way that would be applied to someone in our culture, we should put in some mental effort to understand the role and function of that tradition or behavior in its cultural context.

A classic example of ethnocentrism versus cultural relativism is ritual cannibalism, which was still practiced in some traditional hunter-gatherer societies when they came into contact with Western colonial powers. This behavior was sensational to many Westerners, but sociologists sought to understand under what circumstances, and for what purposes, people in those societies engaged in cannibalism. By the way, ritual cannibalism is also a topic with an interesting medical connection, since it was found to be the mode of transmission of kuru, a prion disease affecting brain tissue.

9. Must-Knows

- Groups affect individual behavior through social facilitation, social loafing, and the bystander effect.
- Psychological arousal modulates performance. Yerkes-Dodson law: optimal arousal = optimal performance.
- Deindividuation: loss of self-awareness in groups; high psychological arousal and low perceived responsibility
- Group polarization: a group's opinions becoming more extreme than those of their individual members, due to group dynamics such as informative influence and normative influence
- Groupthink: theory of why groups sometimes make very bad decisions
  —Eight factors: illusion of invulnerability, illusion of morality, illusion of unanimity, self-censorship, pressure on dissenters, collective rationalization, excessive stereotyping and mindguards
- Conformity: lining up our behaviors or beliefs with the perspective of others
  — Internalization: completely changing our beliefs for this adjustment; compliance (as a subtype of conformity): adjusting our behavior, but internally dissenting; identification: middle ground
- Solomon Asch experiment: people will conform to group pressure even when group is very wrong.
- Compliance: obeying requests from someone who has no power to enforce them. Techniques include the foot-in-the-door technique, the door-in-the-face technique and the low-ball technique.
- Obedience: obeying requests from someone who has the power to enforce them (Stanford Prison & Milgram)
- Social control (through sanctions) is how all our norms are taught, enforced, and perpetuated.
  — Formal norms: encoded in laws or regulations and have specific penalties for violating them.
  — Informal norms are not written down, unlikely to have fixed penalties for violations (folkways, mores, taboos).
  — Anomie: mismatch between stated norms and the norms an individual responds to; often precedes the breakdown of traditional systems of moral regulation.
- Deviance: not following norms; differential association theory: learned by association; labeling approach: deviance increases in frequency in response to being labeled deviant; primary deviance: acts committed before receiving the label; secondary deviance: acts after the fact
  — Fads: behaviors with intense, brief popularity. Mass hysteria: irrational, overblown response to a perceived threat. Sometimes the effects of the mass hysteria are more harmful than those of the threat
- In explaining people's behavior, we make dispositional attributions (inherent factors) and situational attributions (external/temporary factors)
  — Consistency and distinctiveness cues influence which attribution to use, as well as cultural influences (collectivistic - favors situational, individualistic - favors dispositonal)
- Heuristics: mental shortcuts to navigate social environments, can lead to errors or be subject to bias
  — Fundamental attribution error: making preferentially dispositional attributions of other people
  — Actor-observer bias: dispositional attributions for others, situational attributions for ourselves.
  — Self-serving bias: making dispositional attributions for our own good outcomes, and situational attributions for our own poor outcomes
- Internal and external locus of control: focus on own actions or circumstances to explain life outcomes
- Halo effect: perceptions of success/attractiveness spill over into our evaluations of them in other domains.
- Just-world-hypothesis: cognitive error of assuming good outcomes occur in good people and vice-versa.
- Prejudice: feelings and attitudes towards groups, people, or objects
- Stereotypes: contain specific content (paternalistic, admiration, contemptuous, and envious)
- Discrimination: actions taken to treat somebody differently based on their group or demographic category membership and/or existing prejudices. Can be individual discrimination or institutional discrimination.
- Self-fulfilling prophecies are ways in which we alter or sabotage our behavior in response to stereotypes.
- Stereotype threat and stereotype boost refers to how even subconscious stereotypes can alter performance.
- When society strongly disapproves of something, it is said to be stigmatized or have stigma.
- Ethnocentrism: viewing all phenomena through one's own cultural lens, while cultural relativism suggests we can take the perspective of different cultures with different normative behaviors from our own.

End of Chapter Practice

The best MCAT practice is **realistic**, with a focus on identifying steps for further improvement. For those reasons, we recommend completing practice questions in an online setting that simulates the real MCAT interface, and taking advantage of advanced analytic features to help you determine how best to move forward in your MCAT study journey.

With that in mind, **online end-of-chapter questions** are accessible through your Next Step account.

As a further supplement, given the importance of active learning for effective studying, we also suggest that you consult the Must-Knows as a basis for creating a study sheet, in which you list out key terms and test your ability to briefly summarize them.

This page left intentionally blank.

Social Interactions

CHAPTER 10

0. Introduction

Although social psychology as a field encompasses a broad range of very distinct phenomena, the nuts and bolts of social psychology are rooted in our social interactions with each other; in this chapter, we will discuss various aspects of how that happens.

1. Expressing and Detecting Emotion

Although our interactions with other people are shaped by a broad range of factors, emotional signaling is arguably one of the most omnipresent aspects of how we interact with each other. This is true even though—or, on further thought, maybe especially since—a lot of that signaling happens at a subconscious level. Every time we interact with each other face to face, we're constantly signaling our emotional state through our choice of words, tone, facial expressions, body language, and so on. Technological advances have shifted a lot of communication into the form of text, which would seem not to allow such emotional subtleties, but the development of hundreds of emojis helped fix that. Fun fact: in 2015, the 'Face with Tears of Joy' emoji was actually selected as the word of the year by Oxford Dictionaries. This sort of phenomenon does underscore how important emotions are for our ability to communicate.

Not only are emotions important, but we're fine-tuned to pick up **emotional signals** couched in even very small changes in physical stimuli. The subtle way that someone might raise an eyebrow, or the tone of voice in which someone uses, or doesn't use, a word, the way someone leans back in a chair and crosses his or her arms, and even the way someone breathes in and out can be stimuli that we can pick up on as indicating something about their emotional state. This isn't just a set of cliches, it's a very real and remarkable aspect of how we're wired neurologically, and like with many other basic aspects of psychology, there are some variations across individuals in this capacity. One axis of variation has to do with sensitivity and skill picking up these signals. On one hand, certain people may be especially good at observing emotional signals, which might be associated with particularly strong tendencies towards empathy, or sharing someone's emotional perspective. On the other hand, individuals with autism spectrum disorder may have difficulties perceiving such stimuli accurately. Interestingly, although some emotions may be universal—as proposed by Paul Ekman and discussed elsewhere—it is definitely the case that many specific emotional cues are learned in childhood during the socialization process.

This realization points us in the direction of two other factors that shape the expression and detection of emotion: culture and gender. To a certain extent, these are actually two ways of looking at the same basic issue, which is that the details of emotional signaling are shaped by **socialization**. However, looking at emotions through the lens of culture focuses on how emotional signaling practices vary across the world, while looking through the lens of gender focuses on how different groups within a society participate in this process in different ways.

In any case, remarkably different cultural norms exist regarding which emotions are considered appropriate to express under which circumstances. To some extent, this tracks with broader differences in cultures, so in individualistic cultures—most often exemplified by the United States—public and open expression of emotions is relatively encouraged, while that's not the case in more collectively-oriented cultures. Cross-cultural variations also exist with regard to specific emotional signals. For instance, in the United States, smiles can be taken as indicating a general positive attitude or openness, and as such it can be quite appropriate to smile at strangers, whereas in some other cultures, smiles are specifically linked to substantive reasons for being happy that you wouldn't normally share with strangers. In turn, smiling at everyone you meet is felt to be somewhat insincere, almost as if you are oversharing in a way that suggests you're trying to trick people. Eye contact is another good example. In the US, it tends to be associated with a sense of straightforward, sincere trustworthiness, while in certain Asian cultures, eye contact—especially in situations where there's a social hierarchy between speakers—can be seen as a somewhat aggressive signal.

> **MCAT STRATEGY > > >**
>
> Although expressing and detecting emotion isn't an area with a ton of specific terminology, it's an excellent laboratory for the MCAT to test ideas related to the effects of culture on measurable behavior.

Gender is another axis along which emotional signaling varies. One issue here is that certain emotions are associated with certain gender roles. For example, anger tends to be classified as a more masculine emotion, while emotional states indicating vulnerability, compassion, and concern are interpreted as feminine emotions. These points are particularly true for American and Western cultures, at least traditionally, but the broader point still holds true that in general, gender is a way that culture-specific attitudes towards emotion are organized.

Social sanctions are a way in which certain patterns of emotional expression can be indexed to gender. For instance, women who express anger in ways that would be acceptable for men often encounter sharply negative pushback, especially in workplace or otherwise public-facing settings. Analogously, a man who opens up too much about emotional vulnerabilities and worries might create a negative impression. On the flip side, behaving in ways that resonates with gender-specific expectations about emotional signaling can yield positive results for people. Of course, none of this should be taken as either set in stone or a recommendation for your behavior. Gender-specific expectations differ both culturally and in time. As you may be aware many current sets of expectations are not at all as crude as what we outlined above, but the point remains that gender-specific expectations still exist. Another way that gender-specific ideas about emotions can manifest is through experimental findings. For example, when images are constructed with facial expressions that are ambiguous in terms of whether they show anger or sadness, male faces are more likely to be interpreted as showing anger, and female faces as showing sadness.

In addition, there may be gender-specific differences in how emotions are detected—in particular, women may be more sensitive either to emotional signals in general, or to certain signals in particular. However, the scientific literature for this topic is still very inconclusive, despite a lot of researchers having looked into it. If you think about it, this is a legitimately tricky issue to study. As a researcher, how do you set up the stimuli? How do you measure the detection or identification of emotions—that is to say, how do you operationalize such a variable? And if you do get significant results, how do you interpret them? It's possible that such findings could suggest some hard-wired differences between the sexes, but we also have to account for the possibility that women might be socialized to pay more attention to emotional signals than men, and it wouldn't be particularly surprising for that to result in better performance at detecting emotions. In any case, though, this is a topic that's attracted a lot of attention, but not yet yielded a lot of firm conclusions..

We detect emotions through both verbal and nonverbal communication. **Verbal communication** refers to the literal words that we say, either by speaking with our mouths, sign language, writing, texting, or any other medium. **Nonverbal communication** is everything else—tone of voice, eye contact, body language, and so on. Nonverbal communication is not only fundamental for humans, but it also extends into the animal kingdom.

Animal communication is a deeply interesting topic, but the MCAT is a test for future human doctors, and as such, the primary focus will always be human-related physiology and psychology. Nonetheless, it's worth being aware of a few examples of how animals communicate nonverbally. Facial expressions are an area with some overlap between animals and humans. Signals like bared teeth in a dog, for instance, are an indication of readiness to defend. Bright coloring patterns can function like a signal saying "Hey, I'm dangerous! Stay away!" Animals also use scent to communicate; for example, certain animals mark their territory using urine, and pheromones help mediate sexual behavior. Bees use rhythmic "dances" as a way to communicate information through movement, and many different animals can also use vocalizations for different purposes.

To summarize, there's a lot going on in terms of how we as humans express and detect emotion. We pick up on many different, often very small signals, and we do so in ways that are shaped by factors like culture and gender. What's more, zooming out a little bit, the ways that humans do this forms a continuum with how animals signal emotion, attitudes, and information in general. Although expressing and detecting emotion can often fade into the background of our attention as we go about our daily lives, these are common themes that shape just about every social interaction we have, be it with our friends, with colleagues, or even in settings like doctor-patient interactions.

2. Self-Presentation

Whenever we interact with other people, either directly or through more indirect connections like email or social media, we're making choices about how we present ourselves.

Our choices about **self-presentation** can be based on how we envision our authentic self and on how we think it will be advantageous to appear in a certain situation. Although self-presentation is a very broad concept, there are five specific strategies that researchers have identified as especially noteworthy. These are self-disclosure, managing appearances, ingratiation, aligning actions, and altercasting.

> **MCAT STRATEGY > > >**
>
> As is typical with lots of sociology on the MCAT, the terms can start to blur together, especially when they all seem to use ordinary conversational English. But the Psych/Soc section demands that you memorize the exact, technical definition, especially for terms involving "self."

Self-disclosure, is fairly clear based on its name: It refers to what you disclose to others about yourself. This can be really obvious and in-your-face, if, for example, you were to say, "As a premed student,   ..." Alternatively, it can be slightly more subtle, like how mentioning that you did something with your significant other is a way to signal that you have a significant other or that you want to present yourself as such.

Next, **managing appearances** refers to how you groom yourself, how you dress, and how you act. As always, specific strategies are context-specific, so being perfectly put-together, wearing business attire, and exuding a positive, can-do, friendly but not too friendly attitude will communicate one thing on your first day at a new job, and another thing entirely at a punk rock show.

These first two strategies—self-disclosure and managing appearances—are things that we do all the time, even if we don't think about it. Even being careless about one's appearance is a choice that sends a certain signal, and even if we don't put a lot of thought into what we share about ourselves, we still can't avoid making choices about what to put out there and what to keep to ourselves. The next three strategies, though, are a little bit more deliberate.

Ingratiation is just a fancy word for sucking up. As we've seen with some of the other strategies, this can be obvious, as in "Ohhh, professor, your hyper-specialized research project is *so* fascinating, I would love to explore it in a way that would conveniently lead to a good letter of recommendation and a publication." Or it can be less in-your-face, if you just choose to highlight, or even fake, aspects of your personality in a way that you think will improve likeability. If your boss is excited about how the local football team is doing in the playoffs, that might not be the time to talk about how their quarterback is overrated, or how football is linked to high rates of traumatic brain injuries and chronic traumatic encephalopathy, or whatever other adversarial opinion you may have. Instead, projecting excitement about the local team's playoff chances might benefit you more.

Aligning actions refers to presenting your actions, especially those can might seem a bit questionable, in a light that makes them more appealing in a certain setting. Put simply, this can even mean making excuses. But more generally, it can refer to various ways in which we explain what we choose to do. So, for example, imagine you're working in a lab and you figure out a way to do something that's both easier and quicker, but your supervisor needs to sign off on doing it the new way. You're probably going to explain it like "Hey, I came up with this great technique that will improve our efficiency by 20%!", instead of "Can we do it this way because it's easier for me?"

Finally, **altercasting** flips the focus onto other people. In this technique, you project an identity onto someone and then create the expectation that he or she should act the way you want. A blatant example of altercasting would be if a professor told you something like "As a premed student, you shouldn't have to be reminded to turn your lab reports in on time." In a less obvious way, advertisers and marketers do this all the time. For instance, an advertisement for a really fancy watch might try to make the viewer identify as the kind of person who really cares about quality and elegance in timekeeping devices - a natural consequence of which is buying an expensive watch.

Throughout this discussion, we've been talking about various ways that we act. That word was not chosen arbitrarily -- it turns out there's a deep similarity between how we act in certain social situations, particularly in stressful or public situations with real consequences at stake, and the experience of acting on stage or on TV. Based on this insight, in the 1950s a sociologist named Erving Goffman developed the **dramaturgical approach** to self-presentation, and even published a book-length analysis based on this analogy. The most influential theoretical proposal Goffman made is the distinction between the **front-stage self** and the **back-stage self**. The front-stage self refers to how we present ourselves in front of an audience, following certain scripts and expectations, like the more deliberate aspects of impression management that we talked about earlier. The back-stage self refers to our more authentic self, when we're no longer in front of an audience, and we can relax and not worry so much about acting in a way that aligns with our public image.

3. Social Behaviors

Sociologists have identified certain kinds of behavior as being especially characteristic of humans as social beings, called social behavior. Now, by social behavior here, we don't mean things like partying, or gossiping, or study sessions, or meeting up with friends to see a movie. Instead, social behaviors in this context are more general phenomena, or patterns of interaction that pervade many different activities.

I. Attraction

One major social behavior is **attraction**, both in the sense of wanting to be someone's friend, or just to hang out with them, and romantic and sexual attraction.

The first factor contributing to attraction is—perhaps not surprisingly—**physical attractiveness**. This is kind of an obvious point, but there are a few interesting wrinkles here. One possibility to consider may be that physical attractiveness is just a social construct. In fact, it *is* true that beauty standards vary across time and across cultures. However, researchers have identified some objectively-measurable correlates of attractiveness that seem to hold up across cultures, such as facial symmetry. An influential hypothesis is that physically attractive traits are those that indicate suitability as a mate, either by reflecting what we could really simplistically call "good genes" or by serving as a proxy for cultural or economic indicators, like how in some cultures, pale skin may be valued as an indicator that one is affluent enough not to have to work outside. Interestingly, the major histocompatibility complex, an important component of our immune system, may mediate the degree to which people find potential partners' body odor to be attractive, suggesting that scent signals may lead us to be attracted to people who would be good mates from an immunological perspective. This whole issue is far from settled science, though, so beware of pop-science-style generalizations.

Proximity is another factor that contributes to attraction. In other words, we're more likely to be attracted to people who we happen to interact with on a daily basis. There's also a related concept called the **mere exposure effect**, which says that we also eventually develop preferences for familiar people and things.

This brings us to our third factor that contributes to attraction: **similarity**. All things being equal, we're more likely to be attracted to people who are similar to us in terms of various demographic factors, including but not limited to age, socioeconomic status, and educational level, as well as general worldview and cultural background. Well, you might think, what about the saying that opposites attract? First off, "opposites attract" is not exactly an actual scientific principle, and second, to whatever extent it's true, it's true only within a limited scope; for instance, if one partner likes to cook and the other would prefer to do the dishes, that's nice, but it pales in comparison to all the similarities that promote close bonding. That said, of course people can vary in terms of which similarities they find to be important and which differences they find intriguing versus off-putting.

II. Aggression

Although we don't usually think of it as a good thing, **aggression** is also a basic aspect of the human condition. Evolutionary theorists point to the importance of aggression as a way to defend against threats and to obtain greater access to various resources. As such, it shouldn't be a huge surprise that we can frequently observe aggression in the animal kingdom. Interestingly, many "fights" between animals within the same species tend to be almost ritualistic, with a clear and predictable pattern of behavior, and end with the defeated animal submitting and retreating, but usually not being killed. In some social animals, aggression plays a role in reinforcing and maintaining hierarchies.

Evolutionary details aside, aggression is definitely shaped by biological factors. For instance, testosterone levels—in both sexes—have been positively associated with aggression. In the brain, the prefrontal cortex helps to regulate and restrain impulsive behaviors (including aggressive ones) that stem from emotional arousal mediated by the limbic system. Aggression is also shaped by one's personal experiences, potentially including situations where aggression has worked as a way to reach certain goals, or has been fostered by traumatic experiences. Furthermore, although the details are contentious, there's no real doubt that patterns of aggression are also molded by society-wide norms and expectations.

III. Attachment

A third important behavior is **attachment**. This refers to the bonds that form between children and their caregivers, and it can manifest in several distinct attachment styles. The presence of a consistent, responsive, comforting caregiver promotes **secure attachment**. An infant with a secure attachment style feels some distress when the caregiver leaves, but then adjusts to circumstances, knowing that the caregiver will return, and a happy response when they do return. In contrast, **ambivalent attachment** occurs when the caregiver responds to the child inconsistently. This leads to the child not being able to rely on the caregiver, and manifests as a pattern of intense distress when the caregiver leaves, followed by a more mixed and unclear response upon return. In **avoidant attachment**, the child will seem not to really care one way or the other when the caregiver leaves or returns; this is thought to stem from a neglectful relationship. Finally, **disoriented attachment**, which is sometimes also referred to as **disorganized attachment**, manifests as hesitant, contradictory, and confused behavior upon the caregiver's departure and return. This pattern can be a warning sign of abuse.

IV. Altruism

Altruism refers to helping other people at some cost to yourself, even if only in terms of time and energy. From a certain perspective—and we will leave it up to you to decide what this says about modern scientists—this is a puzzling behavior, because it's not exactly obvious how to accommodate self-sacrificing behavior within frameworks like rational choice theory. Some have suggested that maybe we do get something from altruistic behavior: maybe a warm fuzzy feeling inside, or maybe we're building social connections that will pay off later when we need a favor. As a potential example of that latter point, structured gift-giving and generosity played a major role in some indigenous societies in the Pacific Northwest, a fact that provoked much theorizing among anthropologists. Others have suggested that altruistic behavior may have evolutionary benefits in itself.

IV. Social Support

The final major social behavior we need to look at is **social support**. Emotional support is an important form of support that comes to mind, but this category also includes a few other types of support as well. Informational support means providing people helpful information, and as the name implies, material support (or tangible support) means giving someone money or items they need. Finally, companionship support refers to just being with someone in a way that fosters a sense of belonging. Social support has been increasingly linked with positive health outcomes, and this finding has been influential in recent years for how people have been thinking about the aging process.

So, for social support in particular, but really for all of these behaviors, your future career in medicine will be rich in examples of how careful consideration of these factors can shed light on why people behave in certain ways, and which behaviors tend to promote better health in the long term.

4. Biological Explanations of Social Behaviors in Animals

As we've seen, several important social behaviors in humans have biological roots. This is worth focusing on a little bit more. Although the MCAT doesn't generally expect you to have much knowledge about the animal kingdom, social behaviors are actually a bit of an exception, perhaps because this is an area where zooming out to take a broader look at evolutionary history can help yield some insights into ourselves as humans.

The first such behavior worth discussing is **foraging**, which describes how animals search for food. It's hard to get much more basic than the biological imperative for food and water; but not only is foraging important, it's also interesting, because it's not always an easy task for various reasons, so organisms have evolved many different strategies for foraging. Some of these behaviors are learned, making foraging an excellent laboratory for studying the interplay between instinctive and learned behaviors in animals, which is also an area of interest for humans. What's more, researchers often use economic models to make sense of foraging, because there's a tradeoff between getting energy from food and spending energy to do so. Interestingly, some researchers have linked our tendency as humans to overconsume high-fat, high-salt, and high-sugar foods to our history as foragers, essentially suggesting that we evolved these tastes back when such foods were rare and valuable, and that we eat too much of them now because our brain wiring hasn't caught up with the emergence of processed food.

Moving on, we previously discussed attraction in humans, and it turns out that **mating behavior** and **mate choice** are also quite interesting in animals. Mating behavior includes a frankly astonishing diversity of different behavioral patterns, but for our purposes, the core idea is that animals have a wide range of ways of engaging in courtship, copulating, and raising offspring. Patterns of mate choice are similarly diverse. On one hand, mating can be random, as the Hardy-Weinberg model of genotype frequency assumes, but more often, animals respond to highly specific cues, like phenotypic signals, as a way of choosing potential mates. In some cases, attractive traits within a species may be those that directly signal genetic fitness, while in other cases, certain features seem like they're attractive, well, just kind of because. The latter phenomenon is known as Fisherian selection, with the vibrant and otherwise pointless tails of male peacocks being a well-known example. Initially, patterns like this struck evolutionary biologists as wasteful and kind of exceptional, but the point has also been made that a male peacock's ability to grow an eye-catching, colorful, ginormous feathery tail could be a proxy signal for being well-nourished, genetically fit, and generally an awesome candidate for a mate. When you think about how flashy status symbols, expensive clothes, and the ability to follow ever-changing beauty patterns influence how humans find mates, the parallels seem almost too obvious to call out.

> **MCAT STRATEGY > > >**
>
> Get personal! It can help you memorize the various terms related to social interaction if you put those terms in the context of your own life. Think about how these terms relate to your own life, and how you interact with friends, family, and coworkers.

We've already sort of touched on the idea that certain behavioral choices reflect an optimization between competing pressures. More broadly, **game theory** is a branch of applied mathematics that deals with decision-making under circumstances of incomplete information where there are other actors who are also making similar choices, like in a game. A well-known example of game theory is the **prisoner's dilemma**, which asks us to imagine a situation where two members of a criminal organization are caught and interrogated. The idea is that the prosecutors have some evidence against the criminals, but not enough to convict them for the full crime. For that, they'd need one criminal to cooperate and testify against the other. So the prosecutors offer them a deal: if either criminal cooperates, he or she would go free, while the other would get a long prison sentence. If neither cooperates, both will get a lighter sentence. But if both denounce each other, both get the long sentence. So for either criminal individually, the rational choice is clearly to cooperate, but if both criminals behave rationally, both get the long sentence, which could have been avoided if they had both kept quiet.

This apparent paradox is what initially got researchers interested in game theory, and the theory has developed in much greater depth, with more complicated games, variations on what information the players get, and so on. Game theory is relevant to biology because this framework can be extended to model ecological interactions. For example, should an animal engage in predatory or cooperative behavior? There's not really a single answer to this question. It's complicated, and it depends on the circumstances and how other animals in that ecological context interact. The key point for the MCAT is to broadly understand what game theory is interested in and to have a sense of what it can be applied to. Beyond that, if you're asked about game theory in a specific context on the exam, you should be able to get the information you need from the passage or question.

Next, altruism, as we've mentioned, refers to doing something helpful for someone else at a cost to oneself. This makes it sort of a puzzle for schools of thought that conceptualize behavior as a rational optimization guided by one's self-interest, as well as some models of evolution that view natural selection in a very narrow and antiquated sense. But what if we take a view of evolution that focuses on the genes in a population, implying that the mechanism of evolution involves different genetic variants propagating themselves over time? Well, any given individual will share much of their genotype with their close relatives. Therefore, from a genotype-centric point of view, it might make sense for an individual to engage in self-sacrificing behavior to promote the survival of a group of relatives. A pioneering researcher in evolution, J. B. S. Haldane, captured this idea by joking that he would give up his life for two brothers or eight cousins. This basic concept—that is, that natural selection can operate on the group level—is known as **inclusive fitness**.

Inclusive fitness is one way to try to explain altruism, particularly in animals that don't have the cognitive capacity to engage in more elaborate justifications of altruism in terms of morality, like humans can do. Nonetheless, be careful not to confuse altruism with inclusive fitness. They aren't the same thing. Inclusive fitness is just one explanation for the more general phenomenon of altruism, and for it to be the correct answer to a question, it has to involve self-sacrifice on the behalf of related individuals.

5. Definitions and Types of Identity

A relatively straightforward way to approach identity is to see it as how we view ourselves. And that works as a first approximation, but it's ultimately too simple. For one, it's important to distinguish between different ways that we conceive of ourselves on a purely personal level—whether as a good karaoke singer, or a serious chess player, or whatever else—and ways in which we see ourselves as embedded in broader social categories, like as a young adult, or a Spanish-speaker, and so on. The former type of identity is sometimes referred to as **personal identity**, while the latter type is referred to as **social identity**. Generally, though, when we just hear the term "identity" without any further clarification, we can assume that social identity is being discussed.

The concept of identity becomes even more complicated once we recognize that identities can be negotiated and contested in a complex play of personal perceptions and perceptions projected by other people. In simple terms, this means that someone might try to apply a certain identity or label to you that you think is either inaccurate, or doesn't resonate with you or match up with your concept of yourself. For example, very few people find that the label of "millennial" appropriately describes them, but there's absolutely no shortage of media coverage trying to apply that label to anyone in the corresponding age group or beyond. Again, identity does involve some interplay between internal perceptions and external social categories and structures.

In general, any important demographic category can be a form of identity. Although we described a distinction between purely personal identity and social identity, in reality, there's not a completely fixed boundary between the two domains, or a single, short, finite list of relevant social identities. So with that in mind, let's focus on some of the most important categories of identity for the purposes of the MCAT. Note that we cover these social categories in more depth in Chapter 12, which discusses demographics, so our goal in this section will only be to present a brief overview with a focus on the broader theme of identity.

As we mentioned in the example of "millennial" as a contested identity, **age** can be an important form of identity. This is true both in absolute terms—like teenager, young adult, middle-aged, and elderly—and in terms of age-related social categories like **generations**.

Likewise, race, ethnicity, and nationality are important categories of identity, although it's important to remember that they are not equivalent. **Race** itself is not very precisely defined, and it's not at all clear to what extent it's a scientifically valid concept, but insofar as it is a meaningful idea, it refers to physical characteristics. For what it's worth, the United States Census Bureau officially distinguishes the following racial categories: White American, Black or African American, Native American and Alaska Native, Asian American, and Native Hawaiian and Other

Pacific Islander. This categorization is not necessarily the final word on the topic, but it's worth knowing about. **Ethnicity** is a much more specific concept that refers to one's cultural background. Language is sometimes used as a marker of ethnicity, but there's not a one-to-one relationship. **Symbolic ethnicity** refers to contexts where people invoke ethnic identity under specific and limited circumstances; the classic example in the United States is how many people project Irish-American ethnic identities on St. Patrick's Day, even if that ethnic identity might not be particularly relevant to them in their everyday life.

Finally, **nationality** is a political and legal concept that is independent of both race and ethnicity. The simplest way of thinking of nationality is in terms of citizenship status, although in reality, that's an oversimplification, both because of more nuanced statuses like permanent residency and because of more complex legal situations. For example, recognized indigenous groups retain distinct national status in the United States, while maintaining a complex balance of sovereignty with the US government. In other words, for instance, the "Nation" in "Navajo Nation" is meant very literally and entails specific legal obligations. To summarize, the MCAT certainly does not expect you to be a legal expert, but you should be aware of the idea that race is a physical category, ethnicity is cultural, and nationality is legal.

Next, **gender identity** refers to how people perceive themselves relative to the social categories of masculinity and femininity. It's extremely important to distinguish gender, which is a social construct, from sex, which refers to biological categories of male and female. Male and female are traditional and commonly encountered categories of gender identity, but gender identities such as nonbinary, genderfluid, genderqueer, and agender have received greater recognition in Western cultures in recent years. Gender categories beyond the male/female dichotomy have also long been recognized in many other traditional cultures throughout the world. Such categories are often grouped together as **third gender**, although it has been pointed out that this blanket term runs the risk of erasing important culture-specific aspects of how these categories are constructed. The category of **cisgender** refers to people whose gender identity matches the biological sex and gender that they were assigned at birth, and the term **transgender** refers to people for whom that is not the case: that is, their gender identity does not match their birth-assigned sex and gender.

Sexual orientation, in contrast, describes who people are attracted to as sexual partners. **Homosexuality** means being attracted to the same sex or gender, **heterosexuality** to the opposite sex or gender, and **bisexuality** to both sexes and genders. **Pansexuality** has also been defined as an orientation involving attraction to all genders, more explicitly including non-binary gender identities. **Asexuality** refers to a lack of attraction to others and low or no sexual interest. A distinction is sometimes made between sexual orientation and **romantic orientation**, to reflect the fact that some individuals experience an asymmetry between the individuals who they want to have sexual relationships with and those who they want to have romantic relationships with, but romantic orientation is currently not universally distinguished in society as a distinct category. This is an excellent example of how socially-relevant categories of identity are in a constant process of construction, negotiation, and flux.

Socioeconomic class and **religion** are also important categories of identity, although the relative importance, or salience, of these categories differ across people and among societies. For instance, in some societies, religion is felt to be a deeply personal or private characteristic, to the point that one might know someone for years, and never know their religious beliefs or identities. In other societies, religion can be so prominent as a marker of community affiliation that it's even included on someone's identification papers. We see a recurring theme here of variation across cultures and over time in terms of what categories of identity are considered to be salient, and disputes about identity can often be linked to political engagement. For example, disability rights activists might argue that instead of being seen as isolated medical conditions, disability status—that is, disabled, differently-abled, or temporarily able-bodied—should be acknowledged more broadly as a crucial part of a person's identity. However, it's worth noting that the MCAT will not expect you to be up-to-date on every recent development in American culture related to identities, or for you to take specific sides on topics that are still a matter of wide debate. Instead, you should have a good sense of what identity means from a sociological perspective, and understand how identity reflects a balance between internal perceptions of oneself and social categories that exist outside of oneself. Furthermore, being aware of some of the issues at stake regarding especially important categories of identity, such as gender, race, and ethnicity, will help prepare you for related passages.

6. Identity Formation

Now that we've talked a bit about what identity means, a logical follow-up is to ponder how it is that our identities develop. Just as social categories relevant for identity shift over time, and can even be contested, our own personal and social identities change over the course of our life. A tricky aspect of this topic, though, is disentangling developmental processes that are specific to identity formation from the broad range of closely-entwined psychological processes that occur as an individual matures and develops a stable personality. So, to put it very simply, we're talking about identity versus personality. Although it is the case that identity and personality are different terms, with subtle but important differences in meaning, this distinction has not always been clearly made, both by researchers investigating the topic and in materials presenting this information to students. However, in this discussion, we'll focus on identity, and provide pointers as appropriate to areas where this material intersects with topics more closely related to personality.

Social factors are extraordinarily important in the development of identity, because throughout the process of growing up, children receive a nearly constant barrage of input about who they are themselves and how they relate to others. Sometimes this input can be explicit, like when a parent tells a child about who their family is and where they come from, and sometimes it can be implicit, like in the form of behaviors to emulate. This input can shape how children relate to virtually every category that's relevant for identity, but it's worth making a special note of how children receive intense **socialization** about gender norms and roles, shaping their gender identity. This can start as early as infancy or early childhood. A common example is how children are dressed differently and encouraged to play with different toys depending on gender, but this also manifests by gendered language in praise that sets expectations regarding behaviors and values. For instance, even at a very early age, girls might start receiving praise for being pretty or beautiful, while boys might be praised for being brave.

Relatedly, the **psychosexual perspective** proposed by Freud—which we discuss in more depth elsewhere in the context of personality—has implications for identity development. Recall that from the Freudian point of view, sexuality is an omnipresent aspect of human psychology, with relevance for all developmental stages and impacts on virtually every aspect of life. The connection with identity development is that, from a Freudian perspective, conflicts or complexes that remain from various developmental stages can be so pervasive as to impact a person's identity in many different ways. On a similar note, Kohlberg's theory of moral development is also relevant for identity, since our viewpoints about morality in light of social conventions can shape our political identity and sense of ourselves.

That said, focusing so much on the influence of society on identity is all well and good, but after all, many of our experiences with "society" boil down to experiences with people, and interactions with other people therefore shape how our identity is formed. As we already briefly alluded to, imitation is an important mechanism through which our identity is formed. In recent decades, the concept of a role model has gained attention as a way to explain how children internalize and imitate the examples set by adults in their surroundings.

However, our perceptions of ourselves are shaped not only by the actions of other people, but also how they perceive us, because other people in our surroundings send us messages—explicit and implicit—about who they consider us to be. The concept of the **looking-glass self** was coined to describe this effect. To make this metaphor clearer, it's worth remembering that in old-fashioned language, looking-glass meant mirror. Thus, the looking-glass self refers to how we build conceptions of ourselves based on what other people reflect back at us. More precisely, our perceptions of how other people perceive us shape how we see ourselves. Framing it this way, in terms of multiple layers of perception, might sound pretty convoluted, but it gets to an important point, which is that we are sensitive both to how others see us and that it's ultimately our job to interpret signals that other people send us, and we can do so in either healthy or unhealthy ways. We then integrate those signals into our perceptions of self through a process known as internalization.

The term looking-glass self was coined in 1902, but the American philosopher George Herbert Mead developed this idea further. For the MCAT, it's usually more effective to summarize sociologists than to quote them, but Mead articulated his perspective quite clearly in his 1934 work "Mind, Self and Society", so we can make an exception here. Mead wrote "When a self does appear it always involves an experience of another; there could not be an experience of a self simply by itself. The plant or the lower animal reacts to its environment, but there is no experience of a self [...]. When the response of the other becomes an essential part in the experience or conduct of the individual; when taking the attitude of the other becomes an essential part in his behavior — then the individual appears in his own experience as a self; and until this happens he does not appear as a self."

Mead viewed **role-playing**, or **role-taking**, as an essential part of how we gain the ability to inhabit and understand others' perspectives. He pointed out the importance of children's games in this regard, focusing on how even seemingly simple games like "playing house" require children to inhabit specific roles with the corresponding points of view, like that of a mother or a newborn baby. In these games, the roles are structured in ways that replicate social expectations regarding those roles in society. From a test-taking perspective, the key point about role-taking is that the end point of this process is ultimately targeted towards the self. As such, it can be contrasted to similar-seeming concepts like impression management, which is more oriented towards impacting how others see us in specific social settings.

6. Facets of the Self

The topic of identity is especially challenging from a terminological perspective because we have to navigate a ton of different terms that all start with "self-". The goal of this discussion, therefore, is twofold: first, to help you distinguish among several similar-sounding terms related to the self; and second, to explore how our broad concepts of ourselves depend upon more specific perceptions of our ability and value.

As the name implies, **self-concept** refers—in very general terms—to how we perceive ourselves. So, for instance, a person might conceive of herself as a middle-class Pakistani-American young adult who has a good sense of humor, is a good big sister to her siblings, and is better at math than at history. Concepts about oneself along these lines are known as **self-schemas**. Now, it would be reasonable to wonder why we also need a term like self-schemas -- what does this technical term add? It turns out that self-schemas, even very simple-sounding ones like having a good sense of humor, reflect more complex conceptual structures than might be obvious at first glance. That is, how would you even explain everything that goes along with having a good sense of humor? What's more, self-schemas impact our behavior, in that we tend to behave in ways that are consistent with our self-schemas. This latter point leads into a concept known as **self-verification**, which is more of a theoretical proposal than a descriptive term. In any case, it states that we seek to have others perceive us according to how we perceive ourselves. So, to summarize, our overall self-concept is structured in terms of self-schemas, which affect how we behave in accordance with self-verification.

As if we hadn't encountered enough terms related to the self yet, we should also mention the term **self-identity**. Self-identity is generally used as a synonym to self-concept, but with the slight difference that self-identity places a greater emphasis on self-schemas that are relevant for social identity—like belonging to the middle class—rather than on more personal characteristics, like having a good sense of humor.

Now let's turn to some more specific aspects of how we view ourselves. **Locus of control** describes how we tend to assign responsibility for events that occur in our lives. People with an **internal locus of control** tend to see themselves as being responsible for those events, and people with an **external locus of control** tend to focus on outside factors. Common examples are drawn from the world of academic achievements; someone with an internal locus of control might explain a good grade as having resulted from their innate intelligence or their exceptional preparation, and a bad grade as being the result of a failure to prepare or as a sign of being inherently no good at the subject. In contrast, someone with an external locus of control might perceive a good grade as a sign of just having been lucky on the test, whereas a bad grade might be explained as due to getting a poor night's sleep, or having a bad teacher, or the test being unfair, or just plain old bad luck. Now, something to note here is that neither type of locus of control is inherently right or wrong or healthier or better than the other. For instance, someone with an internal locus of control might interpret failure as an indicator of their inherent inability to handle a given subject, like they just aren't capable of it, and this would be less healthy. Alternatively, they might interpret it as a sign that it's time to hit the books, which would be more productive.

It's been pointed out that high self-efficacy tends to be associated with an internal locus of control, because in order to have a high level of confidence in one's ability to take action effectively, you've got to view the relevant situation as being under your control. It's not necessarily true, though, that the converse holds: that is, an internal locus of control may or may not lead to a high level of self-efficacy.

A further important point about self-efficacy is that it's defined in relatively narrow terms. It doesn't necessarily correlate to one's overall sense of worth, which is summed up by the term **self-esteem**. In fact, the well-known psychologist Albert Bandura developed the concept of **self-efficacy** specifically with the goal of developing a more specific and operationalizable concept. Perhaps surprisingly, self-efficacy and self-esteem really don't have to go together with each other at all! We've probably all met low-achieving people who have a fantastic opinion of themselves despite never really taking any actions to move their lives forward, illustrating a combination of high self-esteem and low self-efficacy. It's also completely possible for high self-efficacy to overlap with low self-esteem, for example if someone recognizes that they have the skills to be effective in a certain domain but still thinks poorly of themselves in general. It's been suggested that perfectionists may be vulnerable to this dynamic.

In any case though, locus of control, self-efficacy, and self-esteem are distinct concepts. However, they work together to shape our self-concept and self-identity. Circling back to how we previously illustrated self-concept with some very specific self-schemas, like being middle class, having a good sense of humor, and so on, we can now appreciate how the concepts of locus of control, self-efficacy, and self-esteem add to our understanding by allowing a level of generality that goes beyond specific self-schemas to describe overall trends in how we perceive ourselves. The power of locus of control, self-efficacy, and self-esteem to shape self-concept is part of why these concepts receive so much attention from psychologists.

So let's now step back and illustrate how these terms fit together. The term at the center of this discussion (i.e., what we're building up to) is self-concept, which we can treat as synonymous with self-identity. Our self-concept can be broken down into multiple self-schemas, and then the related but distinct phenomena of self-esteem, self-efficacy, and locus of control can be seen as off to the side, affecting that relationship between self-concept and self-schemas. We can then relegate other "self-" terms, like "self-verification", off to the side, as concepts that are relevant for this discussion, but don't directly participate in the structural relationships we've identified, and are more likely than not to appear on the MCAT as distractor answer choices rather than as core concepts that the test is trying to evaluate.

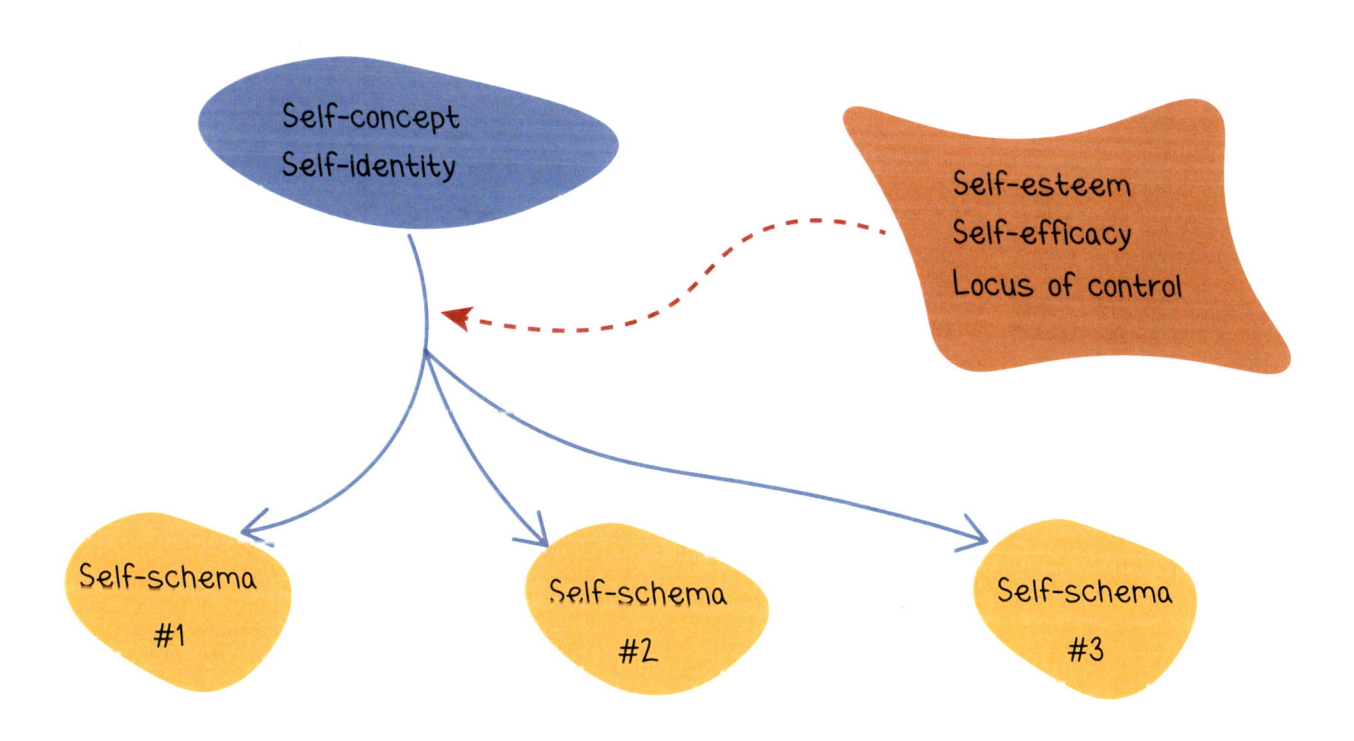

Figure 1. Terms related to the self.

7. Must-Knows

> - Verbal communication: literal words that we speak, write, sign, text or otherwise use
> - Nonverbal communication covers everything that is not verbal communication and is a fundamental form for communication for both humans and animals
> - Self-presentation strategies: self-disclosure, managing appearances, ingratiation, aligning actions, and altercasting
> - Dramaturgical approach to self-presentation or impression management states that we maintain both a front-stage self and a back-stage self
> - All human interactions are effectively social behavior
>   - Attraction is influenced by physical attractiveness, proximity and similarity
>   - Aggression: often found in hierarchical environments and regulated or restrained by the prefrontal cortex.
>   - Attachment: bond between children and their caregivers (secure attachment: only mild distress when caregiver leaves, quickly self-regulating and happy on return; ambivalent attachment: intense distress when caregiver leaves, followed by mixed signals on return; avoidant attachment: no apparent concern for caregiver leaving or returning, thought to stem from neglectful relationships; disoriented/disorganized attachment: hesitant, contradictory, and confused behavior both on the caregivers departure and return).
> - Altruism: helping other people at some cost to oneself. Altruism may help genetically similar organisms, such as kin, survive. The idea that natural selection can act on groups is known as inclusive fitness
> - Social support: emotional support, informational support, material support, or companionship support.
> - Mating behavior is the description of mate selection in a species and believed to often be non-random
>   - Fisherian selection: preference for physical traits or behaviors that have no use besides attracting mates, such as peacock feathers
> - Game theory: simulating games where all players are acting on incomplete information to make a similar set of choices. This has been used to model ecological interactions
> - Identity can refer to both personal identity and social identity, with the latter being the default
>   - Demographic identity contains race, ethnicity and nationality
>   - Gender identity as a category contains both sex and gender
>   - Gender is a social construct by which we identify ourselves
>   - Sex refers to biological categories
>   - Sexual orientation describes attraction to sexual partners and includes homosexuality, bisexuality, heterosexuality, asexuality, and pansexuality
>   - Socioeconomic class and religion are also categories of identity
>   - Identity formation is mediated by social factors
> - George Herbert Mead coined the term looking-glass self to describe the process by which we build conceptions of ourselves by what is reflected back at us about our behavior from others. Integrating this feedback into our perception of self is called internalization.
> - Role-playing or role-taking: putting oneself in the role of others, while impression management describes how we seek to control how others see us
> - Reference groups are groups we compare ourselves to, whether we are a part of the group (more in Ch. 11)
> - Self-concept: in broad terms, our perception of ourselves. This is made up of several self-schemas, which are traits we ascribe to ourselves.
> - Locus of control: whether a person thinks their actions and qualities dictate outcomes, or whether their circumstances do
> - Self-efficacy: the degree to which people perceive themselves as being effective

End of Chapter Practice

The best MCAT practice is **realistic**, with a focus on identifying steps for further improvement. For those reasons, we recommend completing practice questions in an online setting that simulates the real MCAT interface, and taking advantage of advanced analytic features to help you determine how best to move forward in your MCAT study journey.

With that in mind, **online end-of-chapter questions** are accessible through your Next Step account.

As a further supplement, given the importance of active learning for effective studying, we also suggest that you consult the Must-Knows as a basis for creating a study sheet, in which you list out key terms and test your ability to briefly summarize them.

This page left intentionally blank.

CHAPTER 11
Social Structures

0. Introduction

Nearly 400 years ago, the English poet John Donne wrote,

> "No man is an island, entire of itself;
> every man is a piece of the continent,
> a part of the main. [...]
> And therefore never send to know for whom
> the bell tolls; It tolls for thee."

This sentiment has long since become a cliche, but for good reason, since humans are defined in many ways by the groups that they belong to and/or identify with, and by their ability to cooperate. All of these topics will be major themes of this chapter.

1. Status and Roles

Status and role are two broad concepts that help describe how we situate ourselves within groups and the ways that we function in the setting of social groups.

I. Status

When you hear the word **status**, you might immediately associate it with so-called status symbols, like sports cars, fancy watches, and so on. Well, we're not going to be studying bling here, exactly, since the concept of status in sociology is a little more technical. But the point nonetheless holds that there are a lot of different ways that we can choose to signal to society who we are, or who we aspire to be, and the ways in which we do so are closely related to social perceptions that we can't exactly control. To put it in a more down-to-earth way, you might choose to have a mullet because you want to signal to the world that you're all about that "business in the front, party in the back" attitude, but the end result might not be as impressive as you would hope. That is, people might have negative stereotypes about mullet-wearers that don't align with the image that you, the mullet wearer, wanted to project.

In sociology, status refers to any social category that is used to identify people. This is extremely broad. So "physician" is a status, but so is "mullet-wearer." What's more, statuses aren't mutually exclusive—you can be a physician *and* have a mullet (dream big, right?). However, social status in this sense is almost so broad as to be useless. To say anything interesting about society, we have to narrow our scope. So, for this reason, there are a few different types of status to be aware of.

An **achieved status** is one that a person works to attain. "Physician" is a perfect example of an achieved status, because there's no way to become a physician without working really hard. Again, though, the possible scope of achieved statuses is huge, and they don't have to be fancy and prestigious. From the point of view of sociology, "high school senior" is just as much as an achieved status as "physician" or "NBA champion." In contrast, **ascribed statuses** are those that come from outside of ourselves, that we don't attain based on our actions, but rather just have involuntarily. Classic examples include demographic categories like race, ethnicity, and gender.

In some cases, a certain status can play such a dominant role in someone's life that it crowds out other statuses that apply to them. This concept is referred to as a **master status**. So, for example, if you've ever met an old-school surgeon who lives at the hospital and thinks that work-life balance is an insult, you've probably met someone for whom "physician" is their master status. The concept of master status also often applies to celebrities. There's no objective cut-off for when a status becomes a master status, and it might even be possible for someone to disagree with what others perceive as their master status; for example, if someone was a well-known actress but personally felt like her role as a parent is the most important part of her life.

> **MCAT STRATEGY > > >**
>
> On the MCAT, you won't run into ambiguous situations regarding status; whether a status is achieved, ascribed, or master should be clear from context if you know how these terms are defined.

II. Roles

Statuses aren't just empty labels. They come with expectations. A physician has to maintain accreditation, treat patients, and so on. A student has to take classes and try to do well in school. A sibling should try to look out for his or her siblings. You get the idea. Now, of course, if we're in an argumentative frame of mind, we could come up with exceptions to all of these generalizations -- what about a retired physician, or a physician who is no longer in clinical practice? What about a lazy student? What about siblings who don't get along? Well, okay, fine, all of those scenarios occur in reality, but it doesn't change the fact that society has some general expectations of people who have those statuses. That is, just because your buddy Jim is a bad student who skips class doesn't mean that students in general aren't expected to go to class.

These expectations are known in sociology as **roles**. Not surprisingly, sociologists have developed various technical terms to describe some of the experiences that people have with roles. There are four such terms that you should know, and all of them are similar-sounding two-word phrases that start with "role." Therefore, as you can imagine, they provide wonderful material for multiple-choice questions.

As we hinted at with the example of being a physician, a single role can involve many different tasks and responsibilities. Physicians have to care for their patients and fill out paperwork and negotiate with insurance companies and supervise staff members and trainees and complete continuing education and so on. So it's not surprising that sometimes people experience difficulty handling the multiple responsibilities associated with a certain role. This is known as **role strain**.

People might also experience difficulty because they have different roles that are pulling them in different directions, and it's hard to balance them both. For example, it's notoriously difficult—although certainly not impossible—to balance the roles of physician, spouse, and parent. Experiencing difficulties balancing multiple roles is known as **role conflict**, because it's like the different roles are fighting with each other for priority.

We can't emphasize enough how important it is to be able to distinguish role strain from role conflict. They're both similar concepts in that they involve someone experiencing difficulty in connection to one or more social roles, and the difference between them isn't completely obvious based on their names. This makes these terms common material for multiple-choice questions designed to trip up students who forgot to study this topic carefully—so don't fall into that trap! Remember, role strain has to do with the strain a given role places on a person, and role conflict has to do with conflict between different roles that are each fighting for priority in a person's life.

> **MCAT STRATEGY > > >**
>
> You feel strain when a single role creates a strain in you. Roles can conflict when multiple different roles place conflicting expectations on you. Remember, conflict happens between two or more things (people, roles, etc.)

Moving on to some other role-related concepts, **role exit** is the process that one goes through when disengaging from a role. For instance, ceasing to be a college student isn't something that just happens one day. You start making your post-graduation plans, finish up your classes, make sure that everything is lined up in terms of paperwork, and then there might be the culminating event of graduation, after which you move onto other things. But it's a process. The details of role exit are different for each role, and even for different individuals, but the underlying idea is that role exit is what happens when you're stepping out of a role.

In contrast, **role engulfment** occurs when a role expands to dominate someone's life. This is similar to what we talked about before with master status, although master status has more to do with how the rest of society sees someone, and isn't necessarily connected with a person's daily actions. In contrast, role engulfment is more closely related to what someone does with their time or energy. A classic example related to the field of medicine is the way in which the role of a patient—for example, a patient with a chronic illness such as cancer—can expand to fill up someone's life, both because of the psychological impact of the disease and because of the very real logistical burden that a complex treatment regimen can place on a patient.

4. Groups, Networks, and Organizations

Since groups make up a core part of human society, it's not surprising that sociologists have sought to understand different types of groups and to analyze the inner workings of larger, more complex groups. We'll start with smaller groups, covering a few key terminological distinctions, and then zoom out to larger-scale organizations.

I. Groups

There are several ways in which groups are typically defined for the MCAT, and it's important to note that these definitions are generally not mutually exclusive. Keep that in the back of your head for now, and once we review their definitions, we'll illustrate this point more concretely.

First, an important distinction is made between **primary groups** and **secondary groups**. In a nutshell, primary groups are long lasting, with deep bonds formed among members, while secondary groups are short-lasting and more superficial. Family is a common example of a primary group, along with religious organizations and so on. On the other hand, classes in school and work colleagues are common examples of secondary groups. The trick here is not to confuse these examples with the definitions of primary and secondary groups. In particular, keep in mind that a primary group is defined by enduring relationships, even if these relationships don't make you feel warm and fuzzy, or even if they cause significant distress, whereas a secondary group is defined by superficial, more transient relationships, even if those relationships are very positive. Of course someone might have difficult relationships with family members, and there are definitely tightly-knit, stable workplaces where people get to know each other really well. Examples like this might seem to blur the distinction between primary and secondary groups, but that's not really true; they just illustrate how hard it can be to find universal examples of sociological phenomena. The fundamental distinction is always that primary groups are deep and long-lasting, and secondary groups are superficial and short-lasting.

> **MCAT STRATEGY > > >**
>
> If primary vs. secondary groups are tested on the MCAT, you'll be given a clear example, not an unusual borderline case, but be vigilant for traps that rely on the incorrect assumption that primary groups must always foster positive relationships.

To get even more specific, we can also distinguish between **peer groups** and **family groups**. Peer groups are made up of people who are often similar in terms of age, status, background, interests, and so on, and we usually think of those groups as being self-selected. So, while age is definitely a component, peer groups aren't quite as simple as just groups of people of the same age. For example, if you went to a large public high school, your high school class might not be a peer group in that sense—it might actually be hundreds of people from vastly different backgrounds. Extracurricular organizations in a high school can be better examples of peer groups, since you choose to join them, they're defined by a shared interest, and they might tend to attract people from similar backgrounds, even if that's not a defining feature of the group. Family groups, on the other hand, are what they sound like: groups defined by genetic relationships and/or relationships like marriage, partnership and adoption. These are groups that you're typically born into or marry into. In some ways, family groups are more tight-knit than are peer groups, but they also involve people of very different ages, and may span different cultural backgrounds as well, all of which can lead to some degree of tension.

Next, a distinction is also made between **in-groups** and **out-groups**. In-groups are categories that someone identifies as a member of, or feels that he or she belongs to, while out-groups are the opposite. Examples of in-groups can be down-to-earth and small-scale—that is, someone's extended family, school, or workplace can be in-groups—but most commonly, this distinction is applied to broader demographic categories, like local identities, race, gender, sexual orientation, culture, religion, profession, and so on. With this in mind, the concept of in-groups versus out-groups becomes relevant for phenomena like stereotypes, prejudice, and discrimination, which we've covered in another chapter.

All three categories of groups that we've discussed—that is, primary versus secondary groups, peer versus family groups, and in-groups versus outgroups—on some level involve distinguishing between people who are close to us and those who are more distant. Our final term that includes the word "group," **reference groups**, is a little bit different. These are the groups that we compare ourselves to.

This is probably the category of groups that causes students the most confusion, despite its simple definition, so let's pause to think through the implications of how we define a reference group. We can start off with a simple question: does someone have just one reference group? The answer is no, because people can have multiple different reference groups for different aspects of their identity. To take a simple example, think of someone who is both a physician and a serious runner. For things relating to medicine, patient care, and so on, his or her reference group will consist of other physicians. But when it comes to running a 10k, other runners will be the reference group. Now, here's a question that's a little bit trickier. In the example we just worked through, our physician/runner belonged to both of the reference groups. Is that necessarily the case? Again, no. You can certainly compare yourself to groups you don't belong to. You may have on occasion found yourself comparing yourself to students who have been accepted to medical school, even though you haven't been accepted yet. There isn't really a technical limit for who or what a reference group can be. It is much more commonplace for someone to use in-groups as reference groups, but there's no real reason why someone couldn't compare themselves to members of an out-group.

The key point for the MCAT is that for reference group to be the correct answer, there *has to* be an explicit indicator that someone evaluates his or herself with reference to that group. So let's imagine a very simple multiple-choice question: *Leila works at a large retailer. Her co-workers form a: primary group, secondary group, peer group, or reference group?* Let's think this through based on our definitions of these concepts. We can securely eliminate primary group, because secondary group is almost always going to be a better fit for workplace environments, where relationships tend to be more superficial and transient. Secondary group therefore seems like a good choice. But what about peer group or reference group? Her workers could be a peer group, if this retailer hires people of similar age and background and people opt to work there at least partially for those reasons. But we just don't know whether that's true based on the information that we're given. It could just as easily be the case that the retailer hires people of all ages and backgrounds, and their employees really have nothing in common with each other besides the fact that they work at the same place. So we shouldn't pick "peer group." How about reference group? Leila's co-workers *could* be a reference group, for example if she's trying to measure up to their work performance to get a promotion or bonus, or if she thinks they're cool people worth emulating for whatever reason. But we have no evidence for this. Leila could just show up at work, punch the clock, do her job, and leave, and never give her co-workers any particular thought beyond the bare minimum. So we just don't know, and we therefore can't pick "reference group." We only have evidence for one thing: that Leila's coworkers are unambiguously her secondary group. Whether or not they could be anything else is irrelevant.

What's more, it's worth noting that depending on the circumstances, Leila's co-workers could be a secondary group *and* a reference group *and* a peer group *and*, for that matter, an in-group. These categories aren't mutually exclusive at all. We just have to pick the answer that's best supported by the information that we're given. When studying this material, many students ask questions like "is XYZ group a reference group?" or "is ABC group a peer group?" The answer is almost always that it depends. The way to think about these definitions is not to create a list of groups and memorize which category each group belongs to. Instead, the goal should be to understand that these definitions of groups are based on how people experience them, which can show tremendous variation, because everyone's different! Therefore, the examples we give just reflect typical situations. Instead of relying on these examples, try to understand how each group is defined, and then apply those definitions based on the information you're given in a passage or question. So with our example, even though overlap between these different types of groups is quite possible, and it certainly remains possible that Leila considers her colleagues both a peer group and a secondary group, we should only select the answer choice that we have best evidence to support.

> **MCAT STRATEGY > > >**
>
> Groups are a paramount example of how important it is to carefully analyze the context provided by a given passage or question, a pattern that some students find similar to CARS.

Groups come in many different sizes, of course, ranging from as few as two members—think a small study group, or a tight friendship—to over a billion for categories like Muslims or Catholics. In many contexts, groups made up of two people, or **dyads**, are thought to be less stable than groups made up of three people, or **triads**.

II. Networks

Another way of looking at groups is through the perspective of networks. In everyday speech, we'd say that a person's network is the set of people they're connected with, and we might make distinctions between friend networks, networks of colleagues, networks of alumni, and so on. If we were to zoom out to aggregate those individual-level relationships, we can create a social network map, where each circle, or node, is a person, and each connecting line is a relationship between them. In **social network analysis**, researchers can apply various mathematical techniques to analyze the connections among people in networks, allowing them to identify the most central nodes, to predict how information might move through networks, to characterize how spread-out or centralized a certain group is, and so on.

III. Organizations

Organizations are a subset of groups. As we've seen, groups can be extremely broad categories that just kind of emerge from our social interactions. **Formal organizations**, on the other hand, are strictly defined. For example, according to our broad definition of groups, New Yorkers certainly qualify as a group. But who defines whether someone is or isn't a New Yorker? No one, really. Is there a single boss of all New Yorkers? Not exactly. Is there any structure to this group? Nope. In contrast, the city government of New York is a very different story. A person is or isn't employed by the New York city government—it's not a question of self-identity. The New York city government has a boss (the mayor). It definitely has a specific structure. Importantly, it also has defined rules for entering and exiting the organization, and the organization will continue to exist even when all of its current members are long gone. These are all important characteristics of a formal organization.

There are three major types of organizations: coercive, normative, and utilitarian. A **coercive organization** is one that you don't choose to be part of, but have to anyway. Prison is a classic example. So is the military in countries that have a mandatory draft. **Normative organizations**, in contrast, are ones that people join because of some shared ideal or ethical goal. At least in theory, most volunteer organizations fall under this rubric. Finally, **utilitarian organizations** are ones that people join to make money or be compensated for in some direct way. So employees of a company are part of a utilitarian organization, to give just one example.

Organizations can be structured in various ways, but **bureaucracies** are the most well-known example. In fact, bureaucracies have been studied for well over a century, and researchers have argued that they are the most representative type of modern political and commercial organization. A bureaucracy is a rational, well-organized, impersonal, and typically large administrative system. Bureaucracies are things like governments, hospitals, schools, corporations, and courts, just to name a few examples. Bureaucracy was most famously studied by Max Weber, a pioneering sociologist who worked in the late 1800s and early 1900s. According to Weber, an **ideal bureaucracy** has the following major characteristics: It has a hierarchical structure, with well-defined roles, responsibilities, and chains of command; it is organized by specialization, with each role corresponding to a clearly-defined skill; it is run impersonally; recruitment and employment are grounded in technical, merit-based qualifications; a predictable career path; and political neutrality. Note that when we say these are characteristics of an ideal bureaucracy, we aren't using the word "ideal" to indicate "good" in the sense of quality or morality. An ideal bureaucracy isn't necessarily better than any other group; instead, "ideal" just means it fits the definition of "bureaucracy" as closely as possible. And as the word implies, not all bureaucracies live up to the criteria of an ideal bureaucracy, but the idea is that these general principles usually hold in most such organizations. Weber's thoughts about bureaucracy were interesting in that he thought that it provided the most efficient rational basis for modern society, but he was also aware that bureaucracies could be stifling, and he even coined the phrase "iron cage of bureaucracy" to describe this sense of stagnation in a bureaucratic system.

Not surprisingly, people have thought about other ways to structure organizations. To take an example, the Berkeley Free Clinic has functioned as an anarchist collective, or a group without bosses and with group-based, consensus-oriented decision-making, for decades. In the world of business, entrepreneurs are continually experimenting with lean, flat organizational structures that minimize hierarchies, and there are certainly organizations—especially volunteer and political organizations—that try to take on some form of democratic governance. However, the so-called **iron law of oligarchy**, which was first proposed over 100 years ago, in 1911, posits that any organization that starts off with democratic decision-making will ultimately wind up being dominated by a smaller group of decision-makers, or an oligarchy. The word "oligarchy" technically means "rule by a few," with the same "oligo" prefix that you might have seen before in scientific concepts (e.g., *oligo*peptides).

The final bureaucracy-related term that we need to cover is **McDonaldization**. This term was coined after McDonald's had swept the world with what really was a revolutionary new way (for better or worse) of delivering and marketing food. McDonaldization refers to an organizational approach that focuses on efficiency, calculability, uniformity, and technological control, which are the factors that go into making a McDonald's hamburger that can be profitably sold at very low prices, but also make the experience much less personal than dining out at a local restaurant. While the word may sound goofy, discussions about the McDonaldization of healthcare frequently pop up on the MCAT, so be prepared!

5. Theoretical Approaches to Social Structures

On a higher-scale level than groups, a number of different institutions shape and regulate our actions, including education, family, religion, the government, the economy, and health care. For the MCAT, you don't need to know everything about these huge topics. Instead, the goal is to have a general idea of what these structures are, to understand some specific issues related to them that the AAMC has identified as important to study, and to recognize how major theoretical frameworks in sociology apply to these areas.

Before we dive into the details of theoretical approaches to sociology, let's start out with a quick general point. Sociology isn't physics. This is obvious, but what we mean is that there's not a right theory of sociology and a wrong theory of sociology, so don't get too caught up in wondering which theory is objectively the most correct. In fact, most of these theories aren't even mutually exclusive. Instead, think of them as being like different lenses that we can wear to view society in a certain way.

The names of theoretical approaches usually give at least some indication of what they're about, which is a double-edged sword. On one hand, the name of a theory can be a valuable hint when you're taking the test, but on the other hand, the test writers don't really want to write questions that most test-takers will answer correctly just by going by the sound of the name. Therefore, you have to be on the lookout for less obvious ways that theories can be applied, as well as ways that similar-sounding theories can be distinguished from each other. As we describe these theoretical approaches, we'll weave in some tips for organizing your studying with this goal in mind.

> **MCAT STRATEGY > > >**
>
> The MCAT will not ask you to decide which sociological theory is right; instead, you'll often be asked to identify a certain perspective on an issue, or to predict what someone working within a certain theoretical framework might choose to focus on, but you won't be asked whether a certain finding proves a given theory.

To start with, a distinction is made between **microsociology** and **macrosociology**. *Micro* means small, and *macro* means large, so microsociology tends to focus on smaller-scale interactions, like how individuals navigate society, while macrosociology focuses on larger-scale interactions, like those involving major social institutions.

I. Functionalism

A good place to start exploring theoretical frameworks of sociology is **Emile Durkheim**'s **functionalism**. As the name suggests, functionalism focuses on the functions of various structures and institutions. So schools are for educating children, hospitals are for treating sick people, and so on. Functionalism provides a very useful point of view for studying other cultures with institutions that might seem unfamiliar to an outside observer. An important distinction is made between **manifest functions** and **latent functions**. The manifest function (or functions) of an institution are its intended functions—basically, what it's supposed to do. Latent functions, in contrast, are unintended functions. For instance, a private four-year college might have the manifest function of providing a liberal arts education to its students. Its latent functions could include being a credential for getting a job after college, connecting students with its alumni network, and so on. Arguably, four-year private colleges also give young adults a space to experiment with living independently before having a full-time job. However, that point doesn't apply to all college students—some college students work full-time, others live at home, and so on—so it depends on socioeconomic status and other factors. With that in mind, we could suggest that another latent function of private four-year colleges is to reinforce patterns of social inequality, because not everyone can afford that opportunity, which does open important doors in the future. Well, now we have a latent function that doesn't sound great—and in fact, unintended negative consequences of a structure or institution can be referred to as **latent dysfunctions**. Generally, the term latent function usually refers to positive or at least neutral unintended consequences.

> **MCAT STRATEGY > > >**
>
> As is often the case for MCAT sociology, context is important to avoid making incorrect assumptions regarding functions. Furthermore, since function vs. dysfunction could be a matter of opinion, watch out for any clues in the question or passage about whether something is presented as positive or negative.

Something else to note about this example is that these distinctions aren't always completely self-evident, or might not apply in all circumstances. So we said that for a college with the manifest function of giving its students a liberal arts education, career success and networking might be latent, or unintended functions. However, a college could choose to emphasize its role in career preparation, making this a manifest function.

II. Conflict Theory

Conflict theory is another major sociological framework with an informative name. It's generally thought to have originated with Karl Marx, but it is not synonymous with Marxism or socialism. Instead, it focuses on the competition between different structures or groups for resources, and the conflicts that arise in that process. This logically entails a focus on power differentials. So, to return to our example of education at four-year colleges, conflict theorists might be interested in how education controls access to various economic opportunities in society, or in how socioeconomic status and pre-existing resources shape access to four-year college education, with all its economic consequences. Again, note the emphasis on access, resources, and power—but a conflict theory analysis doesn't necessarily require a situation in which, to continue this example, lower-status and higher-status groups are literally fighting, or even perceive themselves as adversaries.

On the flip side, as paradoxical as it might sound, not all situations involving conflict are examples of conflict theory. Let's illustrate this with a very microsociological example—imagine that you have a brother, and your relationship with him is complicated. If you get into conflicts with him because he's a jerk, has obnoxious friends, and is generally annoying, that's not really an example of conflict theory. However, if you're competing with your brother for resources—either tangible resources like financial support or intangibles like attention or approval—then conflict theory might apply. This point is worth appreciating because this kind of distinction is a way that the MCAT can test whether you've actually studied conflict theory or are just guessing based on the name.

III. Symbolic Interactionism

Switching gears a bit from the typically macrosociological approaches of functionalism and conflict theory, **symbolic interactionism** tends to take a more microsociological perspective. Symbolic interactionism may sound very theoretical and vague, but it's fairly straightforward when analyzed carefully. As the name suggests, symbolic interactionism is interested in how people interact, using symbols. Although this definition sounds simple, mistakes involving symbolic interactionism are pretty common. So let's dig in a little bit.

There are two main things to keep in mind when navigating this topic. First, *interactions* must be part of a symbolic interactionist analysis. That is, don't focus on "symbolic" to the point of overlooking the other half of the name of this theory. The second key is understanding what *symbols* mean here. This isn't like literature class, where a seemingly straightforward object has some hidden meaning, and you can just make up any claim about it, the more fanciful the better. Instead, in symbolic interactionism, a **symbol** is something that we assign meaning to, but the idea is that we have to have a shared sense of such meanings for society to work. To take a very simple, everyday example, what does it mean to shake hands when you meet someone? It's a pretty weird gesture when you think about it. The idea that hand-shaking is an aspect of greeting is a shared cultural symbol. Moreover, it's culture-specific. In some European and Latin American cultures, people greet each other by briefly embracing and exchanging two or three quick kisses on alternating cheeks. This practice doesn't translate universally, and trying it with someone who's not familiar with it will result in confusion at best. More broadly, for a symbolic interactionist, symbols include rituals and other social practices. For example, Thanksgiving dinner has a certain meaning in American society that's recognized even by people who opt out or celebrate non-traditionally.

IV. Social Constructionism

A follow-up question might be: where does the meaning of Thanksgiving dinner come from? **Social constructionism** emerged to try to answer this kind of question. Social constructionism posits that the meaning of a social structure or concept emerges from how we think about those concepts and communicate with each other about them. Holidays like Thanksgiving are good examples of social constructs, because not only do people participate in holidays when the time rolls around each year, but we also communicate about holidays. We talk about them with friends and family members, and even if we're not really engaged in them, we get messages through social media and mass media reminding us that other people are taking part in them and reinforcing their meaning and significance. The meaning of holidays changes over time, indicating that social constructs can be fluid, because they change as society changes.

Holidays are pretty straightforward examples of social constructionism in action. However, this theoretical framework can also be applied to examples that might feel less obvious. For instance, a social constructionist analysis of the scientific method would focus on the ways that it's taught, the way that it's put into practice (successfully or not) in real-world scientific research, and the ways that scientists communicate with each other about their methods, and maybe even compare the scientific method as we understand it now to ways that scientists have gone about their work in other times in history. This kind of analysis can feel uncomfortable, because as people who have taken science classes and care about science, we might be deeply convinced that the scientific method is an objectively legitimate way to obtain knowledge about reality, not just some made-up thing like Thanksgiving. As always, the MCAT doesn't require you to make a judgment one way or the other—but you should be able to recognize a social constructionist analysis, even if you don't necessarily agree with it. On a similar note, gender roles and concepts like love, patriotism, and respect, just to pick a few examples, are also generally thought to be social constructs.

As a final note on these theories, it can be easy to confuse symbolic interactionism and social constructionism. These approaches sound similar, and they do deal with similar issues. The key to keeping them distinct is to relentlessly focus on what their names imply. Symbolic interactionism focuses on people interacting with each other in symbolic activities, while social constructionism focuses more on how we build, or construct, those symbols in the first place.

V. Rational Choice Theory

Sociologists have also sought to understand how people make decisions. **Rational choice theory** posits that people have certain preferences or goals, and then choose actions based on the pros and cons of various possible choices in a way that maximizes the likelihood of satisfying those preferences or goals. Now, you might think that this is a bit naive, since people make irrational choices all the time! The point of this theory is not so much to argue about what preferences people have, which we might disagree with, but instead to model how they try to accomplish those goals. So, a rational choice perspective on addiction, for instance, might say that for someone addicted to a drug, pursuing intoxication and avoiding withdrawal are very high priorities that they work rationally to accomplish. Now, that's certainly not an adequate explanation for addiction in light of modern scientific research, but it serves to illustrate how rational choice theory isn't about what people value, but how they choose to act in pursuit of their goals.

VI. Social Exchange Theory

A related theoretical approach, **social exchange theory**, builds on this perspective of self-interestedness and views social interactions as involving interchanges with costs and rewards. Commercial relationships are an obvious example, but exchange theory would extend this perspective to even include, say, friendships, since you invest time and energy into a friendship, and then you receive benefits like companionship and support. This might seem a little cold-blooded, but as always for the MCAT, you don't need to completely buy into a theory to be able to recognize it. For our purposes, rational choice theory and social exchange theory are extremely similar, but one way you can think about the difference is that rational choice theory focuses on how people make choices, whereas social exchange theory focuses on actual interactions.

VII. Feminist Theory

The final theory we'll cover here is **feminist theory**. The term is kind of an oversimplification, because there have been multiple different waves of feminist theory, and feminist theorists do in fact disagree about many important issues. However, underpinning feminist theory is the goal of understanding and remedying gender injustices through a focus on both lived experiences and objective data. Despite this focus on inequalities faced by women, some theorists have broadened the scope of their analysis to include critiques of gender inequalities in general, and how such inequalities are shaped and perpetuated by gender roles and power structures. The focus on power and inequality is a similarity between feminist theory and conflict theory, but feminist theory is both more specialized in terms of its focus on gender and somewhat more methodologically diverse, in that not all feminist perspectives are explicitly focused on competition for resources.

6. Education, the Family, and Religion

I. Education

As we've all experienced, **education** is one of the dominant features of life as a child and young adult in the United States. The aspects of education that are tested on the MCAT tend to relate to the unintended consequences of education, or what you could even see as its dark side—that is, ways that the educational system functions that don't match up with its stated purpose of transmitting knowledge and expertise.

The **hidden curriculum** is the first of these concepts, and it's one that should be of interest to anyone contemplating medical school, or any other career in the health professions. The idea here is that in an educational or training setting, we learn all sorts of things that aren't officially included in the curriculum, especially values, norms, and ways of interacting with others. In recent years, particular attention has been paid to how the hidden curriculum of medical school can inculcate toxic or harmful attitudes, like dismissiveness towards other specialities, judgmental attitudes towards patients based on attributes like weight or socioeconomic status, and a tendency to focus on the technical aspects of care instead of patient-centered care. That said, a hidden curriculum doesn't have to be completely negative, or even negative at all: the key things to look out for are any values or attitudes that are transmitted outside of the curriculum.

There are also many ways in which the educational system is affected by inequalities that exist in our society. The concepts of **educational segregation** and **stratification** refer to some ways in which this happens. Segregation and stratification sound similar, and are used to refer to broadly similar phenomena, but let's try to tease these concepts apart.

Segregation in a literal sense means putting different things in different places. It's used in this sense in genetics to talk about the segregation of alleles into different daughter cells. In the sociology of education, it originally referred to a system in which children from different racial groups were legally required to attend different schools. That system ended in the mid-twentieth century in the US, but just ending legal segregation didn't mean that schools were automatically integrated. After all, public school districts draw their student populations based on area of residence, and residential areas often have racially-imbalanced populations, resulting in residential segregation. Therefore, the term segregation has continued to be used to refer to uneven distributions of students in schools, based on parameters like race, ethnicity, or even poverty.

Stratification literally means arranging things in layers. In sociology, it's usually used to refer to levels (layers) of socioeconomic status. Educational stratification is therefore the idea that people with higher status and more resources have more options in terms of access to the educational system. What's more, educational structures that put high-achieving students on a track towards college and lower-achieving students on a track towards more vocational options are also a form of stratification, although such systems aren't strictly defined in terms of socioeconomic status. However, even if such systems claim that they're purely defined based on merit, they do intersect with socioeconomic issues, because all things being equal, people with more access and more resources will be more likely to have children who do better in school. Putting these concepts together, educational segregation and stratification refer to a situation in which poorer students, and students from disadvantaged minority groups, are clustered together in certain school systems, which themselves tend to be poorer and have trouble recruiting high-quality teachers because school systems in the US are generally funded based on property taxes.

On more of a microsociological level, teacher's expectations of their students—which may be rooted in stereotypes—are thought to impact students' performance. That is, students who pick up on high expectations perform better, and vice versa.

II. Family

Family is another institution that defines our early lives. Family bonds involve **kinship**, which sociologists have defined in multiple ways. The first distinction to make is between **kinship of descent**, which is based on shared ancestry, and **kinship of affinity**, which is based on relationships like marriage and adoption. Kinship can also be classified based on degrees of closeness. **Primary kin** are people to whom you're related through a very close bond, like through parent-child relationships, marriage, or siblinghood. **Secondary kin** are primary kin of your primary kin, so for example your sibling's spouse. **Tertiary kin** are either primary kin of your secondary kin, or secondary kin of your primary kin, so like your brother-in-law's parent, or your sibling's sister-in-law. Interestingly, languages show tremendous diversity in the words they use for kinship terms.

Likewise, families themselves come in all shapes and sizes, including families with opposite-sex married partners and children, families with same-sex partners, families with single parents, families that include other members of the extended family, like grandparents, aunts, and uncles, and so on. Family structures also vary across cultures - for example, in many Asian cultures, multigenerational families are more common than has traditionally been the case in the United States. Patterns of family structures also change over time; for example, in the last 50 years in the United States, it has become more common for unmarried partners to form families, and for married partners to get divorced. The divorce rate spiked around 1970 in the US, but since the mid-1980s, both the divorce and marriage rates have declined. In the meantime, families with same-sex partners have become more common.

Unfortunately, as many physicians regularly encounter, the family can also be a structure in which violence takes place. Abuse can be psychological, physical, or sexual, and can also manifest as neglect, or failure to provide the care that someone needs. Abuse can be directed against children, spouses, and elderly family members, and it cuts across all socioeconomic categories.

III. Religion

Over the course of history, and to a great extent still to this day, **religion** has been among the institutions with the strongest impacts on people's lives. Although religions have various beliefs about the meaning of life and death, the nature of the universe, and spirituality, from a sociological perspective, religions also function as institutions that replicate themselves over time and structure people's lives by providing rituals, community, ethical frameworks, and a space for important life events like marriage. The term **religiosity** refers to how religious a person considers him or herself to be, and this is something worth being aware of as a physician, because a patient's religiosity may shape how he or she relates to medical treatment.

Religious organizations come in several forms. Just as a quick note, this is a subfield of sociology that originated with a distinct focus on Christianity as practiced in Europe and the US, so the degree to which these definitions apply to other religious traditions is kind of up for debate. In any case, the German sociologist Max Weber, who worked in the late 1800s and early 1900s, proposed that religious organizations existed on a spectrum, with highly-stable, well-organized, consensus-promoting, and even somewhat bureaucratic institutions called **churches**—like the Catholic church—on one end, and **sects**, which are smaller, dissident split-off groups that advocate for a different form of the religion, on the other end. **Denominations** are somewhere in between. The various types of Protestantism, like Lutheranism, Methodism, and so on, are common examples of denominations. They all have different interpretations of a set of religious beliefs, and different traditions to some extent, but are basically grounded in the same religious context and are stable, consensus-promoting organizations. **Cults**, on the other hand, are small, tightly-controlled groups with novel beliefs that usually involve a charismatic leader and some degree of isolation of cult members from the rest of society.

Finally, given the hugely important role that religion has played throughout history, it's no surprise that religious structures and practices have been affected by social changes. Broadly speaking, **modernization** can be thought of as the cumulative impact of the technological advances that have been made in the last century or so, with corresponding transformations of social structures. Modernization has had interesting, and at times divergent, impacts on religion. On one hand, in some settings, modernization has decreased people's religiosity, a trend referred to as **secularization**. On the other hand, though, modern societies have also seen a swing towards **fundamentalism**, which is a literalist, uncompromising, and extreme approach to religion that emphasizes the superiority of fundamentalist groups over other faith communities. In a certain sense, we can see these trends (secularization and fundamentalism) as two sides of the same coin. Modernization has disrupted traditional social structures and given people many new ways to connect with each other, and that can play out in many different ways.

7. Government and Economy

Now it's time to zoom out to look at some higher-level social structures: the government and the economy. Although we might be able to get through the day without specifically noticing the role of these institutions, they do shape virtually every aspect of our lives. They're also interrelated, in that both the government and economy regulate how we interact with each other. Moreover, the government regulates economic activity, and aspects of the economic system impact the government too, although generally not quite as directly.

I. Government

The government organizes society through a combination of **power** and **authority**. We often use these terms as if they mean the same thing, but that's not quite the case in sociology. The power of a government refers to its literal ability to get things done, including the fact that the government can use force to compel certain behaviors. But the government doesn't usually need to invoke that power directly. Instead, it might rely on its authority, a term which refers to the overall legitimacy of the government, or the degree to which the government is felt to have the right to structure our lives in certain ways, regardless of its power to actually enforce regulations. As an example, let's consider taxes. There are a couple of different reasons to pay taxes. For some people, the only reason to pay taxes is that the government might punish you if you don't, and it's not worth the risk. This point of view focuses on the power of the government. Other people might genuinely feel that paying taxes is the right thing to do as a way to contribute to all the services that the government provides. This point of view focuses on the government's authority. Of course, these viewpoints aren't mutually exclusive. Nothing's stopping you from feeling that the government is a legitimate representative of our collective interest *and* realizing that if you don't pay up, you could face serious consequences. But power and authority do focus on different aspects of the government's role.

Broadly speaking, there are three main types of governmental systems: monarchy, authoritarianism, and democracy. The defining feature of **monarchy** is that rulership, or sovereignty, is passed down in a defined succession, usually through family networks. The United Kingdom is probably the best-known monarchy in the modern world -- but interestingly, there, the monarch doesn't actually make any real decisions about how the country is run. The U.K. is an extreme example of a **constitutional monarchy**, where a constitution puts restrictions in place on a monarch's power. In such systems, a monarch usually coexists with an elected government. On the other end of the spectrum, in **absolute monarchies**, the king or queen is the sole person in charge. While you won't be expected to know the exact structure of government in the U.K., or any other government for that matter, you should understand the basic features of a monarchy and be able to distinguish it from authoritarianism and democracy, which we're about to discuss next.

This leads to **authoritarianism**, in which citizens have no input into the government, and are expected to obey whatever the government decides. So-called soft authoritarian systems are those in which there may be some elections, but usually with a limited choice of candidates. In these systems, the government minimizes its intrusions into citizens' private lives, while repressing outward forms of of dissent that could destabilize the system. In contrast, **totalitarianism** is like authoritarianism on steroids. In such systems, the government regulates every aspect of life, including citizens' communications, and any form of dissent whatsoever can be brutally punished. Famous examples include Nazi Germany and the Stalinist period in the Soviet Union.

Democracy, on the other hand, is a system where people vote. Direct democracies are systems in which people vote for laws themselves, and indirect democracies, or **democratic republics**, are systems where people vote for representatives who then make laws. The federal government in the United States is an example of a democratic republic. The two aren't mutually exclusive, however; for instance, California, and many other places in the United States, have systems where most lawmaking is handled by elected representatives, but citizens do also get the chance to vote on some laws directly through ballot measures.

II. Economy

Our next social institution, the economy, follows closely from the discussion of government that we've just covered. After all, most governments that we are familiar with regulate the economy in some fashion, although the extent and details of that regulation vary. The two main economic frameworks that have influenced the modern world are capitalism and socialism. **Capitalism** is characterized by private ownership, both of property and of companies that produce goods and provide services. **Socialism**, on the other hand, emphasizes social ownership and worker's self-management, whether collectively or through the government, but still maintaining many of the structures characteristic of a capitalist state. **Communism** is formally defined as a utopian society, the end-goal of a transformation that proceeds through capitalism and socialism, in which society becomes class-less, state-less and free of hierarchy. This has never been achieved, and organizations and states that have historically used the name of communism have been far removed from this ideal.

The question of whether certain economic systems go along with specific governmental systems is a thorny one. We can identify some trends, but there are often important exceptions. For instance, communism has generally been implemented by authoritarian, and even totalitarian governments, although some theorists have argued for the possibility of anarcho-communism, or a system of communism that wouldn't have a centralized state at all. Such experiments do exist in a few enclaves around the world. Socialism has been implemented in several countries with authoritarian governments, but many more countries, including Bolivia, Vietnam, and many western European ones, have implemented social democratic systems, which usually involve more private enterprise than would be possible under a "purer" form of socialism. We often associate capitalism with democracy, but the majority of authoritarian and even totalitarian states have had capitalist economies, most famously in fascist governments. On the other hand, capitalism is also sometimes associated with libertarianism, which refers to a movement that tries to completely minimize the role of government. Therefore, it's not really a one-size-fits-all kind of situation.

A principle underlying every modern economic system is **division of labor**. To consider a classic example that's often used in introductory economics classes, think about what goes into making a pencil. Just a simple pencil, nothing fancy, just wood, graphite, and an eraser. Simple as it is, can you even imagine what it takes to produce and sell a pencil like this? You would have to find the right kind of tree, chop it down, somehow make it into the right shape. Then you'd need graphite, which is what the so-called "lead" in a pencil is actually made of. And the eraser? You'd have to figure out how to harvest and make rubber. Plus you'd need that little metal doo-dad that holds the eraser in place. It's frankly amazing that the humble pencil is so cheap and widely-available. Among other factors, division of labor is a huge part of what makes this happen. It allows everyone to be really good at something, and then we can work together to do lots of different things, rather than everyone producing and maintaining every single thing that they own.

Of course, not all skills are equally useful in a given setting. Some skills are in high demand, or highly specialized, while others are less specialized or in low demand. In a capitalist economy, high-demand skills, which are often—but not always—highly specialized, tend to be rewarded with higher wages than are low-demand skills, which are often—but again, not always—less specialized. Whether this is a good or a bad thing is probably a matter of perspective, and both capitalist and socialist systems have sought ways to balance this tendency with the needs of all citizens for a baseline level of living, people's desire to choose their own professions, and the fact that modern society requires a very diverse set of specializations, some of which are less glamorous than others.

8. Health and Medicine

And now, at least from the point of view of future physicians, we get to the good stuff: health and medicine. But we're going to cover health and medicine from a different perspective than you may be used to, because we're going to be discussing the sociology of health and medicine, and some doctors find that to be a bit of a distraction from the sweet, sweet world of blood tests, imaging results, and surgical techniques. But in any case, the idea for the MCAT is that future physicians should have some basic grounding in health and medicine from a sociological framework, since after all, society is where we all live.

We'll start with the concept of **medicalization**. This concept is kind of like social constructionism applied to medicine. It may seem strange to think of medicine made up of social constructs, but there's often no self-evident, objective boundary between things that are medical conditions and things that aren't, and we negotiate and construct these boundaries as a culture. Addiction is an excellent example. Traditionally, addiction was felt to reflect a moral failing, or a simple lack of self-control, and as such it was viewed as a personal or ethical problem, rather than a medical problem. But with our increasing understanding of brain chemistry, stronger evidence has emerged that we should think of addiction as a medical condition. Another example, although it's somewhat controversial, is pregnancy. Some have argued that modern medicine treats pregnancy as a dangerous, pathological condition, managing it in a sterile, top-down, authority-driven way that alienates women from their own bodies. A counterpoint, though, is that modern medicine has led to much lower rates of death in childbirth, both for mothers and for infants. A final example of medicalization to ponder is erectile dysfunction, or ED. Only in the 1990s, after the somewhat accidental discovery of drugs like Viagra, did ED come to be considered a medical condition that could be straightforwardly treated with medication, rather than an unfortunate part of aging or some sort of personal failure. In fact, a couple years after Bob Dole, the Republican candidate for president in 1996, lost the election, he returned to the public eye in a series of high-profile commercials for Viagra that focused on his experiences with ED, urging viewers to talk to their doctors and to seek treatment. This was medicalization in action.

Being sick is both a biological and a social process. People with an illness play something called the **sick role**, which carries with it certain rights and responsibilities expected of sick individuals in society. The sick role reflects a social consensus that it's not someone's fault that he or she becomes sick, and that sickness can make a person exempt from normal social responsibilities as a result, but with the expectation to behave in certain ways—in particular, they should follow the instructions of doctors or other medical professionals, and generally take steps to try to get better. This balance of rights and responsibilities is a key feature of the sick role.

As is often the case with generalizations about roles, we can find some exceptions. In particular, sometimes people are blamed for their illnesses, especially illnesses that result from lifestyle factors. Alcoholics may be blamed for having liver disease, smokers for having lung cancer, obese individuals for having diabetes, and so on. It's also been pointed out that the framework of the sick role works better for acute illnesses, like the flu, than it does for chronic conditions that are usually managed rather than cured. Consider someone who develops type 2 diabetes as an adult—that condition can be managed, and controlled, but it doesn't really disappear from someone's life as an issue, and we don't exempt people with well-managed type 2 diabetes from social responsibilities. What's more, the sick role isn't always consistent, in that different people and organizational cultures can have different expectations about what a sick person should do. So, for example, if you have a cold, your parents may want you to stay home in bed and eat lots of warm soup, but your friends might be irritated that you couldn't join them for some event. More seriously, at least in the United States, some workplaces respect sick days, and others don't. People can even be fired for missing work due to illness, and it's definitely common, even in healthcare, for there to be peer pressure against taking time off due to sickness because it means more work for the rest of the team. Still another issue is that the sick role might be pushed on some people who don't want it. For example, in the United States, homosexuality was officially classified as a mental disorder until the 1970s, so same-sex-attracted people at that time would be considered as disordered, or ill, regardless of whether they agreed with that perspective. This is the flip side of medicalization, which we discussed earlier.

As you've likely seen based on your own experiences, health care is delivered by teams of medical personnel with various specializations and roles, ranging from EMTs who help get acutely sick patients to the hospital, to nurses, who help monitor patients and administer care, to medical assistants, who help take care of routine but important work like taking vital signs in non-hospital contexts, to physicians, who diagnose illnesses and prescribe medications. Additionally, pharmacists specialize in dispensing medications, dentists focus on oral health, and so on. One important concept that provides some organization to this complex system is the idea of increasing specialization. In non-emergency circumstances, patients visit a primary care doctor, who helps take care of various more or less routine health problems, and then provides a referral to a specialist when a patient needs treatment for a more complex condition. For this reason, primary care physicians are often thought of as playing a gatekeeper role in the medical system.

But just as medical care is given by a variety of professionals, it's also administered through a network of institutions. On one end of the spectrum are specialized hospitals that treat the whole spectrum of illnesses, including patients with serious, life-threatening conditions and those with rare diseases. Hospitalized patients are also referred to as inpatients, and hospitals are therefore described as providing inpatient care. On the other end of the spectrum are what we refer to casually as doctor's offices, which provide care to non-hospitalized patients, or outpatients, typically for non-urgent conditions. Acute care clinics are somewhere in between. Such clinics provide opportunities for patients to receive care for conditions that need immediate attention, but aren't actual emergencies.

Medical care can involve highly sensitive, personal, and even life-or-death issues. As a result, medical ethics is a major issue. In the past, physicians often made decisions on patients' behalf, without giving them much input or even information about their conditions. This pattern is known as **paternalism**, because it's like how parents make decisions on their children's behalf, without necessarily giving them background information. In the 1960s and 1970s, there was an intense backlash against medical paternalism in the United States, and the current paradigm of **medical ethics** in the U.S. was formulated in an attempt to avoid this and other potentially unjust or harmful patterns. This paradigm focuses on the following four principles: **beneficence**, **nonmaleficence**, **respect for patient**

autonomy, and **justice**. Let's take these one by one. Beneficence basically means acting for the patient's benefit or in the patient's best interest. Nonmaleficence is the flip side of that principle. It means "do no harm". Well, medical treatment can obviously be harmful in a certain sense—surgery involves literally cutting people open—but according to this ethical framework, the harm of treatment has to be balanced by its benefits. Next, as the name implies, respect for patient autonomy means that patients have the right to make their own decisions, even when those decisions contradict medical advice. For example, Jehovah's Witnesses refuse to receive blood transfusions for religious reasons, and healthcare providers are obligated to respect that. However, there are exceptions to patient autonomy, including children and or other people who may not be fully able to make their own decisions. Finally, justice refers to a doctor's obligation to provide care equally and fairly, and to work for the equitable allocation of healthcare resources.

Pulling these threads together, the **illness experience** describes illness as a social construct, or in other words, how people conceive of and experience the phenomenon of becoming ill, navigating the decision of whether or not to seek care, and the experience of recovery. Researchers who explore the illness experience usually focus on the social context of illness and the meanings that people ascribe to illness, care, and recovery. For example, some people might perceive illness as a punishment, while others might see sickness as a challenge that provides meaning to their lives. For example, we often talk about cancer in particular as being a "battle," in which patients fight their disease and may win or lose. But for all that this metaphor of illness as a battle is pervasive in modern American culture, that's certainly not the only way to look at it—for example, in previous eras, and in other cultures, illness might be thought of as a curse, or a punishment from God.

The field of **epidemiology** deals with who gets various illnesses, and how those patterns are affected by factors like age, sex, where people live, behavioral patterns, socioeconomic status, and so on. By the way, it's worth mentioning that because we often talk about epidemics of infectious diseases, it's easy to immediately think of epidemiology as involving transmissible diseases like the flu, or HIV. And in fact the field of epidemiology did emerge as a result of physicians and scientists trying to understand and prevent infectious diseases, but epidemiology in the modern sense can be applied to all diseases. So you can have epidemiological analyses of heart disease or cancer, for instance.

The field of **social epidemiology**, in particular, focuses on how social factors contribute to illness and health. To take a simple example, lower socioeconomic status is associated both with less access to high-quality health care and with a greater likelihood of exposure to environmental toxins, lack of access to healthy food and opportunities to exercise, and other factors that contribute to illness. Thus, low socioeconomic status is associated with poor health outcomes. For instance, in the US, it's been found that the poorest socioeconomic groups have a life expectancy that is almost ten years shorter than that of the wealthiest groups. This tremendous gap occurs for many different reasons, and it's the job of social epidemiologists to try to figure out why disparities like this exist and how they can be remedied.

9. Must-Knows

- All human interactions are affected by social behavior.
  - Attraction is influenced by physical attractiveness, proximity, and similarity
- Status is any social category used to identify people: achieved status = a person had to work to attain; ascribed status = one that is thrust upon an individual; master status = overshadows other statuses a person holds
- Roles: expectations that come with a certain status; role strain = competing demands within a role; role conflict = competing demands between roles; role exit = process of disengaging from a role; role engulfment = a role dominates someone's life
- Groups and organizations structure our lives to a great extent:
  - Primary groups: long-lasting interactions with deep bonds; secondary groups: short-lasting and superficial
  - Peer groups: self-selected and usually consist of people who are largely similar
  - Family groups: genetic or non-genetic relationships (such as partnerships, marriage or adoption)
  - In-groups: we identify as a members, while out-groups are the opposite
  - Social networks include all connections and relationships a person has, regardless of type
  - Formal organizations: defined rules for entering and exiting, usually have hierarchies, and will continue to exist independent of any member, even all members
  - Organizations can be coercive (must join), normative (shared ideals/goals) or utilitarian ($$$)
  - Bureaucracies are a particular kind of structured organization; Weber's ideal bureaucracy: hierachical structure, well-defined roles, responsibilities and chains of command, organized by specialization, merit-based recruitment and employment, a predictable career path and political neutrality
  - Iron law of oligarchy: decision-making will be taken over by a few people
  - McDonaldization focuses on efficiency, calculability, uniformity and technological control
- Microsociology and macrosociology: small vs. large scale sociology.
- Functionalism (Durkheim): components of society work all perform a function, work together as a whole
  - Manifest functions are intended; latent functions are hidden or unintended; dysfunctions are harmful
- Conflict theory (Marx): social groups compete for resources; focus on power differences and social inequality
- Symbolic interactionism: interactions using shared symbols (things we've collectively ascribed meaning to)
- Rational choice theory: people choose actions to achieve preferences based on pros and cons of each choice
- Social exchange theory: social interactions as exchanges with costs and benefits
- Feminist theory: understanding and remedying gender injustices
- Hidden curriculum: habits, values and norms imparted without being an explicit part of the curriculum.
- Segregation: separation and unequal distribution of people by race, ethnicity, or other demographic factors
- Stratification: division of society into layers of socioeconomic status
- Kinship: descent (shared ancestry) vs. affinity; primary kin: related or very closely bonded, secondary kin: primary kin of primary kin; tertiary kin are secondary kind of primary kin or primary kin of secondary kin
- Religiosity is the measure of how religious a person considers themselves to be
- Religious organizations: churches, denominations, sects, and cults (charismatic leaders and tight control)
  - Secularization: less belief in religion and its institutions; fundamentalism: uncompromising literalism
- Government forms include monarchy, authoritarianism and democracy; economic systems include capitalism, socialism and communism (at least within MCAT-relevant boundaries)
- Medicalization: social construction of illnesses (e.g. addiction as disease vs. moral failure)
- The sick role: rights and responsibilities granted to a sick individual
- Paternalism: physicians not letting patients make their own decisions or deliberately underinforming them
- Modern paradigm of medical ethics: beneficence (acting in a patient's best interest); nonmaleficence (doing no harm); patient autonomy (patients have the right to make their own medical decisions); justice (duty to provide equal care to all)
- Illness experience is the illness as a social construct from the afflicted individual's perspective.
- Epidemiology is interested in the patterns of illness in a population.
- Social epidemiology focuses on how social factors contribute to illness and health.

End of Chapter Practice

The best MCAT practice is **realistic**, with a focus on identifying steps for further improvement. For those reasons, we recommend completing practice questions in an online setting that simulates the real MCAT interface, and taking advantage of advanced analytic features to help you determine how best to move forward in your MCAT study journey.

With that in mind, **online end-of-chapter questions** are accessible through your Next Step account.

As a further supplement, given the importance of active learning for effective studying, we also suggest that you consult the Must-Knows as a basis for creating a study sheet, in which you list out key terms and test your ability to briefly summarize them.

This page left intentionally blank.

Culture, Demographics, and Inequality

CHAPTER 12

0. Introduction

Having reviewed the study of the individual (i.e., psychology) and several concepts in sociology, it's now time to turn our attention to some of the broadest and most intriguing aspects of social structure: culture, demographics, and identity.

1. Elements of Culture

Culture is a word that we use all the time, but rarely stop to clearly define what exactly we mean by it. Sometimes it refers to intellectual and artistic achievements, sometimes to the shared practices and conceptual underpinnings of a society, and sometimes it refers to growing cells in a lab under carefully controlled conditions. It shouldn't come as too much of a surprise that we can put cell culture completely out of our minds when studying sociology for the MCAT. Perhaps less obviously, we can also mostly forget about high culture, used as a synonym for highly-sophisticated works of art and literature, the kind of things that you go to a museum or take classes to appreciate. Instead, for a sociologist, culture has to do with the other idea we mentioned: more precisely, the common practices and shared understandings that bind us together in a human society.

This is a very general concept, so it may help to break it down a little bit. One important distinction is between **material culture** and **symbolic culture.** Material culture is essentially our stuff, ranging from obvious things that come to mind like personal possessions and consumer products, to things like buildings and roads. Symbolic culture is basically everything else, or anything that you can't touch. Art is an enlightening example. The physical aspects of art, like the chemical makeup of pigments or paints, correspond to material culture, while the significance and meaning of a work of art would be part of symbolic culture.

Within the broad domain of symbolic culture, we can differentiate several components of culture. The first is **beliefs**, which reflect a general cultural consensus about how the world works. An example is the belief in some Eastern European cultures that drafts are harmful to one's health. This is actually an interesting example, because it hasn't exactly been proven by modern medical studies, and if you were to ask someone from a culture where that's a belief, they may or may not personally endorse it, but it persists strongly enough that, for instance, people might be reluctant to open a window on a crowded train, even if it's really stuffy and hot inside. A parallel in American culture might be the belief that being cold is what makes you catch a cold.

Values, in contrast, refer more specifically to convictions about how the world should be, how people should act, and what should be prioritized. Values can exist on the community level, in which case they shade into the concept of norms, which we discuss more elsewhere, or they can reflect an individual's personal assessments of what should be prioritized in life and how one should act. Even in the latter case, though, values exist in a broader cultural context - we all receive input from various agents of socialization and media sources about what's worth valuing in life, and we make our choices in that context.

Next, **rituals** can be thought of as actions that have a script. Ceremonies come to mind as examples, including rather formal ceremonies like weddings. But not all ceremonies are equally formal. Think about a kid's birthday party, for example. The actual experience can be pretty chaotic, but there's a sense that at some point towards the middle or end, the grownups should announce that it's time for cake, sing "Happy Birthday," have the birthday child blow out candles, and so on. Holidays can also involve rituals, as can structured events. A person can even create his or her own personalized rituals. For instance, people can have very fixed routines for starting or ending the day. Such routines can even have specific meanings, and people can feel attached to them.

It shouldn't come as too much of a surprise that **symbols** are also part of symbolic culture. Basically, symbols function as a sort of shorthand, and can range from very broad symbols that we readily identify with a culture as a whole, like how a bald eagle symbolizes America, to symbols with narrower scope. An example of the latter might be how inner cities are often used in American culture to symbolize poverty and violence. The fact that many inner-city communities have undergone gentrification and are now quite affluent, while many small towns and rural communities are struggling with poverty, helps underscore how there's a symbolic layer of meaning attached to the concept of "inner city" above and beyond whatever literal demographic trends we can point to.

We should be careful to distinguish symbols from beliefs and values because symbols don't imply that you literally buy into some kind of fact or value statement. Instead, the key is that symbols create a common ground that we can then negotiate based on our personal perspectives. For instance, we could use the symbol of a bald eagle, let's say superimposed onto an American flag, which is another symbol, to create either a patriotic poster or an anti-patriotic poster. Or to return to the example of inner cities symbolizing poverty, if someone says something about "inner-city problems," you can understand what he or she is referring to, regardless of whether you agree. The point is just that regardless of our own personal opinions, we can immediately recognize what a culturally-shared symbol is intended to mean.

Finally, **language** is an important part of culture, not least because it provides the means through which we communicate about various cultural concepts. However, we shouldn't rush to equate languages with cultures. For instance, Spanish is spoken as a first language in many countries throughout the world that have very distinct cultures. Correspondingly, many aspects of American culture have diffused throughout the world without people necessarily shifting to English.

However, an interesting aspect of language in relation to culture is that its lexicon can encode culturally specific concepts, or so-called untranslatable words. Slang furnishes many such examples: what does it mean to call something dope? How would you translate that into German, or Chinese, or Hindi? And what's more, how would you do so in a way that would capture the idea that something being dope is not exactly the same as something being good? Saying that aerobic exercise is good and that aerobic exercise is dope would have different implications, right? At the very least, those statements aren't equally acceptable in all contexts or from all speakers. So all of this reflects how culture is encoded in how we use language, and how our linguistic choices can be emblematic of our culture. Note, though, that whether and how language shapes culture, or how culture shapes language, are much harder questions to explore, and there aren't really any clear-cut answers out there that stand up to careful scrutiny.

To summarize, the various concepts we've just covered, ranging from beliefs to symbols to language, can be thought of as being the ingredients of culture, since they're unique to each culture. For our purposes, it's especially important to understand that all of these concepts have distinct meanings in sociology, because in everyday life we're unlikely to spend a lot of time worrying about the difference between, say, beliefs and values. Plus, with a solid understanding of these basics, we can move on to explore other dynamics and trends involving how cultures are structured, how they develop, and how they interact with each other.

2. Subcultures, Mass Media, and Evolution

So far, we've been talking about cultures as if they were homogeneous entities—as if American culture, for instance, were a single constant thing. That's true to some extent—in other words, there are common reference points shared by the vast majority of Americans—but it's also far from being the whole picture. **Subcultures**, for instance, are groups of people within a larger cultural framework that either have additional cultural practices and norms or certain cultural traits that are at odds with the surrounding society. Many common examples of subcultures are associated with groups defined by affiliations with certain artistic or musical movements, like punks, goths, metalheads, and so on, but the concept itself is very broad. More specifically, **countercultures** are subcultures that orient themselves in opposition to the broader culture that surrounds them. The hippies of the 1960s are the example that everyone gives as a counterculture, perhaps because they explicitly identified as such, but you could also consider survivalists, or even certain religious groups that oppose mainstream cultural trends, to be countercultures, even though they themselves might not choose that term, in part because of the degree to which the term is commonly associated with left-wing movements in the 1960s.

Moving on, in some ways, the history of the last 200 or so years can be thought of as a sequence of improvements in communication technologies. In particular, the term **mass media** refers to the conglomeration of radio, television, and newspapers that dominated how information was disseminated for most of the twentieth century - but more recently, also the internet. A key point here is that these communication technologies allowed a relatively small number of radio stations, TV channels, and major newspapers to reach the vast majority of the public, creating a situation in which people throughout the country—and even, to some extent, throughout the world—were generally aware of the same trends in music, the arts, and entertainment. These shared points of reference became known as **popular culture**, or **pop culture** for short. The word "popular" here means "of the people", not "popular" in the sense of a popularity contest, and, for better or worse, pop culture developed the reputation of being not particularly sophisticated or elegant. Pop culture still exists, of course, but it's worth mentioning that various trends in the last few decades, in particular the emergence of the internet, have decentralized pop culture, creating space for more subcultures to exist and possibly reducing the degree to which all Americans share the same framework in terms of cultural developments.

As a final note, researchers have put quite a bit of thought into culture in the context of human evolution. Humans are deeply cultural beings, so that fact needs to be accounted for in any history of humankind. An influential school of thought in recent decades holds that culture has been a major driver of human evolution, since cultural developments shape the context in which natural selection takes place. That's a very abstract statement, so let me make that a bit more concrete. Tools, for example, are a part of material culture, and the knowledge of how to make and use them is also passed down within a certain culture. So, broadly speaking, any genetic traits that help humans use tools skillfully and participate in the cultural process of passing down that knowledge will be favored evolutionarily. Groups that are good at using tools are more successful than those that aren't, and on an individual level, people who succeed in this context of tool-using are likely to out-reproduce those that don't, especially in settings where resources are scarce. Another way of looking at this is that cultural developments, including technology, can change patterns of reproductive success. To take a very direct example, the development of in vitro fertilization and other forms of assisted reproductive technologies are cultural innovations—using "culture" broadly—that enable people to reproduce who might not otherwise be able to. That is, in at least some cases, physical variations that would otherwise be selected out of the gene pool no longer face those selective pressures.

What's more, cultures themselves can certainly change over time, and researchers have even proposed that those patterns of cultural change can be modeled in evolutionary terms. That, though, is a little bit more speculative, and takes us away from the realm of MCAT-testable content. However, the idea that culture has participated in, and even driven, human evolution is very much in bounds.

3. Interactions Between Cultures

As we've mentioned, cultures aren't static. They change over time, and what's more, they interact with each other.

Culture lag refers to how changes in material culture—particularly technological changes—can happen more quickly than the ability of a society to catch up in terms of nonmaterial culture. For example, after the technology of texting was introduced, it took a little while for social norms about texting to emerge and stabilize. As a less immediately obvious example, the introduction of oral contraceptives—also known as "the Pill"—in the early 1960s was absolutely revolutionary in terms of women's ability to control their own fertility, and this eventually triggered major realignments in sexuality-related norms. However, those realignments didn't happen overnight. The timeline of the resulting cultural changes would better be measured on the scale of decades.

Culture lag can be relevant not just within a single culture, but also for interactions between cultures, since technological developments can diffuse, or spread, from one society to another. Regardless of the context, the key point with culture lag is to always look for a material or technological innovation followed by a time gap for symbolic culture to integrate and make sense of the new development.

Culture shock, in contrast, happens when an individual is immersed in a new culture. Classic examples include immigration, especially in settings where there might not be a community of people from the same cultural background, or anthropologists or Peace Corps volunteers who immerse themselves deeply and intensely in a new culture. In fact, the concept of culture shock was developed by anthropologists, basically as a way of describing their own experiences when doing fieldwork.

> **MCAT STRATEGY > > >**
>
> Culture shock is another classic example of a term where test-writers could set up an incorrect answer choice designed to trap students who apply everyday meanings of words (like being "shocked"), instead of technical definitions.

Sometimes people just think of culture shock as being shocked by a different culture, but that's not quite right. Someone traveling internationally for the first time over spring break and then saying something like "OMG, can you even believe what these people do? Ugh!" isn't quite what the concept is getting at. Instead, it refers to a more deep-seated sense of becoming unrooted and feeling out of place after being plunged into a new, deeply unfamiliar environment and facing the need to navigate new social norms for everything from basic aspects of daily life to higher-level, symbolic issues.

One basic fact about the last hundred or so years of human history is that people have moved around a lot. These migrations, which we talk about more elsewhere in the context of demographics, result in many situations where people from different cultural backgrounds live in the same place. Major world cities like New York, London, and Los Angeles come to mind as example, but cultural diversity is often present in many smaller communities too. In any case, when people from different backgrounds are living in the same space, there are two basic directions in which things can go: assimilation and multiculturalism.

Assimilation is what happens when people are expected to integrate themselves into the predominant culture by learning the major local language and perhaps even no longer using their native language, by adopting various social norms, by becoming familiar with all the cultural references of the predominant culture, and so on.

Multiculturalism, in contrast, happens when people preserve their original cultures in local communities. A common metaphor used for these concepts is to see assimilation as being like a melting pot, and multiculturalism as being like a salad bowl.

Parenthetically, it's worth taking a moment to acknowledge that the distinction between assimilation and multiculturalism is an oversimplification. For instance, people living in America can speak fluent English and fluent Hindi, love Hollywood and Bollywood, and so on. One doesn't exclude the other, and in fact the MCAT can refer to degrees of assimilation. Nonetheless, it's worth being aware of these terms as general descriptors of broad trends that have been relatively emphasized and de-emphasized at various points in history and, of course, for the very practical reason that they're testable content.

A further point here is that the likelihood of assimilation is shaped by factors such as where people live and the degree to which they're accepted into society. The idea here basically is that, on one extreme, a community that lives in a concentrated area and experiences discrimination in the workforce and other social settings is relatively unlikely to assimilate. But on the other end of the spectrum, assimilation is much more likely for a community whose members are all spread out and don't face any particular obstacles integrating into various social settings.

Finally, when thinking about phenomena like culture lag, as well as the other concepts that we've discussed here, it's helpful to make a distinction between transmission and diffusion. **Cultural transmission** describes how elements of a culture are passed down from one generation to another. Rituals are great examples, as are myths, and for that matter even things like values and symbols. **Cultural diffusion**, in contrast, describes how cultural elements and practices can be passed from one culture to another. For examples of this, just think **Westernization**. People throughout the world wear suits, drink certain Western brands of soda, listen to hip-hop, integrate English words into their own language, and so on. There's a lot to think about regarding this theme, but for our purposes, we can keep it pretty simple: transmission, with a *t*, happens over *time* within a culture, and *diffusion*, with a *d*, involves features spreading to *different* cultures.

4. Demographic Structure of Society

Demography is a field of sociology that deals with the various categories we use to describe people, and by extension, to structure society and our perceptions thereof. This is one of those situations where it actually helps to break down the etymology: *demos* is Greek for "people," and *graphy* literally means "writing," but more broadly connotes description or analysis. The Psych/Soc section of the MCAT will expect you to be aware of major demographic categories and some specific points related to them. In this discussion, we'll concisely cover age, gender, race and ethnicity, immigration status, and sexual orientation. This is not an exhaustive list of demographic categories, but these demographic categories are definitely the most important ones that you will encounter for the MCAT.

I. Age

Let's start with **age**. As we've discussed previously, aging itself is associated with a broad range of physical and psychological changes. From a sociological perspective, though, aging also involves progressing through the life course. In other words, different stages of life are associated with distinct sociological roles. For instance, there's a lot more that goes into our understanding of what it means to be "middle-aged" than just physical changes like a slower metabolism or menopause. And it's not just a set of social expectations that we're dealing with -- although yes, everyone's different, on a population-wide level, the lived experiences of middle-aged people tend to be different from, say, that of twenty-somethings in any number of ways, and the experiences of elderly people are different yet. These differences affect virtually every aspect of life, from familial relationships and friendships to occupational and housing patterns. Cultures vary in terms of the most common living arrangements of elderly people and how they are viewed. In particular, many cultures throughout the world view elderly people as highly-respected community members who continue to live with their extended families as long as possible, whereas generally speaking in American culture there exists a tendency to encourage elderly people to live with other elderly people in assisted-living or nursing homes. Researchers in the fields of sociology and public health have sought to identify ways to promote the health of elderly people in various social contexts, so being aware of these general trends provide a baseline for being able to do so. In sociology, a framework known as the **life course perspective** approaches aging in light of these considerations.

In addition to the changes that take place as any given individual reaches various ages, people who are born and grow up in roughly the same period of time might be affected by the same—or at least comparable—historical events and social trends. This is the rationale for identifying specific **age cohorts**, or **generations**. For example, the group of people who were born around 1920, grew up in the Great Depression in the 1930s, and experienced World War II as the defining feature of their young adulthood have been dubbed the **G.I. Generation**—a reference to their military service—or as the **Greatest Generation**. They were succeeded by the so-called **silent generation** born between 1925 and 1945, named after their relatively muted social activism during times of great upheaval like the cold war. After the end of World War II in 1945, there was a baby boom as an increasingly high number of people coming back from the war sought to have children and build stable lives after the chaos of World War II; people born between 1946 and 1964 are thus known as **baby boomers.** Children born in the mid-1960s to early 1980s form **Generation X**, and it's thought that this group was affected particularly strongly by the aftermath of the social changes of the 1960s and 1970s, especially by the social fallout of the war in Vietnam. Next, the **Millennials** are usually defined as including children born from the early 1980s to around 2000 or so; formative events for this generation include the 9/11 attacks and the aftermath thereof, as well as the 2008 economic crisis. The following generation, born around 2000 and later, is most commonly known as **Generation Z**, or less imaginatively as **post-Millennials**, and those born after 2010 are beginning to be called **Generation Alpha**.

II. Sex and Gender

Next, let's move on to two closely related, but crucially distinct concepts: sex and gender. **Sex** is a biological category that we generally subdivide into categories of male and female, although it's also important to note the category of intersex, which refers to a set of physical features—ranging from the chromosomal level to hormonal signaling and factors affecting the development of sex organs—that do not correspond to the typical definitions of male and female bodies. **Gender**, instead, is a social construct that we can think of as all the social baggage that comes with any particular gender identity.

Relatively obvious examples of how gender is a social construct include conventions like associating pink with girls and blue with boys, or stereotypical expectations like "men don't cry." More subtly, though, gender can shape virtually all aspects of how people interact with the world and view themselves. For example, consider the difference between being a good big brother and being a good big sister. These roles carry a range of subtly different implications in terms of which aspects of siblinghood they emphasize, and both terms are not quite equivalent to being a "good sibling." This isn't necessarily a negative thing, in that gendered self-perceptions—including both relatively obvious ones like being a woman or a man, as well as perhaps less obvious ones like brotherhood or sisterhood, or motherhood or fatherhood—can be powerful positive forces in people's lives. But it does remain important to observe that the content of these roles, and the ways that they are associated with gender, are products of a certain social consensus. This observation has a few consequences. First, we would expect **gender roles** to vary across societies. This is certainly true. Second, we would expect gender roles to change over time even within a certain society. This is also very clearly true; even in the last 50 years of American history, many expectations surrounding gender roles have changed dramatically. Third, and perhaps least obviously, we can also predict a certain level of fluidity in individuals' own relationship with gender roles and identifications—and this prediction is also borne out, although the degree of such fluidity certainly varies from person to person.

The concepts of **gender schema** and **gender script** were introduced to systematize some of these observations. Gender schemas refer to how we cognitively organize information about gender, and how we perceive the world through the lens of gender. In other words, gender schemas account for what we consider to constitute maleness and femaleness. In contrast, gender scripts are more concrete, and refer to specific expectations about how an individual of a given gender is expected to act in a given situation. A good example of a gender script comes from sports spectator culture. Traditionally in American culture, there's this ritual where men exchange small talk about sports teams using a pretty predictable set of questions and responses. The key point here is that a gender script refers to a specific scenario. You could imagine the process as giving a script to an actor. A gender schema, in contrast, refers to the ideas about gender that may lie at the root of a gender script.

As a final term that starts with "gender," **gender segregation** refers to social institutions where people are separated by gender. Places like locker rooms are classic examples of gender segregation, as are any organizations that are either female-only or male-only. Gender segregation in many contexts has been the focus of intense debate in recent years; for the MCAT, though, it suffices to be aware of the general concept.

III. Race and Ethnicity

Race is another social construct that is important for demographic purposes. You could easily spend your whole life studying the history and impact of race as a concept, but as always, the MCAT emphasizes understanding a more limited set of core ideas. A rough definition of race is that it refers to physical characteristics associated with descent from certain populations. That definition is admittedly vague, but it has to be for historical reasons: for instance, in the past, legal criteria existed for categorizing people by race according to their ancestry, and those rules had little to do with anything objectively observable about a person. The degree to which race is associated with specific genetic patterns has long been a topic of lively debate in the scientific literature, but it's clear that simple relationships are not supported by the current evidence. For instance, greater genetic diversity has been found within Africa than among different racial groups from other continents. Variations in how race is socially constructed and perceived—that is, who is perceived as belonging to a certain race—further complicate the picture. The following racial categories are officially distinguished by the US government: White American, Black or African American, Native American and Alaska Native, Asian American, and Native Hawaiian and Other Pacific Islander. These categories can be, and have been critiqued, but we mention them to give you some examples of how race is a very high-level, broad, and general categorization of populations throughout the world.

Now, we sort of hinted at this, but let's make it explicit: the fact that race is a social construct means that people can disagree about racial categorizations. For example, in the early 20th century in the United States, some states legally codified a principle according to which anyone with even one sub-Saharan African ancestor was defined as black. When a racial identity is externally imposed on a person, group, or even a certain practice, that process is known as **racialization**. On a somewhat more general level, **race formation theory** describes how processes of racialization are deployed by power structures in society to advance specific political or social goals. For example, a race formation analysis might point out how definitions of blackness in the 1700s and 1800s changed in ways that went hand-in-hand with the economic exploitation of slaves, such that racial definitions reinforced an oppressive economic system

In contrast to race, **ethnicity** refers to someone's cultural background. Language is often associated with ethnicity, but there's not a perfect relationship between the two. For instance, the majority of ethnic Irish people no longer speak Irish Gaelic. Ethnicity can also be considered a social construct, in that it's subject to broad social processes in which meaning is assigned, often subjectively.

IV. Immigration Status

Immigration status is the last demographic category that we should take note of in this discussion. The most important thing to understand about immigration status is that it's not a yes/no category. A variety of legal statuses can apply to immigrants, or people who move from one country to another. On one end of the spectrum, it is possible for immigrants to gain citizenship in their country of residence, although the rules are typically highly complex and differ from country to country. In many countries, such as the United States, it is also possible to obtain permanent resident status; permanent residents do not have all the rights of citizens, such as voting, but otherwise permanent residents face few restrictions. Other immigrants might hold specific visas that impose certain time limits and/or occupational restrictions. Finally, undocumented immigrants are those that have not registered with the host country, either because they are in the process of applying for asylum or refugee status or because they have postponed documentation for any reason, for example fear of deportation. In the US, undocumented immigrants have constitutionally protected rights, but cannot vote. A key terminological distinction is made between immigration, or migration into a certain country, and emigration, or migration out of a certain country.

Immigration status is a legal concept that may not seem to logically entail specific links with race or ethnicity, but historical circumstances have affected trends in migration, so that specific ethnic or racial groups might be disproportionately represented among immigrants at certain historical timepoints. Likewise, immigration laws have varied over time in terms of how they handle migrants from certain countries. In fact, from 1882 to 1965, the United States had immigration laws that specifically targeted certain ethnicities and nationalities. For this reason, even now, in many countries, perceptions of immigration are intimately linked with perceptions regarding race and ethnicity. More generally, we can close our discussion here by noting that demographic categories often tend to show complex patterns of interrelationships; after all, despite all the details that we cover, demographic categories remain relatively crude ways of capturing the complexity of human social existence.

5. Demographic Shifts

Demographic categories are useful for taking a snapshot of a population, but populations do change over time. Various concepts related to demographic shifts have been developed to analyze these changes.

I. Theories of Demographic Change

An English scholar named **Thomas Robert Malthus** is generally credited as the first researcher to have seriously thought about population changes. In 1798, he published a book on the topic, arguing that there exists a fundamental conflict between the exponential process of population growth and the linear growth of means for sustenance. In Malthus's view, human populations would always outstrip the resources necessary to sustain them in comfort, making poverty, violence, and starvation inevitable parts of existence. Pretty grim, huh? Well, advances in agriculture and resource extraction have allowed the population of Earth to balloon beyond Malthus's wildest dreams. When Malthus wrote his book a little over two centuries ago, there were about 1 billion people worldwide, and now there are closer to 7.5 billion people. Score one for humanity; but at the same time, the last 200 years have seen terrible wars and famines, and Malthus's ideas still cast a long shadow, as debates continue about whether humanity's impact on the environment is sustainable.

However, there is at least one development that took place in the 20th century that would have definitely shocked Malthus. Namely, it turns out that once societies hit a certain level of prosperity—especially with access to modern health care and contraception—the rate of population growth slows dramatically. In other words, people have fewer children. This process, in which societies transition from a pattern of high death rates and birth rates to low death rates and birth rates, is known as the **demographic transition**, which takes place over several distinct stages. In **stage 1**, both the death rate and birth rate are high. Depending on the precise balance between the two, the overall population remains stable or increases slowly. This pattern has been present across most of human history. Then, in **stage 2**, the death rate decreases due to advances in medicine, hygiene, and prosperity, but the birth rate remains high. During this period, the population expands very rapidly. In **stage 3**, after a generation or so, the death rate is still slowly decreasing, and the birth rate starts decreasing very abruptly. This slows down population expansion. At **stage 4**, the birth and death rate are both low, and the population again becomes more or less stable. Some researchers have proposed a **stage 5**, in which low death rates coexist with very low birth rates that have dipped below the replacement threshold of slightly over 2 lifetime births per woman. This proposed stage 5 has already occurred in many European and East Asian countries; for example, the fertility rate of South Korea is estimated to have dipped below 1 lifetime birth per woman. This pattern leads to a decreasing population, and also an aging one, as over time, elderly people will become increasingly overrepresented in a population with a below-replacement birth rate.

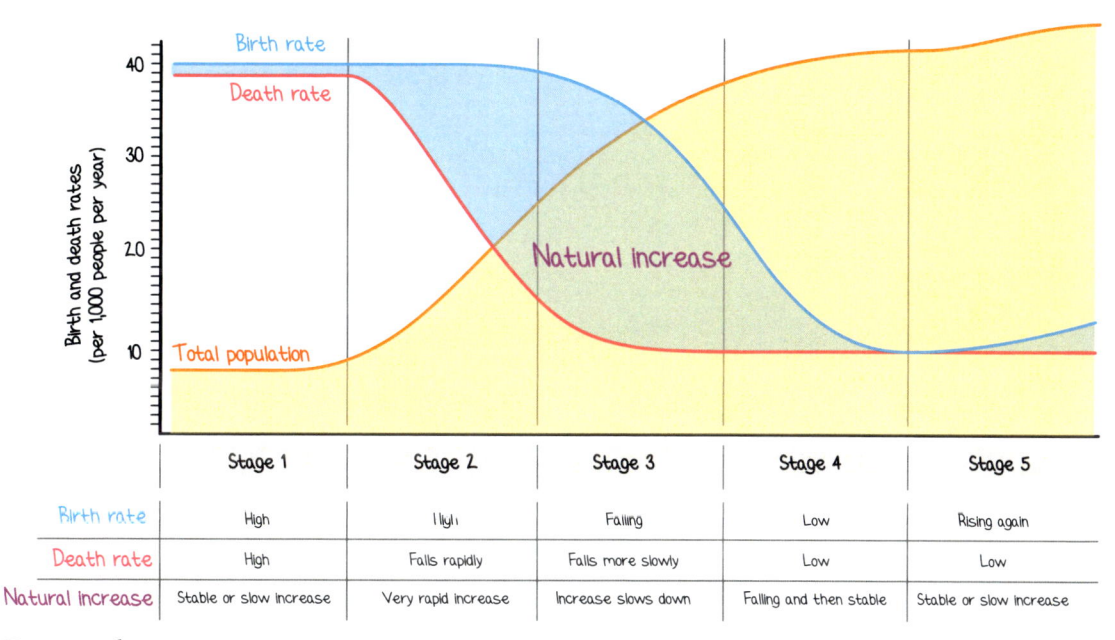

Figure 1. Demographic transition

Predicting future trends in population levels is obviously of major interest for society. The most recent population projections made by the United Nations suggest that the world's population will continue to grow throughout the 21st century, but that the growth rate will become very small by 2100, suggesting that the world's population will increase more slowly over time and reach a peak around 2100 or so. Other demographers have predicted that fertility rates will fall more quickly than anticipated, which would lead to a peak in the world's population occurring earlier. Only time will tell!

II. Population Growth and Decline

Population pyramids are often used to visualize the balance of different age and gender groups in society. Take a look at the population pyramid above. Old age groups are arranged at the top, and younger age groups at the bottom. Men are usually shown on the left and women on the right. Thus, a population pyramid gives us an easy-to-read snapshot of the age and sex structure of a population, and these tools can also be used to track the progress of the demographic transition. In stage 1, the population pyramid is very heavily weighted towards the bottom, to reflect high birth and death rates. Then, in stage 2, the pyramid starts to fill out, becoming more pyramidal as death rates decrease and more people survive to old age. In stages 3 and 4, the base of the pyramid becomes narrower and the top of the pyramid becomes somewhat wider, reflecting both longer life expectancies and a lower birth rate. A somewhat related concept, the dependency ratio, is calculated as the ratio of people aged younger than 14 and over 65—that is, those approximately outside of the workforce—to those aged 14 to 65 years old, who are more likely to be in the workforce. This provides a rough estimate of how many young or elderly people a workforce has to support, and population aging is projected to result in higher dependency ratios in strongly-affected countries.

We've been throwing around terms like **birth rate** and **death rate**, but let's pause to make this discussion a bit more precise. The crude birth and death rates are calculated in a fairly simple way, just by taking the number of births and deaths in a population, in a given year, and dividing that by the size of the population. The value is then multiplied by 1,000 to get a value with units of births/deaths per 1,000 people. These rates can be further broken down by age group and sex to calculate **age-specific birth rates** and **age- and sex-specific death rates**. **General fertility rate** refers to births per year per woman of reproductive age. The **age specific fertility rate** is the number of births per 1000 women of a specific age (for example, 31). The **total fertility rate**, which we mentioned before, is a little bit more complicated, and is presented as the number of lifetime births per woman. It's based on a projection of current age-specific birth rates, measuring how many children an average woman would have if the current age-specific birth rates applied over the entire course of her life. As such, this measure can provide a snapshot of the rate of reproduction, expressed in a way that's easy to relate to. Keep in mind that for any fertility rate measurement, only live births are considered.

III. Key Demographic Trends

The MCAT doesn't expect you to be an expert on American history, but you are expected to be aware of some general demographic trends in the last century. Some points to note include that the Great Depression, which lasted from 1929 to 1939, was a period of serious deprivation and poverty in the United States that is thought to have left a lasting impact on generational cohorts. The fertility rate in the US peaked in the late 1950s to early 1960s at around 3.5 children per woman, but this rate plunged in the 1970s. Since then, the fertility rate in the US has bounced around in the vicinity of 2 children per woman, but it has decreased further since the Great Recession of 2008, paralleling trends found in many other developed countries.

Of course, birth and death are not the only factors that affect population size—migration can be a major factor too. The United States has undergone periods of relatively heavy and light immigration, shaped both by worldwide trends and shifts in the legal landscape surrounding immigration. Immigration was very common in the late 1800s and early 1900s, a period during which immigrants generally constituted 13 to 15 percent of the US population. Starting in the 1920s, more restrictive laws on immigration were put into place, decreasing rates of immigration. Immigration picked up again after legal reforms in the 1960s, and immigrants now again make up roughly 14 percent of the US population.

Sociologists make a distinction between so-called **push factors** and **pull factors** that drive migration patterns. As the name suggests, push factors lead people to emigrate *from* a certain country. Examples of push factors include poverty, war, and violence. Pull factors, in contrast, are those that draw people towards a certain country as a destination. Examples of pull factors might include economic prosperity and social stability. To a certain extent, pull factors can be influenced by deliberate policy choices to either favor or disfavor migration. Circling back to the previous point that we made about population aging and the demographic transition, in some countries, policies have been implemented to utilize immigration as a buffer against some of the negative effects of a rapidly-aging population. A recurring point here is that demographic changes, much like demographic categories themselves, tend to intersect and involve complicated aspects of social structure and cultural perceptions.

6. Globalization, Urbanization, and Social Movements

I. Globalization

In some sense, global history of the last millennium can be understood as involving progressively tighter links between geographically distant regions. But that process has really picked up speed in the last century or so, and the resulting phenomenon, involving ever-closer economic and cultural linkages, is known as **globalization**. Technical advances have been a major contributor to globalization, especially advances in communication technology. Such advances have both facilitated economic interdependence, in that they have made it easy to coordinate industrial operations on intercontinental scales, and have promoted cultural diffusion. Researchers have expressed considerable concerns about the negative impacts of globalization on cultural diversity, especially the viability of smaller cultures and languages. Globalization has also been linked to patterns of civil unrest and terrorism, although of course it's difficult to establish the degree to which globalization as such is responsible for any given event, since it's not like there's a non-globalized alternate universe we can compare things to.

World systems theory is a theoretical perspective that has emerged to help make sense of globalization. This framework divides the world into core, semi-peripheral, and peripheral nations based on the place that specific nations occupy in the global economy. Core nations specialize in higher-skill labor that requires extensive capital investment, whereas peripheral nations focus more on lower-skill production that is labor-intensive. Semi-peripheral countries are somewhere in between. There's no need to memorize an exhaustive list of which countries are which, but just for the sake of providing some examples, as of the year 2000 or so, Canada, the United States, Australia, and Western European countries had core status, China, India, Indonesia, Brazil, Mexico, Argentina, and South Africa were considered to be semi-peripheral, and most other countries were classified as peripheral. Of course, this status is not set in stone, as it is dependant on patterns of economic specialization that are subject to change.

II. Urbanization

For most of human history, urban living was the exception, not the rule. There are a few examples of premodern cities with around a million inhabitants or so, but those were truly exceptional situations. As recently as 1800, there were only two cities on that scale worldwide: London and Beijing.

The first stages of urbanization were driven by the Industrial Revolution, a dramatic transformation in manufacturing technologies that took place in the late 1700s to mid 1800s in England and the United States, and somewhat later elsewhere in Europe and the world. This process was associated with a dramatic growth of urban centers -- for example, the population of London more than tripled between 1750 and 1850, from about 700,000 to more than 2.3 million, and then nearly tripled again in the next 50 years, reaching about 6.5 million by 1900. Similar stories can be told for many cities throughout the world, although the chronology is different due to specific historical circumstances impacting industrialization.

However, in the United States, a process took place after World War II in which large amounts of lower-density housing were built outside of cities. Many families, especially relatively affluent ones, migrated from the cities to these suburbs, drawn by the promise of spacious single-family housing, their own backyards, easier commutes to the city facilitated by advances in roads, and also driven by racial prejudice and fears about crime in the cities. These trends led to a pattern of urban decay, characterized by an economic hollowing out of urban core areas, which in many cases became concentrated pockets of poverty. In recent decades, this trend has reversed, as more well-to-do groups have shown tendencies to move back into cities. The term **urban renewal** is used to refer to the more positive consequences of these changes, but as always in sociology, nothing is simple. This process also involves the displacement of lower-income, working-class communities from neighborhoods where they have deep roots, a phenomenon known as **gentrification**. In neighborhoods experiencing gentrification, the local government's tax base increases, but existing residents are at a high risk for displacement, and very sharp patterns of economic stratification tend to emerge. During periods of gentrification, efforts are likely to be focused on developing luxurious, market-rate housing, rather than affordable housing.

III. Social Movements

So far, we've been talking about demographic and social changes as if they were just things that happened. And this is true, to some extent -- some changes that affect society's demographic structures do seem to just take place gradually, below the threshold of people's conscious awareness. But certain demographic and social changes also occur in response to deliberate social movements. Broadly speaking, we can classify social movements as **proactive** if they seek to make a certain kind of change happen, or as **reactive** if they seek to prevent change. Social movements are generally organized to try to accomplish certain goals, typically by coordinating members to exert political pressure on their government. However, the operational strategies of social movements can be quite diverse, ranging from things like letter-writing campaigns to organizing protests to even direct action. The concept of relative deprivation has often been invoked to explain the motivations for social movements. **Relative deprivation** refers to a situation in which a person or group lacks certain resources in comparison to other groups in society or what they are accustomed to. This concept is very similar to the idea of relative poverty versus absolute poverty. In both contexts, the idea is that psychologically, people are less motivated by their absolute circumstances than by mismatches between their circumstances and their expectations.

7. Social Class

Inequality is an omnipresent feature of the societies that we live in. Inequalities in factors such as access to resources and opportunities, or even in the ways in which our environments promote or negatively impact health, have major impacts on well-being, and the AAMC has identified this as an important concept for future physicians to be familiar with. In fact, roughly 5% of the questions on the Psych/Soc section of the exam will deal with social inequalities, underscoring the importance of this central concept.

The first point that we should appreciate is that inequalities aren't distributed randomly throughout society. Instead, we can group people into classes, which are characterized by similar economic situations, similar access to opportunities, and maybe even similar cultural attitudes. Typically, we view society as being stratified—or divided into layers—into the upper, middle, and lower classes. Defining these classes can be tricky, not least because the tendency has been observed for something like 70% or more of Americans to view themselves as middle class, which is not consistent with the actual income distribution. In any case, the upper class is wealthy and powerful, and at least in the United States, wealth and power increase dramatically moving from the top 10% to the top 5% to the top 1% and so on. The lower class, sometimes called the working class, is on the other extreme of the spectrum. That is, people in the lower class usually work low-paying hourly jobs, often without much stability, and often experience economic insecurity and limited access to opportunities. In between is the middle class, which can be broken down into the upper middle class, the lower middle class, and well, the middle middle class. The upper middle class is usually thought of including successful professionals—that is, people who generally work for a salary and earn enough to live a comfortable life with access to many opportunities and the ability to enjoy various luxuries. The lower middle class includes people who work relatively well-paying hourly jobs or relatively lower-paying salaried jobs, and more or less corresponds to being able to get by, but not in the best neighborhoods and without much margin for error. The middle middle class is again somewhere in between. More precise attempts have been made to define social classes, but they're kind of a moving target because of changing social and economic circumstances, and a rough idea suffices for the MCAT.

Note how we've defined classes in terms of **socioeconomic status**. An individual's socioeconomic status can change over time, and that's not the only way that societies can be stratified. And how this occurs depends on the social system we're talking about. In particular, **caste systems** are different from class systems in that they reflect a hereditary assignment of social status. The term caste system usually refers to the intricate system characteristic of traditional South Asian societies in which movement between castes is nearly impossible, but we can see something similar in traditional European societies too, where nobility was generally inherited, and noblemen or noblewomen would always retain that status no matter how rich or how poor they were. We can still see echoes of that in modern Western societies, where a distinction is sometimes made between the old rich, whose families have been wealthy for generations, and typically show more genteel, refined, and fancy behavior, and the new rich, who are felt to act basically like regular people with a lot of money. Similarly, the term lower-class can be used pejoratively, indicating that our perceptions of class aren't just about socioeconomic status. However, don't let those considerations distract you from the distinction between caste and class systems.

That said, the idea that class isn't purely about money, even in a capitalist class-based society like the United States, is an important one. To further refine this insight, sociologists have developed the concepts of **social capital** and **cultural capital**, based on a parallel drawn with financial capital, which basically refers to monetary wealth. Social capital, instead, is the "wealth" that someone has through their social network and contacts. Cultural capital is a little trickier to pin down, but we can think of it as all the traits that signal membership in a higher class of society. This can include everything from ways of speaking, to credentials like university degrees, to understanding how to dress in a certain way, to being familiar with the right kind of cultural references, like fancy novels and famous writers instead of NASCAR, and so on. Since cultural capital can be so broad, it can be easier to understand in opposition to financial and social capital—that is, cultural capital is not how much money you have or who you know, it's basically everything else that signals prestige.

The differences between these types of capital can be persistently confusing for students, and they come up fairly often on the MCAT, so let's consider some examples of imaginary people who have one kind of capital, but not the others. How about just financial capital? Well, imagine someone who's a loner, works poorly-paid jobs, and is fairly uneducated and unsophisticated—but one day wins millions of dollars in the lottery. That would correspond to financial capital, with minimal social or cultural capital. What about just social capital? Imagine someone who works as a bartender in a fancy resort, and is super-charming, and gets to know all sorts of influential people—but never makes much money in the process, and definitely doesn't come off as fancy, educated or otherwise important. This person would have an awesome social network—hence, social capital—but not really any financial or cultural capital. For just cultural capital, imagine an introverted person from a relatively less-well-off family who goes and gets a PhD in literature or art history, and then has trouble getting a job after grad school. They've got a great credential, and probably have learned all sorts of cultural references and ways to pass as sophisticated, but they might not have much of a social network and definitely don't have financial capital. These are obviously caricatures and exaggerations, but hopefully they help you get the idea.

We mentioned earlier that as of 2018 about 70% of Americans consider themselves as belonging to the middle class, even though this perception might sometimes conflict with income-based definitions of middle class. This raises the question of how people perceive themselves in terms of social class. The degree to which one identifies a member of one's class and advocates for the interests of that class is referred to as **class consciousness**. In contrast, **false consciousness** refers to someone focusing on other parts of his or her identity to the exclusion of class, or buying into incorrect ideas about social class or mobility. False consciousness emerged from socialist and communist theorists trying to account for why the European and American working classes often didn't want to rise up and overthrow the bourgeoisie. The idea is that these workers were basically tricked into participating in a capitalist society, by believing themselves to be of a higher class than they actually were - essentially letting themselves be exploited, because they believed to be beneficiaries. To take a more modern example, if people work hourly jobs but oppose unionization or a much higher minimum wage because they plan on eventually becoming managers or business owners, they might be accused of experiencing false consciousness. That is, someone might say, "you're actually a member of the working class, unionization and a higher minimum wage would be in your interests, and you're just being tricked into thinking that your ultimate interests line up with those of the ruling class." The solution to false consciousness, then, would be to increase someone's class consciousness. As always, you can feel free to decide for yourself what you think about this concept personally—for the MCAT, the key point is to understand what it refers to so that you can answer questions accordingly.

7. Social Inequalities

Now that we've established the basic framework of social class and social stratification, let's take a closer look at social inequalities, both in terms of how inequalities manifest and in terms of specific types of inequalities.

I. Power, Prestige, and Privilege

Three words that all start with "p" are used to describe how inequalities present themselves in social interactions: power, prestige, and privilege. We've got to be careful here, both because these words sound similar, and because they're used in sociology with specific meanings that don't always overlap with how we use them in daily life.

Power, in sociology, basically refers to the ability to get things done, to shape the world according to your decisions. We often think of high-ranking business executives and politicians as powerful, with good reason—they're at the top tier of organizations that are designed to do things, and they therefore have considerable resources at their command. But that's not the only form of power. A cute little aphorism that relates both chemistry and sociology goes like this: "Money is the universal solvent." The analogy here is that money dissolves all your problems, or makes them disappear. Well, whether or not that's true for all problems, it does point to the fact that especially in a capitalist society, financial resources are also a form of power. Social and cultural capital can also be deployed to exert power, for that matter.

Prestige helps explain why cultural capital can be a medium through which power is deployed. That is, certain things—including consumer products, ways of acting, ways of speaking, locations, and so on—can be associated with the higher levels of society to which people aspire, making them prestigious.

Privilege is a concept that we have to be careful about. We often use it in daily life to mean something akin to permission to do something that's not automatically granted to everyone, the ability to do something special, or exceptions that are made to the normal rules. Instead, in sociology, privilege refers to favorable assumptions that are made about someone due to features beyond their control, like race or sex. So, for example, a member of a certain race might be assumed to belong to a prestigious social setting, whereas a member of a more marginalized race might be assumed not to belong. These assumptions have consequences, especially when aggregated over the course of someone's lifespan. In recent years, racial privilege has received particular attention in American society in the context of interactions with police, in that racially-based assumptions about the degree of danger posed by a subject are thought to drive some police officers' decisions about the utilization of force.

In analyses of people's experience of power, prestige, and privilege associated with demographic categories like race, sex, class, and sexual orientation, the concept of **intersectionality** has been proposed. In a nutshell, the idea of intersectionality is that people's lived experience of discrimination is specific to the combination of their various demographic features, and various combinations of discrimination can excarbate each other. In other words, even though sociology isn't math, the idea is that the social experiences of Black women are not equivalent to those of "Black people" plus those of "women."

II. Poverty

Poverty is one of the ways that socioeconomic inequalities manifest. Poverty can be defined as absolute or relative. **Absolute poverty** refers to a situation where someone is not able to obtain the basic necessities of life, like food, water, shelter, and clothing. The threshold for absolute poverty in terms of income or varies from place to place, although the federal poverty line in the United States reflects an attempt to establish a basic minimal standard. As of 2018, the federal poverty line in the continental United States was $12,140 per year for a single person and $25,100 for a family of four. State and federal benefits are often based on this definition. For example, the Affordable Care Act—also known as Obamacare—provides subsidies on a sliding scale to households making up to 400% of the federal poverty line.

Relative poverty, as the name suggests, is when a person has insufficient means to maintain the living standard of the country or community they live in. This doesn't mean they have to be in danger of starvation, but that they make significantly less than their peers. The consequences of relative poverty depend on circumstance and the degree of relative poverty - but they can reach as far as lacking existential safety, living from paycheck to paycheck, having no means to get an education or achieve greater financial stability and so on.

Poverty is also broken down into subtypes called **marginal poverty** and **structural poverty**. Marginal poverty refers to poverty caused by the lack of stable employment. Structural poverty, instead, describes poverty that results from aspects of economic structure that are more general than any one person's individual circumstances. For example, institutions like payroll loan establishments, which charge extremely high interest rates—like 15% on a two-week basis, corresponding to an annual rate of 400%—have been criticized as contributing to structural poverty, in that they reflect something like a "poor tax" compared to the loan options that more affluent people have.

A point worth emphasizing about these types of poverty is that they're not mutually exclusive. Someone could be affected by absolute poverty *and* relative poverty *and* marginal poverty *and* structural poverty, under some circumstances, but the idea is that these terms are helpful for labeling and understanding the different specific experiences that people have with poverty.

The experiences of poor people are also sometimes not very well-recognized by mainstream society. One reason for that is that marginalized people don't have access to resources, opportunities, and even rights that are available to other members of society. This phenomenon is known as **social exclusion**. It results in a degree of isolation and contributes to the persistence of poverty. What's more, its effects aren't strictly limited to poverty—social exclusion can be experienced by any marginalized group. Its effects can also be relatively overt or relatively subtle. Actual laws and regulations, such as legislation aimed at car-camping and loitering, are in-your-face examples, but policies that seem neutral can also have exclusionary effects. For example, many homeless people point to how difficult it is to find a job when one doesn't have an address to list on a job application or paperwork, which then makes it harder to climb out of homelessness. Along those lines, in 1894, the Nobel-prize winning author Anatole France wryly commented: "In its majestic equality, the law forbids rich and poor alike to sleep under bridges, beg in the streets, and steal loaves of bread."

III. Spatial Inequalities

Social inequalities also manifest in terms of where people live and work. This is known as **spatial inequality**. **Residential segregation** refers to situations in which people of certain demographic categories cluster together. At its most extreme, this was enforced by legal and quasi-legal regulations, as well as discriminatory lending practices that affected who could buy homes where, but it can also persist even in the absence of such factors. There may also be a degree to which people choose to live close to people who are like them. Extensive research has investigated the tendency towards demographic polarization, as manifested by residential segregation in America in recent decades, because residential segregation creates closed social networks, which promote the formation of distinct subcultures. This, in turn, has major political and cultural implications.

Other concrete ways that spatial inequality manifests include its connection to inequalities in the quality of public schools, which is partially due to the fact that in the United States, funding and enrollment take place at a local level, and sharp differences in safety and violence across neighborhoods. The latter point is particularly relevant for health professionals, both because violence directly influences people's health and because the safety of a neighborhood can impact the degree to which people are able to follow lifestyle recommendations. For example, it's easier to follow advice about regularly getting out for walks if your neighborhood has sidewalks, and if doing so doesn't put you at risk for being affected by violent crime.

There are also environmental risk factors for many diseases, and those risk factors also aren't distributed equally. To take a simple example, air pollution in the form of industrial emissions and exhaust fumes are definitely a health risk. Poorer and more marginalized people generally live in neighborhoods next to factories and highways, making them more widely exposed to those health risks. Movements attempting to rectify these inequalities describe themselves as fighting for **environmental justice**, which in the context of public health has the specific meaning of spatial inequalities that affect health.

IV. Inequalities: Other Considerations

Another important fact about inequalities is that they persist over time, and that this doesn't happen randomly. The term **social reproduction** refers to the structures and patterns of activity that cause inequalities to persist over time—the idea is that these are social factors that cause inequalities to reproduce over time.

So far, we've been mostly talking about inequalities within societies, but inequalities also exist between various societies. **Global inequalities** affect just about every parameter of social well-being or health that you could think of, with a few examples including income, access to safe water sources, access to health care, educational levels, life expectancy, and so on. Some patterns of global inequality are relatively obvious, like on the level of recognizing that some societies are broadly speaking wealthier than others, but some patterns of inequality might be less evident. For instance, inequalities exist in the degree to which wealth is concentrated among a few people within a society, a parameter measured by something known as the **Gini index**. In 2016, the US had a Gini index of 0.415, with individual states scoring as high as 0.49 for California or 0.52 for New York. This is on par with Brazil or Rwanda. As you can imagine, social inequality plays a large role on the MCAT and in clinical practice.

What's more, a final point to recognize about social inequalities is that they can exist not just in what we have, but what we do. For instance, child-rearing behaviors show a correlation with class in the United States, as more affluent and more educated parents are more likely to rely on a parenting approach involving techniques like time-outs, reasoning with children, and so on, whereas more punitive disciplinary techniques are more common in lower socioeconomic strata.

8. Inequalities in Health and Healthcare

Social inequalities in health and healthcare are an issue of major concern for physicians and health professionals—and, therefore, for the MCAT. An interesting aspect of this topic is that it could be summarized in more or less a single sentence—namely, that inequalities in health and healthcare are pervasive, and can be found according to almost any demographic parameter that you could look at—but it could also be the topic of a book-length treatment. We'll try to strike a balance between these two extremes in this section by pointing out some of the most important patterns in such inequalities, in order to prepare you to encounter related passages and questions on the MCAT.

We'll organize this brief discussion in terms of demographic categories, in order to help identify the specific social patterns at hand more clearly, but before we do so, it's worth taking a moment to tease apart the notions of inequalities in health and inequalities in health care. These concepts are obviously linked, in that inequalities in health care can produce inequalities in health outcomes, but they're not completely equivalent, in that susceptibility to health conditions can vary across demographic categories on a biological level. To take a really obvious example, women are more susceptible to health problems related to pregnancy than men. To build on this example in a less straightforward way, there are sex-specific differences in the levels of circulating hormones throughout the lifespan, and those differences might exert less-than-obvious impacts on various health outcomes.

Cardiovascular disease is an excellent example that helps untangle the difference between inequalities in health versus healthcare. For instance, it is generally thought that the persistence of relatively high estrogen levels until menopause helps explain why women have a later onset of cardiovascular disease than men. That's a biologically-driven health inequality. But it's also been pointed out that misperceptions about women being "protected" against cardiovascular disease, as well as a lack of awareness of how the symptoms of cardiovascular disease may vary by sex, might lead to less aggressive treatment when a woman presents with symptoms of cardiovascular disease. That, in contrast, is an example of inequality in health care.

To get the most out of this discussion, it's also helpful to understand the difference between two terms that are commonly used in epidemiology: incidence and prevalence. These terms are commonly confused, even some doctors get them backwards on occasion. But that's even more reason to get it right. **Prevalence** is a snapshot of how common a given condition is in a population. It's usually used as a point estimate of how many people have a condition divided by the total population, but it can also be expanded to include time intervals. For example, the 12-month prevalence would refer to how many people have a condition over the course of a year. In contrast, **incidence** describes how many new cases occur among an at-risk population over a certain time period.

Now that we've gotten the preliminaries out of the way, let's dig into some of the details relating to health and health care inequalities. **Socioeconomic status** (SES), or to put it bluntly, the difference between being poor and being affluent, is one of the major loci of inequality in both health and health care. In a nutshell, poorer people have worse health and less access to quality health care. This latter factor—unequal access to health care—is more severe in the United States than in other industrialized countries due to certain aspects of our healthcare system. Measures like the Affordable Care Act, popularly known as Obamacare, and programs like Medicaid attempt to rectify these inequalities to some extent, but such programs are still a topic of intense political debate and they have certainly not eliminated income-based inequalities in health care. An important point to note here is that inequalities in health care can manifest both in access—that is, whether someone can see a doctor and receive care—and in quality of care.

However, inequalities in health care are not the only drivers of poorer health outcomes among lower-SES groups. Factors including unequal exposure to environmental risk factors, lack of access to healthy food options, obstacles in engaging in healthy lifestyles, the effects of chronic stress, and so on all collectively contribute to the association between poverty and poor health.

Race and ethnicity are also associated with inequalities in health and healthcare, although researchers must take special care to distinguish factors specific to race or ethnicity as such from those that reflect inequalities in socioeconomic status by race. Interestingly, there are some genetically-driven variations in susceptibility to certain disease that cluster according to race. For example, variation by race exists in the precise locations where melanoma, a form of malignant skin cancer, develops. Broadly speaking, in terms of race and ethnicity, in the United States, Asian-Americans tend to show the best health outcomes, followed closely by white Americans. On the other end of the spectrum, African-American and Native American communities tend to exhibit less positive health outcomes, and Hispanic communities tend to show a mixed pattern. As we've mentioned, socioeconomic status is a major mediator of these outcomes, as are phenomena like social support.

Sex is also a major axis along which health inequalities exist. In industrialized, affluent countries, there's a strong tendency for women to have a longer life expectancy than men. To some extent, biological factors might contribute to this. As we mentioned earlier, for instance, differences in hormone levels might explain why cardiovascular disease tends to occur later in women than in men. This trend might also be related to health care, in that women tend to receive medical care more often and more readily than men. Another possible contributor to this trend is an unequal distribution of risk factors. Traditionally, in many societies, men have tended to engage in risky behavior like smoking, alcohol consumption, dangerous activities and high-mortality jobs more often than women. Of course, some of these trends are changing along with modernization, which has spurred intense interest among public health researchers.

A final point worth mentioning here is that the determinants of health care inequalities include the degree to which people feel that they receive understanding, compassionate, and relevant health care. For instance, if health care is delivered in a way that's not in alignment with a person's cultural background, identity, or personal circumstances, that can be an impediment to receiving high-quality care. Thus, it's important for providers to deliver culturally competent care and to be aware of the specific needs faced by people belonging to various groups defined according to socioeconomic status, race, age, sex, sexual orientation, gender identity, amd cultural background.

9. Social Mobility

In our discussion of social inequalities, we shouldn't lose sight of the fact that people's social status isn't necessarily fixed across their lifetime. The term mobility is used to describe changes in social status. This is yet another one of those sociology topics where various adjectives are put front of the term mobility to generate a range of technical terms that you can be tested on, so it's key to understand and be able to differentiate all the various types of mobility.

The first parameter that we can use to organize our thinking about mobility is time -- that is, how long does it take for mobility from one socioeconomic stratum or another to occur? If it happens across more than one generation, we refer to it as **intergenerational mobility**, and if it takes place within a single generation, the term **intragenerational mobility** is used. Not surprisingly based on this definition, intergenerational mobility often focuses on the changes experienced by a family over longer periods of time, encompassing multiple generations, while intragenerational mobility tends to focus on the changes experienced by an individual.

Mobility can also be defined as vertical or horizontal. In **vertical mobility**, one moves to a higher or lower stratum of the socioeconomic hierarchy, and in **horizontal mobility**, one switches roles within a single class. So, for example, if someone in the lower-middle class won a billion-dollar lottery jackpot, that would be an extreme example of vertical mobility, while embarking on a career retraining program to switch from being an electrician to being a carpenter would be a clear example of horizontal mobility. Something to note here is that the MCAT defines these terms exclusively in terms of income. So if someone went from being an electrician making a certain amount of money to being a college English instructor making the same amount of money—which is not impossible, by the way, especially for entry-level and non-tenure-track college teaching jobs—that would also be an example of horizontal mobility, and the phrase "making the same amount of money" is what allows us to be confident in that decision. You could very reasonably object that, for better or worse, college instructors and electricians have different levels of prestige, which may manifest as inequalities in social and/or cultural capital. This is a legitimate point, but if we go down this road, where would we stop? Different social perceptions exist for just about every single role we could find in society, so who says which is higher or lower and by how much? For the purposes of the MCAT, we simplify things by just focusing on income.

There are also a couple of different perspectives that can be taken on vertical mobility in particular. **Exchange mobility** views the basic socioeconomic structure of society as being stable, so that someone moving up the socioeconomic ladder will be balanced out by someone else slipping down that latter, with the overall effect that the number of people in each class remains similar. **Structural mobility** takes the other perspective, and points out that dramatic changes to society can either enrich or impoverish many people at once. For example, huge economic perturbations like the Great Depression can plunge many people into poverty, dramatically expanding the proportion of people in the lower class. On the other hand, anti-poverty programs and improved systems of distribution might expand the middle class, while shrinking the lower class. Exchange mobility and structural mobility aren't mutually exclusive concepts, but certain periods of a society's history might be characterized by one pattern over the other.

Finally, the question arises of how people manage to move from one social class to another. An ideal that many people strive for is **meritocracy**, in which more capable people are able to experience more success. When framed that way, it might sound like a fantastic idea, but it's also worth keeping in mind that it's not always obvious what "capable" means, and that might vary from one society to another or be both elusive and subjective. Another point to think about regarding meritocracy is that in its ideal form, it involves unequal outcomes that are based on equal opportunities—that is, for a pure meritocracy to exist, everyone would need to have access to the same opportunities to prove their capability and we would have to somehow be able to define merit, or capability, in a fair way. The degree to which that can coexist with dramatic inequalities in outcome is very much up for debate, though, because as we've discussed, social inequalities do tend to be inherited. As with the other terms we've covered here, though, the key for the MCAT is to apply terminology precisely, in order to determine which scenarios could accurately be described as meritocracies.

10. Must-Knows

- Material culture: physical artifacts; symbolic culture: everything else (beliefs, values, rituals, symbols)
- Subcultures: groups of people within a larger cultural framework w/ additional practices, norms, or values
- Mass media: radio, television, newspapers, magazines and the internet; broad diffusion of messages
  - Popular culture: mass media allow centralization and standardization of culture
- Culture lag: delay between changes (e.g. technologies) happening and cultural integration
- Culture shock: disorienting experience of immersion in a new culture
- Assimilation: integration into the predominant culture; multiculturalism: preservation of cultures
- Cultural transmission: cultural elements transferred over time; diffusion: transfer between different cultures
- Key demographic categories include age (absolute years and cohorts/generations), sex/gender, sexual orientation, race, ethnicity, immigration status)
  - Important generations: G.I. Generation or the Greatest Generation: (born around 1920), Silent Generation: 1925-1945; Baby Boomers: 1945-1965; Generation X: 1965-1982; Millennials: 1982-2002; Generation Z: 2002-2010; Generation Alpha: 2010+.
  - Ideas related to race: racialization (imposing a racial identity), racial formation theory (use of racialization for political/social goals)
  - Immigration status: citizenship, permanent residency, visas (temporary/limitations), undocumented
- Demographic transition model: stage 1: high death rate, high birth rate; stage 2: decreasing death rate, high birth rate; stage 3: slowly decreasing death rate, rapidly decreasing birth rate; stage 4: low birth and death rate, stable population; stage 5 (proposed): low death rate, very low birth rate.
- Migration: emigration (out of a country, push factors) and immigration (into a country, pull factors)
- World systems theory: for understanding globalization; core nations: high-skill labor requiring extensive capital investment; peripheral nations: lower-skilled labor and natural resources; semi-peripheral: in between
- Urban decay and urban renewal: economic changes to urban core areas; gentrification: displacement, usually by economic factors, of poorer local residents as an area becomes more affluent
- Class systems: defined largely based on income, mobility possible; caste systems: hereditary membership
- Financial capital = $$$, social capital: social contacts and networking; cultural capital: prestigious signals
- Class consciousness: awareness of class interests; false consciousness: adopting goals of other class
- Power: ability to directly get things done; prestige: signals that appear to correlate with power; privilege: favorable assumptions due to features such as race, sex, and physical characteristics
- Intersectionality: experiences of an individual are more than the sum of component demographics
- Absolute poverty: insufficient means to subsist; relative poverty: poorer than the surrounding community; marginal poverty: caused by a lack of stable employment; structural poverty: overall economic structure
- Residential segregation: clustering of demographic groups
- Social reproduction is the passing of social status (esp. poverty/inequality) from generation to generation
- Global inequalities are those differences between countries and are often measured with the Gini index
- Prevalence: how many people in a population have a particular condition; incidence: how many people get the condition over a given time frame, in a population
- Intergenerational mobility: the ability for successive generations to rise or fall in status or class
- Intragenerational mobility: events within a person's lifetime that change his/her status or class
- Vertical mobility: a rise or fall in income
- Horizontal mobility: keeping the same income, but in a different occupation (including no occupation)
- Meritocracy: promotion, advancement and success are based on capability

CHAPTER 12: CULTURE, DEMOGRAPHICS, AND INEQUALITY

End of Chapter Practice

The best MCAT practice is **realistic**, with a focus on identifying steps for further improvement. For those reasons, we recommend completing practice questions in an online setting that simulates the real MCAT interface, and taking advantage of advanced analytic features to help you determine how best to move forward in your MCAT study journey.

With that in mind, **online end-of-chapter questions** (7 passage-based and 8 discrete) are accessible through your Next Step account—either your course account if you're a Next Step course student, or your free account. (And if you haven't signed up for a free account yet, we highly recommend that you do so, because that will also give you access to valuable resources including a half-length diagnostic exam and a practice full-length exam!)

As a further supplement, given the importance of active learning for effective studying, we also suggest that you consult the Must-Knows as a basis for creating a study sheet, in which you list out key terms and test your ability to briefly summarize them.

IMAGE ATTRIBUTIONS

Chapter 2
Fig 6: https://commons.wikimedia.org/wiki/File:Spike-waves.png by Der Lange under CC BY-SA 2.0

Chapter 8
Fig 1: https://commons.wikimedia.org/wiki/File:DSM-5_%26_DSM-IV-TR.jpg by F.RdeC under CC BY-SA 3.0

INDEX

A

absolute threshold 45, 46
accommodation 54
accuracy 11, 12, 14
acetylcholine 29, 30, 40
achieved status 194, 210
acquiescence bias 13
actor-observer bias 166, 167, 168
addiction 72, 74, 75, 80
adolescence 22, 24, 40
age (demographics) 217, 218, 221, 222, 230, 232
aggression 181
alertness 67, 68, 72, 80
Allport's module resource theory 78, 80
altercasting 179, 180, 190
Alzheimer's disease 111, 112, 151, 152
amnesia 111, 112
amphetamines 72
amygdala 75, 102, 121
anomie 163
anxiety disorders 145, 146, 147, 152
aphasia 96, 97, 98
Asch experiment 160, 174
ascribed status 210
associative learning 112, 118, 121
attachment 182, 190
attention 67, 68, 70, 71, 72, 75, 76, 77, 78, 80
attention-deficit/hyperactivity disorder 78
attitudes 128, 129, 130, 131
attraction 181, 183, 185, 190
attributions 166, 167, 168, 174
authority 205, 207
automatic processing 78
autonomic nervous system 30, 31, 32, 33
availability heuristic 89

B

back-stage self 180, 190
barbiturates 74, 80
baroreceptors 45
behaviorism 83, 94
belief perseverance 87
beliefs 213
B. F. Skinner 138
Big Five theory of personality 139, 140, 142

biomedical approach 145
biopsychosocial approach 145
birth rate 220, 221, 232
blinding 4, 14
Bobo dolls 118, 119, 121
bottom-up processing 50, 64
bottom-up reasoning 86
Broadbent model of selective attention 76
Broca's aphasia 97, 98
bureaucracies 198, 199, 210
bystander effect 157, 174

C

caffeine 71, 72, 75, 80
Cannon-Bard theory 103, 104, 105
case-control studies 5, 14
case series 5, 6, 14
case studies 5
causation bias 88
cause-and-effect relationships 8
central nervous system 29, 30, 32, 34, 36, 38
change blindness 77
chemoreceptors 44, 63, 64
churches 204, 210
class consciousness 226
classical conditioning 113, 114, 115, 117, 118
cocaine 72, 80
cognitive biases 88, 91
cohort studies 5, 14
compliance 160, 161, 162, 174
computed tomography 38, 39, 40
conditioned response 114, 115
conditioned stimulus 114, 117, 121
cones 53, 54, 56, 64
conflicts 106, 111, 121
conformity 158, 159, 160, 161, 162, 174
confounding variable 2, 10
construct validity 10
content validity 10
controlled processing 78
cornea 54, 55, 64
correlational studies 5
countercultures 215
criterion validity 10
critical period 23
cross-sectional studies 5
crystallized intelligence 85, 90, 91, 98

cultural capital 225, 226, 231, 232
cultural learning 19
cultural relativism 173, 174
culture 213, 214, 215, 216, 217, 218, 219, 232

D

death rate 220, 221, 232
declarative memory 108
deindividuation 157, 166
demographic transition 220, 221, 222
dependence 72, 74, 75, 80
dependent variables 1, 2, 8, 14
depressants 74, 75
depression 147, 151, 152
deviance 164, 165, 166, 174
discrimination 169, 170, 171, 172, 174
dissociative identity disorder 148
door-in-the-face technique 161, 174
dopamine 31, 34, 36
dramaturgical approach 180
drift 118, 121
drive reduction theory 126, 127
drives 126, 127, 128, 135, 137
dual-coding effect 110

E

ear 43, 44, 58, 59, 60, 61, 64
Ebbinghaus forgetting curve 111
economy 199, 205, 206, 207
ecstasy 72
education 194, 199, 200, 202, 203
EEGs 38, 39, 40
elaboration likelihood model 130
electroencephalography (EEG) 68, 69
Emotion 177
emotional intelligence 92
emotions 101, 102, 103, 104, 105, 110, 120, 121, 177, 178, 179
encoding 107, 108
endocrine system 17, 20, 25, 26, 27, 34, 40
epigenetics 22
epinephrine 26, 31
Erikson's stages 131, 132, 133, 142
estrogen 26, 27
ethanol 74, 75
ethnicity 184, 185, 186, 190, 217, 219, 220, 230, 232
ethnocentrism 173
eugenics 91

expectancy-value theory 127
experimental studies 1, 3, 4, 5, 14
external validity 10, 14
exteroceptors 43
extrinsic motivation 125, 127, 128

F

fads 165, 166
false consciousness 226, 232
family groups 196
feminist theory 202
fight-or-flight response 28, 31, 32, 33
fMRI 39, 40
folkways 163, 174
foot-in-the-door technique 129, 161, 174
Freudian psychology 135, 136, 137, 138, 139, 141, 142
front-stage self 180, 190
functional fixedness 87
functionalism 200, 201
fundamental attribution error 166, 167, 168

G

GABA 30
game theory 183
gender 178, 179, 185, 186, 190, 217, 218, 219, 221, 230, 232
gender roles 218
gender schema 218, 219
gender script 218, 219
gender segregation 219
gene expression 21, 22
generations 217, 218, 220, 231, 232
generative linguistics 95
gentrification 214, 224, 232
Gestalt theory 50, 51, 52, 53, 64
Gini index 229, 232
globalization 222, 223, 232
glutamate 30
groups 193, 195, 196, 197, 198, 199, 200, 203, 204, 205, 209, 210
groupthink 158, 159
gustatory receptors 44

H

habituation 114, 121
hair cells 44, 58, 60, 61, 64
hallucinations 148, 149, 152
hallucinogens 75
halo effect 167
heritability 20, 21
heroin 74, 80

heuristics 88, 89, 90, 98
hidden curriculum 203
hormones 17, 24, 25, 26, 27, 28, 40
hypnosis 71
hypothalamus 102, 121

I

identity 180, 184, 185, 186, 188, 189, 190
implicit memory 108, 121
incidence 230, 232
inclusive fitness 184, 190
independent variables 1, 2, 3, 8, 14
in-groups 196, 197
insomnia 70, 74, 80
instincts 19, 40
interference 111
internal validity 10, 14
interoceptors 43, 45
intersectionality 227
intrinsic motivation 125, 128, 142
intuition 87
IQ 90, 91, 92
iron law of oligarchy 199

J

James-Lange theory 103, 104, 105
Jungian psychology 137, 138, 142
just-noticeable difference 46, 47, 64
just-world hypothesis 167

K

kinesthetic sense 45
kinship 204, 210
Kohlberg's stages 133, 134, 135, 142
Korsakoff's syndrome 111, 112
Korsakoff syndrome 74, 80

L

language 83, 93, 94, 95, 96, 97, 98, 214, 216, 217
latent functions 200, 210
lateralization 36
law of Prägnanz 53
Lazarus theory 103, 104, 105
learned helplessness 106, 121
lens 54, 55, 64
life course perspective 218
Likert scale 13
limbic system 35, 102
linguistic determinism 96
linguistic relativity 96
lobes of the brain 28, 35, 36, 38
locus of control 167, 174, 188, 189

longitudinal design 5
looking-glass self 186, 187, 190
low-ball technique 161, 174

M

managing appearances 179, 180, 190
manifest functions 200
marginal poverty 227, 228, 232
marijuana 75
Maslow's hierarchy 126, 139, 142
mass hysteria 165, 166, 174
master status 194, 195, 210
material culture 213, 215, 216
mating behavior 183
MBTI 139, 140
McDonaldization 199, 210
MDMA 72, 80
mechanoreceptors 44, 45, 64
mediating variables 2
medical ethics 208, 210
medicalization 207, 208
meditation 71
melatonin 17, 27, 70, 80
mesolimbic pathway 73, 75, 80
meta-analyses 6
method of loci 108, 121
Milgram experiment 161
mirror neurons 120
mixed-methods 4, 9
moderating variables 3
mores 163, 174
morphine 74, 80
morphology 93, 94, 98
motivation 125, 126, 127, 128, 130, 131, 142
MRI 38, 39, 40
multiple intelligences 92
multitasking 78

N

nationality 184, 185, 190
nativist theory of language acquisition 95
nature-nurture debate 7
nature versus nurture 20
negative controls 4
networks 198, 200, 208
neurons 28, 29, 30, 36, 40
neuroplasticity 112
neurotransmitters 17, 28, 29, 30, 31, 36, 40
neutral stimulus 114, 121
nicotine 72, 80
nociceptors 45, 64

norms 160, 163, 164, 165, 166, 173, 174

O

obedience 160, 162
observational studies 3, 4, 5
operant conditioning 115, 117, 118
operationalization 3
opioids 74, 75
opponent-process theory 128
organizations 195, 196, 198, 199, 204, 206, 210
organ of Corti 58, 60
osmoreceptors 45
out-groups 196, 210
oxytocin 26, 27, 40

P

parallel processing 58
parasympathetic nervous system 30, 32, 33, 40
Parkinson's disease 151
peer groups 196
peripheral nervous system 32, 33, 34
PET 38, 40
phonology 93, 94, 98
photoreceptors 44, 53, 56, 64
Piaget's stages 83, 84, 85, 90, 98
pleasure principle 135, 142
pop culture 215
positive controls 4
poverty 214, 220, 222, 224, 227, 228, 230, 231, 232
power 200, 202, 205, 210, 219, 224, 226, 227, 232
pragmatics 94, 98
precision 11, 12, 14
predictive validity 11, 14
pregnancy 22
prejudice 169, 170, 171, 172
prestige 225, 226, 227, 231, 232
prevalence 230
primacy effect 110
primary groups 195, 196
priming 107, 108, 121
privilege 226, 227, 232
problem-solving 85, 86, 87, 88, 90, 98
procedural memory 108, 121
proprioceptors 45, 64
prospective design 5
protective factors 5
psychological arousal 127, 156, 157, 174
psychosexual perspective 137, 142

PTSD 148, 152
pull factors 222, 232
punishment 115, 116, 121
push factors 222, 232

Q

qualitative methods 9
quantitative methods 8

R

race 184, 185, 186, 190, 217, 219, 220, 226, 227, 230, 232
race formation theory 219
racialization 219, 232
randomization 4
randomized controlled trial 4
recency effect 110
reference groups 196, 197
reflexes 22, 23, 29, 30, 40
reinforcement schedule 116
reliability 11
religion 185, 190, 196, 199, 204, 205, 210
religiosity 204, 205
REM sleep 69, 70, 71, 80
representativeness heuristic 89
research ethics 7
response bias 13
rest-and-digest response 33
reticular activating system 67
retina 43, 53, 54, 55, 56, 57, 64
retrieval 109, 110, 111
retrospective design 5
reward 115, 117, 118, 121
reward pathway 72, 75, 80
rhodopsin 54, 64
riots 165
risk factors 5
rituals 214, 232
rods 53, 54, 56, 64
role conflict 195, 210
role engulfment 195, 210
role exit 195, 210
role-playing 187
roles 193, 194, 195, 198, 200, 204, 205, 206, 208, 210
role strain 194, 195, 210

S

Sapir-Whorf hypothesis 96, 98
Schachter-Singer theory 103, 104, 105
secondary groups 195, 196, 210
sects 204, 210
segregation 203

selective attention 76
self-concept 188, 189
self-fulfilling prophecy 172
self-identity 188, 189
self-presentation 179, 180, 190
self-reporting bias 13, 14
self-schemas 188, 189, 190
self-serving bias 166, 167, 168
self-verification 188, 189
semantics 94, 98
sensory adaptation 49
sensory receptors 43, 44, 45, 49
sequential attention 78
serial position effect 110
serial processing 58, 64
serotonin 21, 30, 31, 36
sex 218, 221, 222, 226, 227, 229, 230, 232
shadowing 76
shaping 104, 118
sick role 208, 210
sign languages 94
simultaneous attention 78
sleep 67, 68, 69, 70, 71, 80
social capital 225, 232
social control 163
social desirability bias 13
social epidemiology 209
social exchange theory 202
social exclusion 228
social facilitation 156, 174
socialization 165
social loafing 157, 174
social mobility 226, 231, 232
social network analysis 198
social reproduction 228
social support 182
socioeconomic status 225, 230
somatic nervous system 32, 33
somatosensation 62, 63
spacing effect 110
spatial inequality 228
spine 36
spreading activation 109, 121
Stanford Prison Experiment 161, 162
state-dependent memory 110
status 193, 194, 195, 196, 200, 203, 209, 210
stereotype content model 170
stereotypes 169, 170, 171, 172, 173, 174
stereotype threat 172
stimulants 71, 72, 74
stimuli 43, 44, 45, 46, 47, 49, 53, 54, 58, 62, 63, 64

strain theory 164
stratification 203
stress 101, 105, 106, 107, 121
structural poverty 227, 228, 232
survey methods 13
symbolic culture 213, 214, 216, 232
symbolic interactionism 201, 202
symbols 214, 217, 232
sympathetic nervous system 32, 40
systematic reviews 6, 14

T

taboos 163, 174
testosterone 24, 26, 27
test validity 10, 11
thermoreceptors 45
Thomas theorem 129
threshold of conscious perception 46, 64
thyroid hormone 25, 26, 28
tolerance 72, 75
top-down processing 50
top-down reasoning 84, 86
Treisman's attenuation model 77

U

unconditioned response 114, 115
unconditioned stimulus 114, 121
universal emotions 101, 103, 121
urbanization 223

V

validity 9, 10, 14
values 214, 215, 217, 232
visual pathways 56

W

Weber's law 47
Wernicke's aphasia 97, 98
Wernicke's area 36
Westernization 217

Y

Yerkes-Dodson law 127, 156, 174